Presented To Boston Univ.

With Best compliments

from.

[signature]

10-12-07.

Basic Principles of Clinical Research and Methodology

Basic Principles of Clinical Research and Methodology

Editor

SK Gupta
Dean and Director General
Institute of Clinical Research (India)
New Delhi, India

Formerly
Professor and Head
Department of Pharmacology
All India Institute of Medical Sciences
New Delhi, India

INSTITUTE OF CLINICAL RESEARCH (INDIA)

JAYPEE BROTHERS
MEDICAL PUBLISHERS (P) LTD.
New Delhi

Published by

Jitendar P Vij

Jaypee Brothers Medical Publishers (P) Ltd

B-3 EMCA House, 23/23B Ansari Road, Daryaganj

New Delhi 110 002, India

Phones: +91-11-23272143, +91-11-23272703, +91-11-23282021, +91-11-23245672, Rel: 32558559,
Fax: +91-11-23276490, +91-11-23245683

e-mail: jaypee@jaypeebrothers.com Visit our website: www.jaypeebrothers.com

Branches

- 2/B, Akruti Society, Jodhpur Gam Road Satellite, **Ahmedabad** 380 015
  Phones: +91-079-26926233, Rel: +91-079-32988717, Fax: +91-079-26927094
  e-mail: ahmedabad@jaypeebrothers.com
- 202 Batavia Chambers, 8 Kumara Krupa Road, Kumara Park East, **Bengaluru** 560 001
  Phones: +91-80-22285971, +91-80-22382956, Rel: +91-80-32714073,
  Fax: +91-80-22281761, e-mail: bangalore@jaypeebrothers.com
- 282 IIIrd Floor, Khaleel Shirazi Estate, Fountain Plaza, Pantheon Road,
  Chennai 600 008 Phones: +91-44-28193265, +91-44-28194897,
  Rel: +91-44-32972089, Fax: +91-44-28193231
  e-mail: chennai@jaypeebrothers.com
- 4-2-1067/1-3, 1st Floor, Balaji Building, Ramkote Cross Road, **Hyderabad** 500 095,
  Phones: +91-40-66610020, +91-40-24758498, Rel:+91-40-32940929,
  Fax:+91-40-24758499, e-mail: hyderabad@jaypeebrothers.com
- No. 41/3098, B & B1, Kuruvi Building, St. Vincent Road, **Kochi** 682 018,
  Kerala, Phones: 0484-4036109, +91-0484 2395739, +91-0484 2395740
  e-mail: kochi@jaypeebrothers.com
- 1-A Indian Mirror Street, Wellington Square,
  Kolkata 700 013, Phones: +91-33-22451926, +91-33-22276404, +91-33-22276415,
  Rel: +91-33-32901926 Fax: +91-33-22456075, e-mail: kolkata@jaypeebrothers.com
- 106 Amit Industrial Estate, 61 Dr SS Rao Road, Near MGM Hospital,
  Parel, **Mumbai** 400 012
  Phones: +91-22-24124863, +91-22-24104532, Rel: +91-22-32926896
  Fax: +91-22-24160828, e-mail: mumbai@jaypeebrothers.com
- "KAMALPUSHPA" 38, Reshimbag,
  Opp. Mohota Science College, Umred Road, **Nagpur** 440 009 (MS)
  Phones: Rel: 3245220, Fax: 0712-2704275
  e-mail: nagpur@jaypeebrothers.com

Basic Principles of Clinical Research and Methodology

Institute of Clinical Research India, D-41, IIIrd Floor, Defence Colony, New Delhi-110024.
www.icriindia.com

First Edition: **2007**

ISBN 81-8448-086-5

Typeset at JPBMP typesetting unit

Printed at Gopsons Papers Ltd., Noida

CONTRIBUTORS

Vijai Kumar MD
President and
Chief Medical Officer
Excel Life Sciences, Inc
2 Spreading Oak Court
Durham, NC, USA
Clinical Research—Past, Present and Future

SK Mishra MD
Vice President - Clinical Research and Medical Services
Dabur Research Foundation
22, Site IV, Sahibabad
Ghaziabad - 201010
Drug Development and Discovery

MUR Naidu MD
Professor and Head
P Usha Rani MD
Associate Professor
Department of Clinical Pharmacology and Therapeutics
Nizam's Institute of Medical Sciences, Panjagutta
Hyderabad - 500082
Designing Clinical Trials

Urmila Thatte MD
Professor and Head
Dept. of Clinical Pharmacology
TN Medical College and BYL Nair Hospital Mumbai - 400008
Ethical Issues in Clinical Research

Sonal Vora MD
Director
Sunita Nair MD
Aventis Pharma Limited
Aventis House,
54/A, Sir Mathuradas Vasanji Road, Andheri (E), Mumbai
ICH -GCP Guidelines

Surinder Kher MD
Chief Executive Officer
Jubilant Clinsys Ltd.
D-12, Sector - 59, Noida - 201301
Informed Consent Process: Protecting Subjects Rights

Sauren Das MD
Director Operations, India
ExcelTrials India Pvt Ltd
252, 2nd Main, 5th Cross, RMV 2nd Stage, HIG Dollars Colony
Bangalore - 560 094
Role of CRC and CRA in Clinical Trials

Anish Desai MD
Vice President-Medical Services
Manish Garg MD
Shree Yashraj Apts,
Flat No. 1000, 10th floor
Plot No.29 K.A.Subramaniam Road, Off Bhau Daji Road,
King's Circle, Mumbai 400019
Protocol Designing

Zinobia Madan Ph.D
Associate Vice President
Anil Kukreja MD
Medical Advisor Wockhardt Ltd
Wockhardt Towers
Bandra Kurla complex, Bandra (East), Mumbai - 400051
Sponsor's and Investigator's Responsibilities

Suhasini Sharma MD
Ex-Chief Operating Officer
Rashna Cama MD
Principal Investigator
ICRI Research P Ltd
127, Chintamani Plaza 1
Chakala, Andheri Kurla Road
Andheri Mumbai - 400099
Patient Recruitment and Retention in Clinical Trials

Arun Bhatt MD
President
ClinInvent Research (P) Ltd.
A-302, Everest Chambers
Next to Star TV Office
Marol Naka
Andheri-Kurla Road
Andheri (E)
Mumbai - 400059
Project Management in Clinical Trials

Moin Don MD
Senior Manager - Pharmacovigilance
Dr. Reddy's laboratories Ltd.
7-1-27/1, Srinivasa Complex
Ameerpet
Hyderabad - 500016
Pharmacovigilance in Clinical Research

Chetan Tamhankar MD
Chief Operating Officer
Anand Bidarkar MD
Senior Manager
SIRO Clinpharm Pvt Ltd
DIL Premises
Swami Vivekanand Road
Nr Tatvagyan Veedyapeeth
Ghodbunder Road
Thane (W) 400 607
Role of Contract Research Organizations in Clinical Research Management

Mohanish Anand Ph.D
Senior Manager
Alliances and Outsourced Operations
Pfizer Limited
Pfizer Centre Patel Estate
S.V. Road
Jogeshwari (W)
Mumbai - 400102
Outsourcing Clinical Research

Suresh Bowalekar Ph.D
Executive Director
PharmaNet Clinical Services
Pvt. Ltd.
Marwah Centre 7th Floor
Krishanlal Marwah Marg
Andheri (E),
Mumbai - 400072
Biostatistics in Clinical Trials

Satish Bhatia Ph.D
Chief Executive-CRO
Fortis Clinical Research Limited
Sunflag Hospital and
Research Centre
Sector 16A,
Faridabad- 121002
Bioequivalence Studies in Drug Development

Kiran Marthak MD
Director
Veeda Clinical Research (P)
Ltd., Shivalik Plaza - A
Near IIM
Ambawadi
Ahmedabad - 380015
Finance and Budgeting in Clinical Trials

ICRI Faculties
Institute of Clinical Research
(India)
242, 13th Cross
CMH Road, Indranagar
2nd Stage, Bangalore-560038
Clinical Data Management

CK Katiyar Ph.D
Director - Herbal Drug Research
Ranbaxy Research Laboratories
R and D - II, Plot No. 20
Sector-18
Udyog Vihar Industrial Area
Gurgoan - 122001

P Yadav
Research Scientist
Ranbaxy Research
Laboratories
R and D - II, Plot No. 20
Sector-18
Udyog Vihar Industrial Area
Gurgoan - 122001
Clinical Trials for Herbal Drugs and Traditional Medicines

ICRI Faculties
Institute of Clinical Research
(India), A 201 Okhla Ph I
New Delhi - 110020
Investigational New Drug Applications

ICRI Faculties
Institute of Clinical Research
(India)
C-9, Central Road No. 22
MIDC Industrial Area
Andheri (East)
Mumbai - 400093
Case Report Form

ICRI Faculties
Institute of Clinical Research
(India)
A 201 Okhla Ph I,
New Delhi - 110020
Clinical Trial Logs

ICRI Faculty
Institute of Clinical Research
(India) A 201 Okhla Ph I
New Delhi - 110020
Standard Operating Procedures

ICRI Faculty
Institute of Clinical Research
(India)
A 201 Okhla Ph I
New Delhi - 110020
Audits and Inspections in Clinical Trials

ICRI Faculty
Institute of Clinical
Research (India)
242, 13th Cross
CMH Road
Indranagar
2nd Stage
Bangalore - 560038
Fraud and Misconduct in Clinical Research

Natasha Das MBBS
Consultant Team Lead
and Domain Expert iLogy
4203, Anriya Dwellington
Dollars Colony
Bangalore
An Introduction to Medical Writing

Rajani Mathur Ph.D
Delhi Institute of
Pharmaceutical Sciences and
Research (Delhi University)
Pushp Vihar
New Delhi-110017
Communication Skills

SK Gupta Ph.D
Dean and Director General
Institute of Clinical Research
(India)
A-201 Okhla Phase-1
Industrial Area
New Delhi-110020
Requirements and guidelines to Undertake Clinical Trials In India Schedule Y (Amended Version)

आचार्य एन.के. गांगुली
महानिदेशक
Prof. N.K. GANGULY
MD, D.Sc (hc), FRC Path. (London), FAMS, FNA, FASc, FNASc
FTWAS (Italy), FIACS (Canada), FIMSA
Director General

भारतीय आयुर्विज्ञान अनुसंधान परिषद
वी. रामलिंगस्वामी भवन, अंसारी नगर,
पोस्ट बॉक्स 4911, नई दिल्ली - 110 029
Indian Council of Medical Research
V. Ramalingaswami Bhawan, Ansari Nagar,
Post Box 4911, New Delhi - 110 029

FOREWORD

India is increasingly being recognized as a quality player and a preferred partner for global clinical trials. India has several prized attributes for clinical trial development making it the "Hub for Global Clinical Research". It is certain that as Clinical Research is growing in India, the demand for Clinical Research professionals is increasing. According to McKinsey Report, the global clinical trial outsourcing to India in the pharmaceutical industry is estimated to reach around Rs. 5,000 crores by the year 2010, and there will be requirement of approximately 50,000 Clinical Research Professionals.

Clinical Research requires specific cognitive and communication skills to handle complex issue. Such know-how resides with specialists, such as clinical research associate, clinical team leader, project manager, clinical supply manager, quality assurance manager, medical and regulatory affairs manager, data manager and head of clinical operations. Training of these professionals in GCP standards would go a long way to strengthen the CR industry. Specialized training requirements may include, training on clinical trial processes, development of standard operating procedures and GCP and applicable regulatory guidelines.

India has already demonstrated its capabilities to undertake contract research for compound discovery and development. There is a phenomenal increase in screening capacity of pharma companies and the Process Development and Synthesis. India's expertise in chemical synthesis can be utilized for development of cost-effective processes for new drugs and intermediates. At this stage the operational deficiencies should be defined and appropriate Regulations/Guidelines developed.

Education in Clinical Research Methodology requires the most up-to-date information to achieve the Global Standards. The book on "Basic Principles of Clinical Research and Methodology" contributed by the eminent professionals from Academia and Industry will fulfill the long felt need for such a publication in the country. I congratulate Institute of Clinical Research (India) and Professor S.K. Gupta for bringing out this excellent publication.

N K Ganguly
Director General

PREFACE

In the last decade, there has been a paradigm shift in drug discovery from the days of lab chemistry, isolation of actives and synthesis to clinical research. Clinical trials represent a bridge from early stage drug development to commercialization. It takes over billion dollars to bring a drug from the lab to the market after a time-span - 9 years on average. Traditionally, high quality clinical research has been branded as a "Western capability" as they possessed excellent infrastructure, standardized research processes, mature Government regulations and healthcare systems and intellectual property protection.

India is fast gearing and rising up to the challenge and catering to the needs of the clinical research industry. It is being recognized as "tomorrow"s market". The fast growing private healthcare sector, lower costs for conduct of trials, rapidly increasing awareness of Good Clinical Practice, vast majority of educated, English conversant population, ethno-socio-cultural diversity, Government commitment and above all wide spectrum of disease-conditions, lure top names in the pharmaceutical world to zero-in on India for their pursuits in clinical research. Global consultancy McKinsey and Co estimates that by 2010, global pharma majors would spend around $1-1.5 billion just for drug trials in the country. Many big global pharma names like Novo Nordisk, Aventis, Novartis, GlaxoSmithKline, Eli Lilly and Pfizer have begun clinical drug trials across various Indian cities. Today, about 80 government and private hospitals in India are engaged in global and local clinical trials. The multinationals in the CRO segment include ICON Clinical Research, Omnicare Clinical Research, Pharmanet global, Pharm-Olam, ClinTec International and Quintiles Spectral have already set their eyes on India.

However, there are some burning issues regarding clinical research that need to be addressed such as amendment of regulations, availability of trained and experienced medical staff, ethical considerations, patient education, pharmacovigilance, intellectual property rights etc. Though a gradual change evident, the area is still in its infancy. WHO and ICMR sponsored survey on the issue had shown that there are no standard, consistent, planned teaching programme on the subject. An academic curriculum needs to develop that can mould and inculcate the essentials of the need and methodology of clinical research right at the undergraduate level. This will equip the students of today to become rational, effective and safe clinical researchers of tomorrow and help to launch India as global leader in the field.

Institute of Clinical Research India has made outstanding contributions in education and training programmes by providing structured course to the postgraduate students. Thus, Clinical Research professionals by providing postgraduate education this fulfilling the need of the country. ICRI is the pioneering institute in India which provides Masters in clinical research and postgraduate courses in clinical research, clinical data management and quality assurance.

This book addresses the broad array of essential topics in clinical research and provides a valuable overview of this rapidly evolving field, not only for professionals from academia but also those in the pharmaceutical industry. All efforts have been made to merge the inputs from the stalwarts in the area, and comprehensively provide information in this area, which appears as a maze, hitherto.

S K Gupta

ACKNOWLEDGEMENTS

I first congratulate all the contributors for being a part of this launch venture and secondly, thank them for their outstanding contributions. Despite their busy schedule and pressing commitments, the authors have put their best effort to give shape to this textbook. The practicalities and nuances that they have gained as experience by way of being in the field for decades, have been succinctly described here. My earnest thanks to them once again, for an excellent job done.

Dr. Laxman Prasad, Advisor and Head, Department of Science and Technology and Dr. G. J. Samathanam, Advisor, Department of Science and Technology (DPRP) Programme of the Government of India, has been constant source of inspiration and help for providing financial support for this publication, which has been the part of proceedings of the national conference.

I would like to place on record the constant encouragement and support provided by Mr. Shiv Raman Dugal, Chairman of the ICRI in completing this task.

I wish to acknowledge the exemplary technical assistance rendered by Dr. Sushma Srivastava for bringing the book in its present form. The Jaypee Brothers Medical Publishers have been associated with me for long and have once again given justice to the contents. Lastly, I pay special thanks to my collegues and students at ICRI and DIPSAR for their valuable help in editorial assistance, without which this task would have been meaningless.

CONTENTS

Appendices

1

Clinical Research–Past, Present and Future

Vijai Kumar

View the past, understand the present and predict the future

WHY IS CLINICAL RESEARCH IMPORTANT TO THE SOCIETY?

Clinical Research involves methodical and systematic study of drugs, devices, biologicals, vaccines used in the diagnosis, prevention or treatment of disease. During the process of clinical research, the physician is treating an individual with an aim to develop an intervention for the patient of tomorrow.

Therefore, the broad aims of clinical research are:

i. Improve patient outcomes
ii. Improve quality of care
iii. Enhance efficiency of system
iv. Inform health policy.

Clinical research is central to translating the promise of biomedical research into improved clinical practice the *"neck of scientific bottle"* through which all advances in biomedicine must flow before they can benefit the public.

THE PAST OF CLINICAL RESEARCH

Clinical research has come a long way from the times of The Old Testament bearing reference to a trial of water and bread versus bread and wine. Clinical trials are also discussed in ancient Greek, Roman and, Arab Woks, but it was not until the 12th and 13th centuries A.D. that any ethical codes regarding human experimentation were written down. Moses Maimonides (1135-1204), the Jewish Philosopher, Physician and Rabbi of Cairo, expounded that physicians should seek to help individual patients, and should not use them to further their own knowledge. Roger Bacon (1214-1294), the English Scientist and philosopher and monk, observed that it was difficult for physicians to conduct experiments on living human beings, "because of the nobility of the material in which he works; for that body demands that no error be made upon it."

The 16th century trial of egg yolk + rose oil + turpentine in wound healing when the conventional boiling oil was not available by a French surgeon is another example of early clinical trial.

Although the efficacy of lemon juice in scurvy was first observed in the 17th century, James Lind in 1753 performed the maritime experiment when seamen fell ill.

In this study, there was a balanced allocation of 12 individuals that received

- A quart of apple juice once daily
- Half Pint sea water once daily
- Nutmeg and garlic (dose uncertain)
- Vinegar, 2 tea spoons thrice daily
- Elixir of vitriol, qtr ts
- Oranges (2) and lemon (1).

Complete recovery was observed ONLY in the group administered oranges and lemon.

This was followed by experiments of Mint Water in rheumatic heart disease in 1865, Sanocrysin in TB in 1931. This was perhaps the first randomized clinical trial where 24 patients were divided into two equal groups. One was treated with Sanocrysin and the other with placebo. The treatment order was decided by the toss of a coin. It was also a blind trial.

The first randomized clinical trial where the sample size was statistically determined, and the protocol contained a section on statistical analysis was initiated by the health authorities in UK when they evaluated Streptomycin in Tuberculosis in 1944. It is important to remember that this randomized trial was done NOT to demonstrate efficacy. It was performed to assess the effectives of Streptomycin on the cost of health care delivery, i.e., the pharmacoeconomic aspect of clinical research was the subject of the first randomized trial.

The first multicenter study was also reported in 1944 publication on the evaluation of Patulin in the treatment of common cold (Patulin Clinical Trials Committee). This trial used a common protocol.

The past of clinical research has to be viewed from the perspective of the various stakeholders:

- Regulatory agencies
- Manufacturers
- Medical profession
- Patients
- Ethics bodies.

The level of sophistication–manufacturing technology, medical technology, regulatory science, and patient expectation has been an evolutionary process.

Consequently, the regulatory controls and various other checks and balances have evolved and tried to keep pace with various other developments.

Drug discovery also followed a tortuous path. Essential oils are considered the oldest therapeutic agents known to man besides being used for their fragrance. The Egyptians were the first to discover the potential of these oils. Records show that when Prince Tutankhamen's tomb was opened in 1922, 350 liters of oil were found in alabaster jars. The ancient Arabian people began to study the chemical properties of essential oils. The Europeans began producing essential oils in around the 12th century. It is surprising that there is no mention of any clinical evaluation of essential oils.

For centuries, the history of clinical testing was ruled more by methodological considerations than personal concerns of the research participants. From 1820 to 1906, the US FDA formed a part of various US Government agencies–from US Customs to the Department of Agriculture. In the 1930's the authorities in Great Britain set up the Therapeutic Trials committee to "consider applications by commercial establishments for the examination of new products, submitted with the available experimental evidence of their value, and appropriate clinical trials will be arranged in suitable cases".

While the US FDA approved a drug on the basis of safety alone, it was amended in 1962 to include evidence of efficacy. Since 1900's, the Food and Drugs act of the US FDA has been amended at least one hundred times to reflect increase in complexity of drug development.

It is extremely important and relevant to understand the role responsibility of the national regulatory agency in the oversight of clinical trials. A vital responsibility of the national regulatory agency is to protect the health of the nation. This public health responsibility requires it to review and amend existing regulations and requirements to further its duty towards the citizens. Since the US FDA is regarded a model agency, it will be appropriate to learn briefly its evolution from a public health perspective.

SOME MILESTONES OF DRUG REGULATION IN THE UNITED STATES

- 1820–Eleven physicians met in Washington DC to establish the US Pharmacopoeia, the first compendium of standard drugs for the United States
- 1848–Drug Importation Act passes by the US Congress requires US Customs Service Inspection to stop entry of adulterated drugs from overseas.
- 1850–US Patent Office Commissioner sets up agricultural division, which would lead to the birth of FDA.
- 1862–Federal Government establishes the Division of Chemistry within the Department of Agriculture
- 1883–Dr Harvey Wiley becomes Chief Chemist, expanding the Bureau of Chemistry's food adulteration studies. Campaigning for a federal law, Dr. Wiley is called the "crusading chemist" and "Father of Pure Food and Drugs Act".

- 1902–The Biologics Control Act is passed to ensure purity and safety of serums, vaccines, and similar products used to prevent or treat diseases in humans.
- 1905–Samuel Hopkins Adams' ten part expose of the patent medicine industry, 'The Great American Fraud' begins in Collier's.
  The American Medical Association, through its council on Pharmacy and Chemistry, initiates a voluntary program of drug approval that would last until 1955. To earn the right to advertise in AMA (American Medical Association) and related journals, companies submitted evidence, for review by the Council and outside experts, to support therapeutic claims for drugs.
- 1906–The original Food and Drugs Act is passed by the Congress on June 30 and signed by the then President Theodore Roosevelt. It prohibits interstate commerce in misbranded and adulterated foods, drinks and drugs.
- 1911–US Vs Johnson, the Supreme Court rules that the 1906 US Foods and Drugs Act does not prohibit false therapeutic claims but only false and misleading statements about the ingredients or identity of a drug.
- 1912–Congress enacts the Sherley Amendment to overcome the ruling in US vs. Johnson. It prohibits labeling medicines with false therapeutic claims intended to defraud the purchaser, a standard difficult to prove.
- 1914–The Harrison Narcotic Act requires prescriptions for products exceeding the allowable limit of narcotics and mandates increased record keeping for physicians and pharmacists who dispense narcotics.
- 1930–The name of the Food, Drug and Insecticide Administration is shortened to Food and Drug Administration (FDA) under an agricultural appropriation act
- 1933–FDA recommends a complete revision of the obsolete 1906 Food and Drugs Act. The first bill is introduced into the Senate launching a five year legislative battle. FDA assembles a graphic display of shortcomings in pharmaceutical and other regulation under the 1906 act. Dubbed by one reporter as the Chamber of Horrors, the display is exhibited nationwide to help draw support for a new law.
- 1937–Elixir Sulfanilamide, containing the poisonous solvent diethylene glycol, kills 107 persons, many of whom are children, dramatizing the need to establish drug safety before marketing and to enact the pending food and drug law.
- 1938-The Federal Food, Drug and Cosmetic (FDC) Act of 1938 is passed by the Congress containing new provisions.
  - Extending control to cosmetics and therapeutic devices
  - Requiring new drugs to be shown to be safe before marketing, starting a new system of drug regulation
  - Eliminating the Sherley Amendment required to prove intent to defraud in drug misbranding cases
  - Providing that safe tolerances be set for unavoidable poisonous substances.
  - Authorizing standards of identity, quality, and fill-of-container for foods
  - Authorizing factory inspections

– Adding the remedy of court injunctions to the previous penalties of seizures and prosecutions.

FDA says that sulfanilamide and selected other dangerous drugs must be administered under the direction of a qualified expert, thus launching the requirement for prescription only (non-narcotic) drugs.

Under the Wheeler-Lea Act, the Federal Trade commission is charged with overseeing advertisements associated with products otherwise regulated by FDA, with the exception of prescription drugs.

- 1941–Insulin amendment requires FDA to test and certify purity and potency of this life saving drug for diabetes.

  Nearly 300 deaths and injuries result from distribution sulfathiazole tainted with the sedative, Phenobarbital. The incident prompts FDA to revise manufacturing and quality controls drastically, beginning of what would later be called Good Manufacturing Practices (GMPs)
- 1945–Penicillin Amendment requires FDA testing and certification of safety and effectiveness of all penicillin products. Later amendments would extend this requirement to all antibiotics. In 1983 such controls would be found no longer necessary and abolished.
- 1948–Supreme court rules in US versus Sullivan that FDA's jurisdiction extends to retail distribution, thereby permitting FDA to interdict in pharmacies illegal sales of drugs- the most problematic being barbiturates and amphetamines.
- 1955–FDA denies a new drug application for the cancer drug, Hepasyn, on the grounds that it was not proven safe because it was not proven effective, an important consideration for a serious disease in which other useful therapies existed. In 1961 the agency was challenged in a hearing over the same issue involving an anti-infective drug, Altafur, which was decided in FDA's favor.
- 1962–Thalidomide, a new sleeping pill, is found to have caused birth defects in thousands of babies born in Western Europe. News reports on the role of Dr. Frances Kelsey, FDA Medical Officer, in keeping the drug off the US market, arouse public support for stronger drug regulation.

  Kefauver-Harris Drug Amendments. For the first time, drug manufacturers are required to prove to FDA the effectiveness of their products before marketing them.
- 1963–Advisory Committee on Investigational Drugs meets, the first meeting of a committee to advise the FDA on product approval and policy on an ongoing basis.
- 1965–Drug Abuse Control Amendments are enacted to deal with problems caused by abuse of depressants, stimulants and hallucinogens.
- 1966–FDA contracts with the National Academy of Sciences/National Research Council to evaluate the effectiveness of 4,000 drugs approved on the basis of safety alone between 1938 and 1962.

- 1968–FDA forms the Drug Efficacy Study Implementation (DESI) to implement recommendations of the National Academy of Sciences investigation of effectiveness of drugs first marketed between 1938 and 1962.
- 1970–In Upjohn vs Finch the Court of Appeals upholds enforcement of the 1962 drug effectiveness amendments by ruling that commercial success alone does not constitute substantial evidence of drug safety and efficacy.

  FDA requires the first patient package insert oral contraceptives must contain information about the specific benefits and risks.
- 1977–Introduction of the Bioresearch Monitoring Program as an agency wide initiative ensures the quality and integrity of data submitted to FDA and provides for the protection of human subjects in clinical trials by focusing on preclinical studies on animals, clinical investigators, and the work of institutional review boards.
- 1981–FDA and the Department of Health and Human Services revise regulations for human subject protections, based on the 1979 Belmont Report, which had been issued by the National commission for the Protection of Human Subjects of Biomedical and Behavioral Research. The revised rules provide for wider representation on institutional review boards and they detail elements of what constitutes informed consent, among other provisions.
- 1983–Orphan Drug Act passed, enabling FDA to promote research and marketing of drugs needed for treating rare diseases.
- 1987–Investigational drug regulations revised to expand access to experimental drugs for patients with serious diseases with no alternative therapies.
- 1989–The FDA issues guidelines asking manufacturers to determine whether a drug is likely to have significant use in elderly people and to include elderly patients in clinical trials if applicable.
- 1991–Regulations published to accelerate the Review of Drugs for life threatening diseases.
- 1992–The US FDA with Japan and Europe establish the International Conference on Harmonization (ICH). The ICH works to reduce the burden on regulation by harmonizing the regulatory requirements in the three regions.

  Prescription Drug User Fee Act (PDUFA) requires drug and biologic manufacturers to pay fees for product applications and supplements, and other services. The act also requires FDA to sue these funds to hire more reviewers to assess applications.
- 1993–A consolidation of several adverse reaction reporting systems is launched as Med Watch, designed for voluntary reporting of problems associated with medical products to be filed with FDA by health professionals

  Revising a policy from 1977 that excluded women of child bearing potential from early drug studies, FDA issues guidelines calling for improved assessments of medication responses as a function of gender. Companies are encouraged to include patients of both sexes in their investigations of drugs and to analyze any gender-specific phenomena.

- 1995. FDA declares cigarettes to be 'drug delivery devices"
- 1998. The Adverse Event Reporting System is a computerized information database designed to support the FDA's post-marketing safety surveillance program to approved drug and therapeutic biologic products. The ultimate goal of AERS is to improve public health by providing the best available tools for storing analyzing safety reports.

  The Pediatric Rule requires manufacturers of selected new and existing drug and biological products to conduct studies to assess their safety and efficacy in children.

  The FDA approves the use of Thalidomide for the treatment of Hansen's disease. In tandem with the approval FDA invokes an oversight program designed to help ensure a zero tolerance policy for Thalidomide exposure during pregnancy.
- Clinical Trials. Govt is founded to provide the public with updated information on enrollment in federally and privately supported clinical research, thereby expanding patient access to studies of promising therapies.

  FDA publishes guidance for electronic submissions that provide for the receipt and archiving of a new drug application entirely in electronic format without any accompanying paper archival copy.

  These are some of the milestone amendments and announcements that the FDA made over the years relating to clinical research, protection of subjects in clinical research, steps to ensure wider patient participation in clinical research. This reflects the concern of the regulators and the process to involve all stakeholders in decision making to ensure compliance and effective implementation.

  The pharmaceutical industry also made significant progress from early 20th century and contributed to the understanding of disease and making available many drugs to combat many diseases.

  It will be clear from the following points how the drug development and regulatory requirements progressed in tandem:
- 1921–Insulin was discovered.
- 1928 Penicillin was discovered
- 1938–Anti epileptic drugs without sedating effects
- 1940–Anti coagulant - Warfarin
- 1943–Streptomycin
- 1948–Methotrexate approved as the first anti cancer drug
- 1950–Relationship between Cortisol and inflammation
- 1951–Mono Amine Oxidase inhibitors for Depression
- 1952–Chlorpromazine for psychosis
- 1953–6 Mercapto Purine for leukemia
- 1954–Polio vaccine
- 1958–Thiazide diuretics
- 1960–Benzodiazepines

- 1963–Measles vaccine
- Nalidixic acid – forerunner of quinolones
- 1966–Allopurinol for Gout
- 1967–First beta blocker – Propranolol
- US FDA approves first drug for renal transplant rejection
- 1972–Second generation inhalation anesthetic – Enflurane
- 1973–Progesterone only oral contraceptive
- 1976–First ACE inhibitor captopril
- 1977–First H2 blocker – Cimetidine for acid peptic disease
- 1983–Cyclosporin for transplant rejection
- 1986 Interferon – birth of recombinant technology
- 1986–Monoclonal anti body for renal transplant
- 1987–SSRIs for depression
- 1987–Azidothymidine
- Ciprofloxacin – first quinolone
- 1989–Erythropoietin for anemia of renal failure
- 1990 Atypical anti psychotics for schizophrenia
- 1993–Tetra hydro amino acridine for alzheimer's disease
- 1990s–Nanoparticles and Liposomal entrapped drugs for targeted drug delivery.

CLINICAL RESEARCH IN INDIA — 1950-1987

Regulatory Agency

India has been a branded generic pharmaceutical market. The Patent Act was amended in 1970 to withdraw product patent. Clinical trials were not mandatory to obtain new drug approval. The first amendment to the Drugs and Cosmetics Act relating to new drug approval was made in 1987 by Schedule 'Y', when the first applicant had to conduct clinical trials in 100 patients and, subsequent applicants were required to establish bioequivalence with the first product.

Progress of clinical research is directly proportional to the regulatory requirements laid down by the national agency that in turn reviews and modifies regulations as the drug discovery programs of the pharmaceutical industry become progressively complex.

Institutional Review Boards

There have been islands of excellence and contribution to global knowledge base through clinical trials in India. Examples are, Prostaglandins in Fertility Control and Maternal health, injectable and implantable contraceptives.

Consequently, composition of Institutional Review Boards (IRBs), their perception of responsibilities towards clinical research was not in consonance with international standards. The IRBs were mainly responsible for approving government funded research projects and academic research.

Medical Professionals

Most of the members of the medical community were not engaged in clinical research, especially at an international level. They were involved in a few studies for local regulatory approval. Hence, their exposure and experience with various global guidelines, regulatory requirements, etc. was minimal. Since the average faculty member of any institution in India is inundated with patients, the voluminous source documentation required or global studies were not practical in India. Most of the clinicians were involved in research funded by various government agencies and, a few international agencies like the WHO, World Bank, UNICEF, etc. Medical education in India does not include details of drug development and research methodology as part of curriculum.

The country's medical professionals could not contribute to various globally important clinical trials that significantly changed the concepts of medical practice in the fields of cardiology, metabolic disorders, hypertension, etc. Practice of medicine was based more on individual opinion than evidence-based medicine.

Pharmaceutical Industry

The Indian segment of the pharmaceutical industry was concentrating on process research for Active Pharmaceutical Ingredient, product and formulation development between from 1950 till few years ago. Since there was no requirement and incentive for clinical research and, product registration was not dependent on evidence showing efficacy and safety, there was no impetus for the industry to conduct clinical research.

The indigenous pharmaceutical industry depended extensively on published literature in international journals for product promotion. The multinational segment of the industry hardly carried out any clinical trials of their innovative products because of lack of patent protection and data exclusivity. Marketing of pharmaceutical products in a generic market was mainly driven by pricing and not much attention was paid by either the pharmaceutical industry or the users about the need to generate local data.

The absence of locally relevant clinical data also put the national regulatory agency in difficult situations during the same period. For example, the Drugs Controller General (India) did not have sufficient data to decide on the continuation of quinolines in the management of diarrhea. Similarly, there was no local data when the controversy about the use of Ketorolac in elderly patients arose in mid 90s. More recently, the national regulatory agency had to depend on data from outside India on the banning of prokinetic agents. Evidence based decisions could have been taken if there was sufficient local clinical data to help the national regulatory agency take decisions on matters relating to public health. Although this prompted the Drugs Controller's office to issue instructions to conduct post-marketing trials to document safety, this is followed more in breach than practice.

This led to a chronic neglect of building a cadre of professionals to manage various aspects of industry-sponsored research. There was minimal awareness of clinical research as a career option for both medically qualified persons and professionals of other disciplines.

Media and Society

The Media was not covering the clinical research area since its attention was more on drug pricing, availability of drugs and, quality control standards of drugs. Medical research connected with family planning methods, control of national programs like TB and Malaria received more attention.

There were no attempts to educate the society at large about the complexities involved in drug research and development. The lay public was not aware of the cost and time taken to discover, develop and introduce a new drug. It was not found necessary to educate the public on various aspects of human research. No attempt was made to communicate constantly the need of the medical community to undertake research to make therapeutic interventions available to the society. It was also not found necessary to involve the society to enhance the public trust and confidence in medical research.

The Present Global Scenario of Clinical Research

The present scenario has evolved over the last thirty years because of:

i. Tremendous progress of understanding the pathophysiology of diseases
ii. Opening of new frontiers in medicine – Immunology, Cellular basis of Malignancy, Cardiovascular diseases, Metabolism, Psychiatry and Neurology
iii. Discovery and development of drugs with precise and complex mechanism of actions and use of rDNA technology in treatment of a multitude of conditions
iv. Development of surrogate markers
v. Advances in regulatory science
vi. Change in societal expectations
vii. Change in IRB norms
viii. Media explosion
ix. Incidents of fraud, misrepresentation of results in clinical research
x. Increasing costs of drug development
xi. Shrinking patient base in traditional areas of research – US, Western Europe, Japan, Canada
xii. Need to reduce the cost and time of drug development

There are currently 23,168 drugs in various phases of development–Cancer 24.95, CVS 7.95, Infectious Diseases 10.95, CNS 10.5 percent, Immune System 5.1 percent, Hormonal 5.3 percent, Miscellaneous 6.1 percent and others 29.2 percent.

Out of the more than 90,000 trials performed globally, more than 60 percent are performed in the US. While the US FDA accepts foreign data to approve US FDA NDA's, it is interesting to recount that, while the number of foreign clinical trials submitted to US FDA as part of NDAs has increased from 43 clinical trials in 1980 to 5777 in 1990s, this number is still less than 10 percent of all global trials. It is very clear that the majority of clinical trials are still performed in the US, because the country accounts for approximately US $ 350 billion out of a global pharmaceutical market of US $ 500 billion.

The FDA recently reported (2003) that 25 percent of investigational new drug applications include critical data from studies conducted outside US. In 2001, the Department of Health and Human Services (US Government) office of the Inspector General reported that the number of foreign investigators conducting research under US FDA IND rose from 41 in 1980 to 271 in 1990 and 4,458 in 1999 (Fig. 1.1).

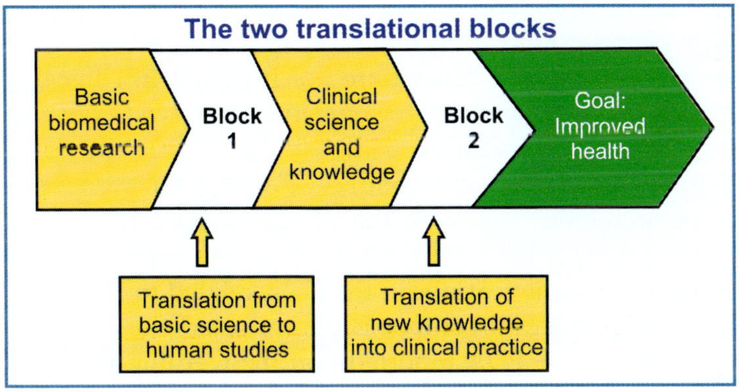

Fig. 1.1: Objectives of progress in medicine

However, if the twin objectives of progress in medicine as depicted above are to be met, it is interesting to consider the following facts to determine if these could be met with efforts to expedite drug development are confined to the US and a few other countries.

The number of patients required per NDA has gone up from approximately 2800 patients in the 1970s to over 6300 in the late 1990s. While the US FDA review time for NDA is reducing (depending on the therapeutic category of drugs), the clinical development time is increasing from about 4 years in the 70s to over 6 years currently.

Some other facts also indicate that clinical development has to be globalized in order to meet the objective of getting the drugs to the patients in a timely manner at manageable costs.

While the USA remains an important geography for conduct of clinical trials of new drugs, the enrollment pattern and time taken to complete the same are not satisfactory.

- 35 percent of delays due to patient recruitment
- 15-20 percent of investigators DO NOT enroll ANY patients
- 30 percent enroll 5 percent of evaluable patients

- 20 percent of the investigators are average performers
- 30 percent are top performers – consistently enroll up to 70 percent patients in phase II and III trials
- Patient retention rate in phase II and III trials – 70 percent
  (Ken Getz at the 2006 ACRP Annual meeting in Phoenix, AZ)

It is also important to remember that every patient not completing the study and lost to follow-up costs the pharmaceutical company approximately US $ 44,000 A DAY.

If one considers the pipeline of biotechnology and device industry, it is easy to recognize that clinical research confined to the US and Europe will not serve the interest of all the stakeholders. According to CenterWatch, 82 percent in Europe and 94 percent in the US miss the enrollment deadlines.

In a survey by Harris poll in 2004, it was noted that in the US, one in eight (13%) physicians is an investigator, 87 percent are not involved in clinical trials, about 34 percent participated in the past but not currently involved. With the continuous increase in the number of clinical trials being conducted and the number of subjects required for each trial, the demand for clinical investigators is increasing.

The clinical research environment in the US and Europe has had its fair share of problems.

One of the most worrisome features in the US is related to Phantom Investigators. Center Watch as early as in November 2001, reported the presence of Phantom Investigators. In 2000, the US FDA reported that the warning letters to investigators contain more citations of failure to personally conduct and supervise the clinical trials. In 2000, approximately 19 percent of investigators receiving warnings or the more serious Notice of Initiation of Disqualification and Opportunity to Explain (NIDPOE) were cited for failing to supervise their trials. Figures for 2001 indicate a three-fold increase in the number of investigators cited for improper/ insufficient supervision of clinical trials.

According to Center Watch (November 2001), an anecdotal analysis of 20 cases where principal investigators received warning letters from the FDA, the PI rarely accepted responsibility for failure to supervise the study. In 39 and 17 percent of the cases, study coordinators and nurses, respectively, received the blame.

Phantom Investigators are people who are delegating work to clinical staff. This is allowed, and individual staff responsibilities may be reflected appropriately in regulatory documents and site signature responsibility logs. However, the ability to delegate many aspects of clinical trial execution does not relieve the PI from fulfilling the principal responsibility of overseeing the conduct of the trial.

The same Center Watch article goes on to add that several major sponsors have also noted investigator absence. The FDA has observed that a number of investigators do not comprehend their extent of commitment while signing the 1572. It appears that many investigators do understand their responsibilities, but are too busy and must therefore delegate extensively. According to Center Watch, "there are a lot of overworked and undereducated people in the clinical research enterprise". Gary Chadwick of University of Rochester IRB has the impression that the problem occurs in large research mills or dedicated clinical trial centers. Stan Woollen, former Acting Head of the US FDA's BioResearch Monitoring Information Service says that the FDA gets concerned when there is a long list of sub investigators in the 1572.

Before 2000, ORPP (office of Research Participant Protection) only supervised NIH funded studies in the USA. However, when OHRP (office of Human Research Protection) was formed in 2001, its charter included oversight of NIH funded and FDA regulated studies. This has led to a perceptible fall in the number of investigators cited for improper/insufficient personal supervision of clinical trials.

It must also be pointed out that the proportion of Academic Medical Centers involved in pharmaceutical industry sponsored clinical research fell from 63% in 1994 to 265 in 2004. One of the important reasons is the complex bureaucracy and delays in initiating clinical trials in academic trial centers. In a personal conversation with the author, a medium sized biopharmaceutical company mentioned that the average time for a local IRB was 280 days.

The UK does not seem to free of problems either. The cost of doing trials in the UK is among the highest in Europe and around ten times higher than in emerging areas in Eastern Europe, India and China (New Scientist, March 2006). Nevertheless, big pharmaceutical companies have preferred UK because of the heritage. According to a report by management consultancy firm McKinsey cited in New Scientist, the UK is squandering its best selling point. The massive patient base that the National Health Service (NHS) offers is a powerful research resource, but red tape and bureaucracy during trial approval are causing disruption and longer start-up times compared with many other countries.

The evidence is easy to find. If a company wants to set up a large trial across 30 different NHS sites, it needs to agree honorary contracts with each primary car trust. This means that a researcher working on the trial needs to have 30 different police checks, health checks, etc. Patient recruitment delays are also a problem. This is the result of a stretched NHS, where there are too few specialized clinical trial nurses, where clinicians fear they will slip in their career paths if they take time out for clinical research, and where foundation hospitals and GPs have no easy way of finding trials that are recruiting patients.

It must be conceded that the UK government has responded to calls for action with unusual vigor. In 2004, it created the UK Clinical Research Collaboration (UKCRC) to make the necessary changes, bringing together the NHS, funding and regulatory bodies, academic or voluntary sector organizations, academia and industry.

One of the UKCRC's first jobs was to find a better way to coordinate trials nationwide, so it set up the Clinical Research Network (UKCRN). The research network controls a number of smaller networks specializing in specific disease areas. The first of these, set up before UKCRC, focuses on cancer research. It has doubled patient recruitment in just three years. This was followed by mental health network focusing on dementia and neurodegenerative disease, diabetes, strokes and medicines for children.

Another idea under consideration is the introduction of research "passport". It means that researchers need complete honorary contracts with one primary care trust for it to be recognized by all the others.

Meanwhile, academic clinicians are being encouraged to get involved with clinical research with a new career track, which has been developed in under a year. This means doctors wishing to pursue clinical research will not be penalized on their route to achieving consultant status. It should also speed up patient recruitment by meeting the shortage of skilled researchers.

There is also a plan for new R and D strategy for the NHS that proposes to tackle red tape and access to funds for the researchers. The potential is enormous – 52 million patient records will allow for phenomenal research that could benefit society, for example enabling active surveillance of drug safety.

However, this strategy and action plan does have its critics who label it as "incoherent" and biased towards the industry.

The present is merging imperceptibly with the future. There is no time for any one to wait to prepare for the future. The future is now and, many stakeholders at many places are gearing to meet the challenges of increasing complexity of drug development in the future.

Some important developments have already begun in clinical development. These include.

ADAPTIVE TRIAL DESIGN

Adaptive Sampling Designs

Adaptive sampling designs, also called response adaptive designs, for statistical experiments are ones where the accruing data from trials (i.e., the observations) are used to adjust the experiment as it is being run. Typically, decisions as how to sample during an experiment are made and fixed in advance. For example, in a classical clinical trial, patients are allocated to one of two different treatment options with half being assigned to each therapy. At the end of the experiment a decision is made as to which treatment is more effective. In contrast, in an adaptive clinical trial, patient outcomes can be used as they become available to adjust the allocation of future patients. This allows one to improve expected patient outcomes during the experiment, while still being able to reach good statistical decisions in a timely fashion. Thus adaptive procedures can offer significant ethical and cost advantages over fixed standard procedures. A situation in which adaptive procedures have become particularly relevant are AIDS clinical trials, since many new drugs come to market, yet classical randomized studies may pose ethical dilemmas and time delays.

Unfortunately, adaptive procedures are more complicated to design and to analyze, and in some settings more difficult to implement. Notwithstanding this and other issues, the US FDA has given is considering adaptive clinical trial designs for AIDS. The objective is to strengthen ethics while expediting drug development (Janis Hardwick and Quentin F. Stout – Computer Science, University of Michigan, Ann Arbor).

Translational Research

Translational Research is already happening in oncology. Attempts are made to discover sensitive and predictive biomarkers for various cancers. Predictive biomarkers are supposed to identify patients that will improve with continued therapy.

Translational research is really about trying to bring together the progress we are making in the laboratory with the progress we are making in the clinic – Robert C. Bast Jr. Vice President of the office of Translational Research – University of Texas M.D. Anderson Cancer Center in OncoLog, March 2004.

Translational research focuses on identifying new drugs, antibodies or genes that would either neutralize the oncogenes, the 'accelerators" that turn tumor growth, or would replace the "brakes" on cell growth, the dysfunctional tumor suppressor genes. Targeted therapy can also intervene in the signaling pathways of cancer cells so that cancer cells would be stimulated to self-destruct, whereas normal tissues would be spared.

GLOBALIZATION OF CLINICAL RESEARCH

In the existing scenario, globalization is inevitable. Drugs will be made for patients all over the world and, while clinical trial subjects will continue to come form traditional areas of the US and Europe, many emerging countries like India, South Africa, Latin America, Thailand, etc. will contribute patients for a large number of clinical trials.

With globalization we need to consider some important factors, especially those relating to patient demographics. For example, in a study among participants in AIDS clinical trials in Canada revealed that the number of women was gradually increasing.

One of the best illustrations of the lack of inclusion and representation of target populations in drug trials is the common practice of excluding elderly subjects. This group, the most rapidly growing segment of the population, is often underrepresented in clinical research. For example, NSAIDs are commonly used in elderly because of the high prevalence of musculoskeletal disorders, especially in women. However, in the major drug trials evaluating NSAIDs, only 2.1 percent of patients were 65 years of age or over and less than 0.1 percent were over 75. In practice, elderly people are among the largest users of drugs and have the highest incidence of drug related side effects.

Elderly people who are included in clinical trials are generally younger and predominantly male. The inclusion of older, frailer individuals in drug trials presents investigators with challenges, including the increased likelihood that these patients may be unable to complete the trial for a variety of reasons. At the same time it must be borne in mind that it is these patients who are commonly prescribed drugs for hypertension, heart failure, arthritis, etc.

FUTURE TRENDS

India can exploit the following attributes to play a meaningful role in global clinical development programs:

- Legal system
- Regulatory mechanism
- Exposure to basic and industrial research
- Growing pharmaceutical sector

However, it is extremely important to pay attention to the expectations and needs of all the stakeholders.

REGULATORY AGENCY

The office of the Drugs Controller General (India) recognized in time the growing importance of clinical research and took appropriate steps to ensure synchronization of the regulatory systems with ICH requirements. The regulatory agency needs to implement its plans to conduct regulatory inspections of clinical trial sites. It may be appropriate to initiate this program by identifying studies conducted by Indian companies. The global pharmaceutical companies have tried and tested quality assurance, audit and inspection mechanisms. The Indian sector has embarked on a serious clinical trial program and, regulatory inspection of these trials will certainly go a long way to enhance the credibility of such studies.

Pharmaceutical Industry and Service Providers

The pharmaceutical industry has enthusiastically welcomed the government's announcements about intellectual property and permission to conduct simultaneous phase global clinical trials. In a country like India that is democratic, it is essential for the sponsor to:

- Exhibit consistency and uniformity of practices globally
- Train the physicians and IRB members in all aspects of drug development and, not only clinical research and GCP
- Eliminate conflict of interest by people involved in conducting clinical research. Maintain respectable·investigator-sponsors relations
- Do not use clinical research as a weapon in the public relations armamentarium. Use it to promote credible evidence
- Let patient well being be the prime objective and responsibility of the physician
- Make informed consent "truly informed".

Institutional Review Boards

Perhaps the toughest function among all stakeholders is that of the IRBs. The ethical issues surrounding:

- Personalized medicine
- Gene therapy
- Early stage Translational clinical trials in cancer and HIV infections pose ethical, legal, intellectual, scientific and administrative issues. It is extremely important for the IRBs to engage in constant dialogue with the other stakeholders to enable them to protect participants while promoting science.
- It might be useful if the IRBs review ongoing translational studies in oncology and HIV infections to appreciate the complexities relating to informed consent, patient well being, etc.
- Accreditation of IRBs to national and international bodies must be actively encouraged.

Medical Profession

Currently, there is a dearth of physicians capable of conducting clinical trials. In such situations, the clinicians need to guard their professional integrity to maintain the confidence of the public in medical research in general and, clinical research in particular. The road of clinical research is strewn with examples of scientific misconduct and fraud. It will be useful for the investigators to remember.

Feasible
Interesting
New
Evaluable
Relevant

when evaluating a clinical trial protocol. This will help them to provide valuable inputs to the sponsors to develop appropriate protocols.

It will also benefit if the medical curriculum includes research methodology and statistical basis of clinical research in undergraduate courses. Medical students can inturn with pharmaceutical companies and CROs to gain practical insight into various aspects of drug development and clinical research and consider clinical research as a career option.

Media

Media does play a significant role in all walks of life. However, we cannot expect media to play the role of "patient educator". It will continue to look for slips and falls. Will continue to ignore and downplay success stories and the positive contribution. All the stakeholders will have to continue to work at achieving success and progress despite the media and, not because of their help. Efforts should continue to educate the media. We should encourage participants of clinical trials to recount their experiences. The patients should be mobilized and invited to speak at clinical trial meetings.

Society

Progress is possible when there is active participation of the community. Currently, the efforts are scattered and not visible. In a highly literate country like the US less than 5 percent of the population participates in clinical research. If 5 percent of the Indian population participates in clinical research, we shall have 50 million patients. If we have modest targets, we can work towards achieving it. Even if we target 2 percent of the population in the next five years, it will take considerable planning and efforts to accomplish this. Progress without societal involvement is unthinkable. It is time for appropriate persons among various stakeholders to get together to involve the society on a proactive basis. A well-informed society is the best spokesperson for this endeavor to succeed.

Training

Training is the most crucial and rate limiting step in the process of clinical research. India can outperform China if we have a sound training program in place.

Various estimates by investment bankers, analysts and others put the figure of patients participating in clinical trials in India by 2010 at 2 million. To achieve this, we need at least 40,000 clinicians (each investigator enrolling 50 patients. This is a far cry from the current rate of about 15 all over the world and, at the most 30 in India) and 200,000 clinical research professionals to manage this enterprise. This appears almost impossible. Even if one targets at 10 percent of this number, India can provide up to 200,000 patients by 2010. This would need about 4,000 physicians and 20,000 clinical research professionals such as CRAs, CRCs, Project Managers, Biostatisticians, Medical Writers, etc.

It is imperative for a collective effort to achieve this in a credible manner. All the stakeholders should supplement the very laudable efforts of Institute of clinical Research, India, Academy of Clinical Excellence and others.

SUMMARY

Indian clinical research enterprise can play a significant role in expediting global drug development if we identify the mistakes of the past committed around the world. We need to pay attention to:

- Training
- Prevention of fraud
- Involve the society on a proactive basis
- Pay attention to good science and sound ethics and commerce will follow.

We need to view the past, understand the present to be able to predict the future.

Success in clinical research is a challenge to the professionalism, integrity and trust of all the stakeholders.

SUGGESTED READING

1. Center Watch – Chasing Away Phantom Investigators, November 2001
2. Ethical and Policy Issues in Research involving Human Participants. National Bioethics Advisory commission. Bethesda, Maryland USA., August 2001
3. FDA Centennial. Exclusive Executive Report by FDA News. 2006
4. James Love. The Scientist. Vol. 17, issue 7. p 46. April 11, 2005
5. Janis Hardwick and Quentin Stout. Computer Science, University of Michigan, Ann Arbor, MI, ISA e mails: jphard@umich.edu and qstout@umich.edu
6. Kenneth A. Getz. In Center Watch, Applied Clinical Trials, etc.
7. New Scientist, March 2006
8. OncoLog. M.D. Anderson's report to physicians about advances in cancer research
9. Richard A. Rettig Industrialization of clinical Research. Health Affairs, March/April 2000
10. Richard Horton. Controlled Clinical Trials. 2001;22:593-604
11. Scott Gottlieb, MD. Deputy Commissioner US FDA. Speech before 2006 Conference on Adaptive Trial Design, Washington DC., July 2006
12. The Globalization of Clinical Trials. A Growing Challenge in Protecting Human Subjects. Janet Rehnquist, Inspector General, Department of Health and Human Services, September 2001.

2 Drug Development and Discovery

S K Mishra

INTRODUCTION

The drug development is a scientific endeavor and is highly regulated due to public health concern. The discovery of a new molecule and its development in to a new drug is complex, expensive and time-consuming process. The cost of new drug development is also critically dependent on the proportion of new molecules that fail in clinical testing. Coupled with the extremely high failure rate hundreds and thousands of chemical compounds are made and tested in an effort to find one that can achieve desirable results. Only one in about 10000 compounds can ever reach market. In general, it takes about 8 to 10 years and about $ 900 million to bring the drug to the market. This estimate includes early laboratory and animal testing, as well as later clinical trials using human subjects. This may vary depending on the type of molecule, targeted disease etc. In view of the high cost of the drug development process, the industry has to be very careful and has to look in to the factors that have significant impact on the process and should form basis for allocation of resources.

The decision to develop a new drug by a pharmaceutical company depends on the various factors and one of the key factors is to review and find out the unmet medical needs in the specific therapeutic area in which the company is interested due to strategic reasons. Sometimes, scientists like to pursue an interesting or promising line of research. In some cases there may be industry- university or industry – government scientific institutes collaboration that may help to develop a new molecule. New and interesting findings may also come from University, Institutes and the lead may be taken over by Pharmaceutical companies for further research. There are a number of research companies, which are comparatively small in their size, but they are contributing a lot in the new drug research. New molecules are being in-licensed by big pharmaceutical Companies to develop them further as they have technical and financial resources.

The drug discovery and development process is designed to ensure that only those pharmaceutical products that are both safe and effective are brought to market for the benefit of the patients.

HISTORICAL ASPECTS

The Renaissance surgeon Ambroise Parè conducted the first clinical trial of a novel therapy unintentionally in 1537. He used a concoction of turpentine, rose oil and egg yolk to prevent the infection of battlefield wounds. He found that the new treatment was much more effective compared to the traditional formula.

James Lind is considered as the father of clinical trials, since he was the first to introduce control groups into his experiments. He documented the fact that citrus fruits in the diet could prevent scurvy. Lind carried out trials while at sea on board the Salisbury in 1747. All scurvy patients were given the same general diet but this was supplemented with various additional items, including oranges and lemons. In just six days, those patients taking citrus fruits were fit for duty.

The focus on the concept of study design began in the nineteenth century and placebos were first used in 1863, and the idea of randomization was introduced in 1923 (Fisher and Mackenzie, 1923). Amerson et al (1931) first considered randomization of patients to treatments in clinical trial to reduce the potential bias and consequently to increase the statistical power for a detection of clinically significant difference.

However, the first trial using properly randomized treatment and control groups was carried out in 1948 by the Medical Research Council, and involved the use of streptomycin to treat pulmonary tuberculosis. This trial also featured blind assessment (researchers and the patients did not know as to which treatment groups each patient was in) enabling unbiased analysis of the results.

Since 1945, the ethical impact of clinical trials has become increasingly important, resulting in strict regulation of medical experiments on human subjects. These regulations have been enshrined in documents such as the Nuremberg Codex (1947) and the Declaration of Helsinki (1964, amended in 1975, 1983, 1989, 1996, 2000, 2002 and 2004).

Clinical trials have thus evolved into a standard procedure, focusing on patient safety and requiring informed consent from all participants. There will always be a balance between medical progress and patient safety, and the regulation of clinical trials helps to ensure that this balance is acceptable.

Regulatory

Earlier availability of drugs and medicines were based on the ancient art of pharmacy. In the nineteenth century pharmaceutical industry has come in to being. Since 1950, the randomized controlled clinical trials have become a definite tool to evaluate safety and efficacy. There was exponential growth in the pharmaceutical legislation after the Thalidomide disaster in the early 1960s.

The process of the clinical evaluation of drugs continues to evolve as a result of many factors including attempts at global harmonization.

The concept of testing marketed drugs in human subjects became a public issue after Elixir sulfanilamide disaster occurred in the late 1930. The disaster was a safety concern and this liquid formulation caused about 100 deaths. This drug had never been tested in human. *Federal Food, Drug and Cosmetic Act* (FD and C Act) was passed in 1938 due to this concern. In 1962, a significant Kefauver-Harris Drug Amendment to the FDandC act was passed. This amendment not only strengthened the safety requirements for new drugs but also established efficacy requirements for the new drugs.

We understand that the drug development is lengthy and costly process. But this lengthy process is necessary to ensure the safety and efficacy of the drug product under investigation. FDA review process for marketing authorization used to take long time about 2.5 years, however, this time was required to review the application thoroughly.

US Congress passed the *Prescription Drugs User Fee Act* (PDUFA) in 1992 and FDA was authorized to utilize the user fee for enhancement of their resources.

This decision helped FDA to reduce the average time required to review the new drug application from 30 months to about 15 months.

In India, earlier there was no review fee when the application for clinical trial/ marketing permission used to be submitted to the Drugs Controller's department, but now there is a defined fee structure.

In Great Britain a committee on clinical trials was formed in early years by Medical Research Council of the Great Britain (Medical Research Council, 1931) to promulgate good clinical practice by developing guidelines governing the conduct of clinical studies. Significant historical events have been mentioned in the Table 2.1.

Table 2.1: Significant historical event in clinical trials and regulations

Year	*Significant Historical Events*
1906	Pure Food and Drug Act (Dr. Harvey Wiley)
1912	• Sherley Amendment
1923	• First randomization to experiments (Fisher and Mackenzie, 1923)
1931	• First randomization of patients to treatments in clinical trials (Amberson, et al., 1931)· Committee on clinical trials by the Medical Research Council of Great Britain (Medical Research Council, 1931)· Formation of U.S. Food and Drug Administration
1937	• Formation of National Cancer Institute and First Research Grant by National Institutes of Health (National Institutes of Health, 1981)
1938	• U.S. Federal Food, Drug and Cosmetic Act (Dr. R. Tugwell)
1944	• First publication of results from a multicenter trial (Patulin Clinical Trial Committee, 1944)
1947	• Introduction of Nuremberg Codex
1952	• Publication of Elementary Medical Statistics (Mainland, 1952)
	• FDA makes designation of Prescription Drug or OTC

Contd...

Contd...

1962	• Publication of Statistical Methods in Clinical and Preventive Medicine (Hill, 1962)· Amendment to the US Food, Drug, and Cosmetic Act
1964	• Introduction of Declaration of Helsinki
1966	• Mandated creation of the local boards (IRB) for funding by US Public Health Service
1975	• Declaration of Helsinki revised
1976	• Medical Device Amendment to the US Food, Drug Cosmetic Act (1976)
1977	• Publications of General Considerations for Clinical Evaluation of Drugs (HEW (FDA), 1977)
1983	• Declaration of Helsinki revised
1984	• Drug Price Competition and Patent Term Restoration Act (Waxman and Hatch, 1984)
1985	• NDA rewrite
1987	• Treatment IND (FDA, 1987)
1988	• Publication of Guidelines for the Format and Content of the Clinical and Statistical Section of an Application (FDA, 1988)
1989	• Declaration of Helsinki revised
1990	• Publication of Good Clinical Practice for Trials on Medicinal Products in the European Community (EC Commission, 1990)
1992	• Parallel track and accelerated approval (FDA, 1992)· Prescription Drug User Fee Act
1996	• Declaration of Helsinki revised.
1997	• Publication of Good Clinical Practice: Consolidated Guidelines (ICH, 1996) • U.S. FDA Modernization Act
1998	• FDA promulgates Pediatric Rule
1999	• ClinicalTrials.Gov founded
2000	• Declaration of Helsinki revised
2001	• Under "accelerated approval" regulations, the FDA approves Gleevec, a promising new oral treatment for patients with chronic myeloid leukemia in less than three months - a record for this sort of therapy.
2002	• The Best Pharmaceuticals for Children Act improves safety and efficacy of patented and off-patent medicines for children. • Declaration of Helsinki revised.
2003	• FDA is given clear authority under the **Pediatric Research Equity Act** to require that sponsors conduct clinical research into pediatric applications for new drugs and biological products.
2004	Declaration of Helsinki revised.
2006	FDA approves first cervical cancer vaccine, Gardasil in just 6 months as a part of FDA's new priority-review system.

BASIC PRINCIPLES

The pathway of new drug development generally is same worldwide. In the new drug research process, there are three broad stages, which have been shown in the Table 2.2.

Table 2.2: The pathway of new drug development

Discovery		*Pre-clinical Development*		*Clinical Development*	
Target identification and validation	**Hit Identification**	**Lead Optimization**	**Drug Candidate Development**	**Clinical Testing**	**Post Marketing Studies**
Target Identification and validation	-Assay development	-Medicinal Chemistry	-Toxicology	-Phase I	-PhaseIV
	-High Throughput Screening (HTS)	-Structure Activity Relationship (SAR): Analog design and synthesis driven by data from *in vitro*, cell-based and animal models of disease	-Pharmaco-kinetics	-Phase II	
	-Hit validation		-ADME (Absorption, distribution, metabolism and excretion)	-Phase III	

- Discovery
- Pre-clinical development and
- Clinical development.

Drug Discovery

New drug discovery begins in the laboratory with scientists of various functional areas working together to identify cellular and genetic factors that play a role in specific diseases.

Most new drug candidates are identified through one or more of the following approaches:

i. Chemical modification of an already known molecule;
ii. Screening for biologic activity for large numbers of natural products, data mining of previously discovered chemical entities or large libraries of peptides, nucleic acid or other large organic molecules;
iii. Rational drug design based on an understanding of biologic mechanisms and chemical structure;
iv. Biotechnology and cloning using genes to produce larger peptides and proteins. Moreover, automation has generated the process known as "high throughput screening" which permits millions of assays per month.

There are following steps of research activities which begins the process and results in the development of new drugs:

Target Identification

Drugs usually act on either cellular receptor or genetic chemicals in the body, known as targets, which are believed to be associated with disease. Various methods are used by the scientists to identify and isolate a target, and learn more about its functions and how these can affect disease. Compounds are then identified that have various interactions with the drug targets, which are helpful in treatment of a specific disease.

Target Validation

In order to select the most useful target among the identified targets, scientists analyze and compare each drug target to others based on their association with a specific disease and their ability to regulate biological and chemical process/molecules in the body. Various studies are conducted to confirm that interactions with the drug target have demonstrated a desired change in the behavior of diseased cells. The data from these studies help the research scientists to identify compounds that have an effect on the target selected.

Lead Identification

A molecule that is believed to have potential to treat disease is a lead molecule. The scientists in the laboratory compare standard drug in that specific disease with new molecules to determine their likelihood of success. Leads are sometimes developed as collections, or libraries, of individual molecules that possess properties, which are required in a new drug. Thereafter evaluation is done on each of these molecules to confirm its effect on the drug target.

Lead Optimization

While working on the lead optimization, properties of various lead compounds are assessed which help to select the compound or compounds with the greatest potential to be developed into safe and effective medicines.

Pre-clinical Development

In the preclinical stage of drug development, an investigational drug is tested extensively in the laboratory under *in vitro* and *in vivo* conditions to ensure that it would be safe to administer to humans. It is important to have the information about the pharmaceutical composition of the drug, its safety, how the drug will be formulated and manufactured, and how it will be administered to the first in human.

Pharmacology and Toxicology

Pharmacological studies reveal the effects of the candidate drug on the body. Toxicity studies in animal models are conducted to identify potential risks to humans.

Results of all these studies are included in the Investigational New Drug (IND) application in order to obtain permission from FDA / DCGI or other appropriate regulatory agencies to begin clinical evaluation in humans. Regulatory agencies review the submitted data so as to permit the organization to proceed to the next stage of development.

Clinical Development

Investigational New Drug (IND) application in India, US, and Clinical Trial Authorization (CTA) in Australia and UK are examples of requests, which are submitted to appropriate regulatory authorities for permission to conduct investigational research.

Clinical evaluation of an investigational new drug begins only after permission to begin administration in healthy volunteers or patients is granted.

This research can also include evaluation of a new dosage form or new use of a drug already approved for marketing.

In addition to obtaining permission from appropriate regulatory authorities, an institutional or independent review board (IRB) or Independent ethics committee must approve the study protocol as well as the Informed Consent Documents (ICD) along with the applicable translated version of ICDs in relevant languages.

Clinical development is carried out in different phases consisting of Phase I, Phase II and Phase III clinical studies. Each phase of clinical development has different objective and in each successive phase, increasing numbers of patients are enrolled.

Phase I Clinical Studies

Phase I studies are designed to verify safety and tolerability of the candidate drug in humans and find out maximum tolerated dose (MTD). These studies take about six to nine months and are the first studies conducted in humans. A small number of subjects, usually from 20 to 100 healthy volunteers, take the investigational drug for short periods of time. Testing includes observation and careful documentation of pharmacodynamic and pharmacokinetic properties of the drug. How the drug acts in the body — how it is absorbed, distributed, metabolized and excreted.

Phase II Clinical Studies

Phase II studies are designed to determine effectiveness and further study the safety of the Investigational New Drug in humans. Depending upon the type of investigational drug and the condition it treats, this phase of development generally takes from six months up to three years. Testing is conducted with up to several hundred patients suffering from the condition the investigational drug is designed to treat. This testing determines safety and effectiveness of the drug in treating the condition and establishes the minimum and maximum effective dose. Most Phase II clinical trials are randomized, or patients are randomly divided into groups, one of which receives the investigational drug, and the other gets a placebo containing no medication and sometimes a third that receives a current standard treatment to which the new investigational drug will be compared. In addition, most Phase II studies are randomized and double-blinded (neither patients nor researchers evaluating the compound know who is receiving the investigational drug or placebo).

Phase III Clinical Studies

Phase III studies are conducted in large patient population to assess the efficacy and safety of an investigational drug, usually in randomized and blinded clinical trials. Depending upon the type of investigational drug and the condition it treats, this phase usually requires one to four years of evaluation. Several hundred to thousands of patients suffering from the condition the investigational drug treats are randomized in phase III. In this phase the investigational drug is compared with the one of the currently available standard treatments.

New Drug Application (NDA) /Marketing Authorization Application (MAA)

NDAs (in India, US) and MAAs (in the UK) are examples of applications, which are submitted to regulatory agencies in these countries for obtaining approval to market a new drug. Such applications document safety and efficacy of the investigational drug and contain all the information collected during the drug development process. At the conclusion of successful preclinical and clinical evaluation, all documents are submitted to "The Drug Controller General of India" or "The FDA in the U.S." or to "The applicable regulatory authorities in other countries". Substantial evidence is presented that the drug will have the desired efficacy and safety in the disease condition for which it has been developed. It takes about six months to two years to take the marketing authorization and varies from country to country.

Phase IIIb/IV Studies

Phase IIIb studies, usually begin before marketing authorization and may provide additional safety data or they may evaluate the approved drug for additional conditions for which it may prove useful. Phase IV studies of a marketed drug expand testing to broader patient populations and compare the long-term efficacy and/or cost of the drug to other marketed drugs available to treat the same condition.

Ethics

Ethical concerns about human experimentation have resulted in enactment of codes, guidelines, and laws, including the Nuremberg code, the Declaration of Helsinki and Federal Regulations. In India there are ethical guidelines for "Bio-medical research on Human Subjects" released for Indian Council of Medical Research.

Informed Consent

This is a process by which a subject voluntarily confirms his or her willingness to participate in a particular trial, after having been informed of all aspects of the trial that are relevant to the subject's decision to participate. Informed consent is documented by means of a written, signed and dated informed consent form.

Informed consent forms are to be in languages, which can be read and understood by the patients. Hence translations to relevant languages are equally important. In the situation where the patient is illiterate, thumb impression and signature by the impartial witness is required. In case of children, their patients or legal representative can sign the informed consent documents. In other circumstances, where time and situation do not permit informed consent (e.g. during cardiac arrest) separate rules have been developed in some countries to allow research.

Institutional Review Board / Independent Ethics Committee (IRB / IEC)

This is a procedure for protecting patient and subject safety and requires an independent body to review and approve a study before it can begin. In the Untied States, this independent body is an Institutional Review Board (IRB). For trials under the purview of the US Food and Drug Administration (FDA) such boards must satisfy a number of federal regulations (that carry the force of the enabling law). In addition, experiments involving investigational new drugs, biologics (that is drugs that are compounds naturally occurring in the human body), and devices must have the experimental protocol approved by the FDA as well as an IRB before implementation. In approving experiments with investigational new drug, both law and the Declaration of Helsinki mandate that appropriate pre-clinical studies be performed before beginning human experimentation.

In India there are ethics committees in various hospitals/medical institutions, which are constituted as per the ICMR "Ethical guidelines for Biomedical Research on human subjects" and ICH GCP guidelines. It is the responsibility of ethics committee to safeguard the rights, safety, and well-being of all trial subjects. Special attention is to be paid to trials that may include vulnerable subjects (e.g. prisoners, cognitively impaired persons, terminally ill patients, etc.).

The IRB/IEC should consist of a reasonable number of members, who collectively have the qualifications and experience to review and evaluate the science, medical aspects, and ethics of the proposed trial. It is recommended that the IRB/IEC should include: (a) At least five members. (b) At least one member whose primary area of interest is in a nonscientific area. (c) At least one member who is independent of the institution/trial site. Only those IRB/IEC members who are independent of the investigator and the sponsor of the trial should vote/provide opinion on a trial-related matter. A list of IRB/IEC members and their qualifications should be maintained.

The IRB/IEC should perform its functions according to written operating procedures, should maintain written records of its activities and minutes of its meetings, and should comply with GCP and with the applicable regulatory requirement(s).

The IRB/IEC should obtain and review the following documents: trial protocol/amendment (if any), written informed consent form and consent form updates that the investigator proposes for use in the trial, subject recruitment procedures (e.g. advertisements), written information to be provided to subjects, Investigator's Brochure (IB), available safety information, information about payments and compensation available to subjects, the investigator's current curriculum vitae and/or other documentation evidencing qualifications, and any other documents that the IRB/IEC may need to fulfill its responsibilities. The IRB/IEC should review a proposed clinical trial within a reasonable time and document its views in writing, clearly identifying the trial, the documents reviewed and the dates for the following: - approval/favorable opinion; - modifications required prior to its approval/favorable opinion; - disapproval / negative opinion; and - termination/suspension of any prior approval/favourable opinion.

The IRB/IEC should retain all relevant records (e.g., written procedures, membership lists, lists of occupations/affiliations of members, submitted documents, minutes of meetings, and correspondence) for a period of at least 3 years after completion of the trial and make them available upon request from the regulatory authorities. The IRB/IEC may be asked by investigators, sponsors or regulatory authorities to provide its written procedures and membership lists.

METHODOLOGY

Non-clinical Development

A new chemical or biologic molecule can be a drug candidate if it demonstrates some desirable pharmacological activities in the laboratory. At such an early stage of drug development the focus of work is mainly on cells, tissues, organs, or animals. Experimentation on human subjects is performed after the candidate passes these early evaluations and looks promising. Non-clinical development may also be referred to as *preclinical* development, since these experiments are performed before clinical trials are performed on the human subjects.

One of the most important properties to be studied at the non-clinical development stage is whether there is a dose-response relationship for the drug candidate. Pharmacokinetics and toxicokinetics are to be studied in the appropriate animal models. Figure 2.1 shows two curves describing these relationships. The x-axis represents the doses of the drug candidate (can be linear scale or logarithmic scale), and the y-axis represents the responses. Suppose the y-axis allows 0% responses at the bottom and 100% responses (both efficacy response and toxicity response) at the top, then as dose increases, the response also increases. The curve on the left represents the desirable response (potency, efficacy); the curve on the right represents the undesirable response (toxicity). The area in between those two curves would be the doses at which the drug works and is safe. Theoretically speaking, the best drug candidate would be one for which the drug potency (efficacy) increases very rapidly while the toxic response does not increase much as the dose increases. Under this ideal situation, a wide range of doses can be prescribed to treat patients. However, in reality these two curves can be close to each other. When this is the case, there is a narrow range of doses that will be both potent and safe, and dose selection must be very careful. In the process of developing a certain drug candidate, should these two curves become too close to each other, or should the toxic response curve locate to the left of the efficacy curve, then the strategy may be to stop development for this candidate.

At the preclinical stage, the study of drug potency or efficacy is part of pharmacology, whereas the study of toxicity is part of drug safety. In addition to pharmacological activity and toxicity, another important process at this preclinical development stage is the formulation of the compound or biologic into a form that can be consumed by humans (for example tablet, capsule, injectable).

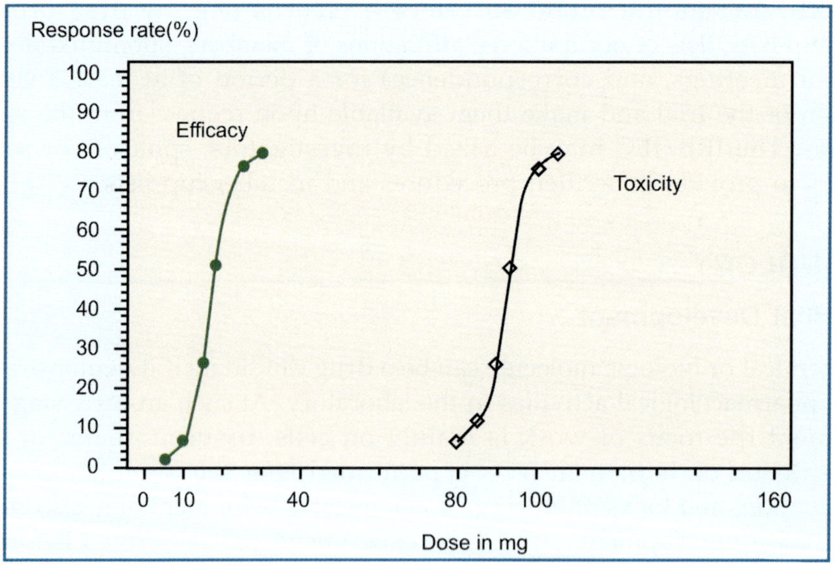

Fig. 2.1: Efficacy and toxicity response curves at different doses of drug candidate

Clinical Trial Design

Parallel Group Design

The most common clinical trial design for confirmatory trials is the parallel group design in which subjects are randomized to one of two or more arms, each arm being allocated a different treatment. These treatments will include the investigational product at one or more doses, and one or more control treatments, such as placebo and/or an active comparator. The assumptions underlying this design are less complex than for most other designs.

Group Sequential Design

In-group sequential design, a number of subjects are entered and studied. During the study an interim analysis of the data is conducted, and if the results are significant or if the treatment groups that is non-significant (statistically) or if the treatment groups are totally alike, then the clinical trial is stopped. If there is a difference between the two groups that is statistically non-significant, then a second group of subjects is enrolled, and the same type of randomization is used as was employed for the original group.

Factorial Design

In this design two or more treatments are evaluated simultaneously through the use of varying combinations of the treatments. The simplest example of 2 ´ 2 factorial design in which subjects are randomly allocated to one of the four possible combinations of two treatments, A and B are A alone; B alone; both A and B; neither A nor B. In many cases this design is used for the specific purpose of examining the interaction of A and B.

Another important use of the factorial design is to establish the dose-response characteristics of the simultaneous use of treatments C and D, especially when the efficacy of each monotherapy has been established at some dose in prior studies.

2 ´ 2 Cross- over Design.

Crossover designs are very commonly used for bioequivalence studies. In chronic conditions disease also this design is used (Fig. 2.2).

The most commonly used statistical design for comparing average bioavailability between two formulations of a drug probably is a two-sequence, two-period,

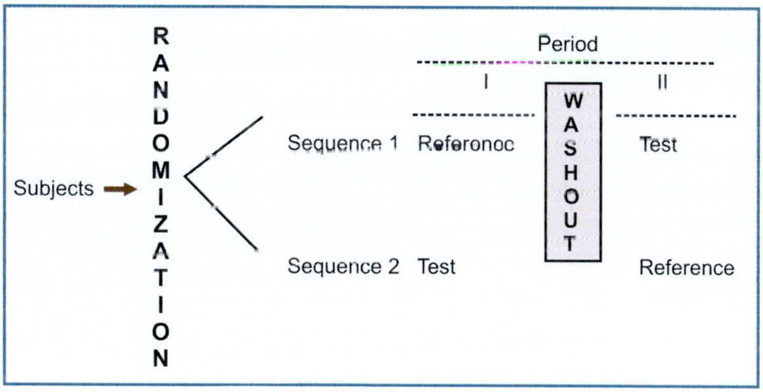

Fig. 2.2: Cross-over design for two formulations

crossover design (2 x 2 Crossover design). For a standard 2x2 crossover design, each subject is randomly assigned to either sequence RT (Reference Test) or sequence TR (Test Reference) at two dosing periods. In other words, subjects within RT receive formulation R at the first dosing period and formulation T at the second dosing period. The dosing periods are separated by a washout period of sufficient length for the drug received in the first period to be completely metabolized or excreted from the body.

Trial Objectives

The trials, when are designed to compare an investigational new drug with an active comparator may have one of the following objectives-

- The superiority of the IND
- Non inferiority of the IND
- The equivalence of the two

Superiority Trial

Efficacy of investigational new drug is most convincingly demonstrated by showing superiority to placebo, active comparator or in dose response relationship studies.

Equivalence Trial

Equivalence trials are those when investigational new drug is compared to reference treatment with the objective to demonstrate that both the treatments are equivalent.

Bio-equivalence studies i.e. absence of meaningful difference between the treatments (test and reference) fall under this objective.

Sometimes clinical equivalence trials are also carried out. A margin of clinical equivalence is chosen by defining the largest difference that is clinically acceptable, so that a difference bigger than this would matter in practice. If the two treatments are to be declared equivalent then the two-sided 95% confidence interval – which defines the range of plausible differences between the two treatments – should lie entirely within the interval – to +.

In the case of bioequivalence studies a coverage probability of 90% for the confidence interval has become the accepted standard when evaluating whether the average values of the pharmacokinetic parameters of two formulations are sufficiently close.

Non-inferiority Trial

There are many active control trials, which are designed with the objective to show that the efficacy of investigational new drug is not inferior (no worse) to that of active comparator.

In Phase III drug development, non-inferiority trials are more common than equivalence trials. In these trials it is shown that a new treatment is no less effective than an existing treatment – it may be more effective or it may have a similar effect. Again a confidence interval approach is the most straightforward way of performing the analysis but here we are only interested in a possible difference in one direction.

Clinical Operations

Understanding and implementation of Good Clinical Practices (GCP) is very essential in the conduct of a clinical trial.

GCP is defined as, "A standard for the design, conduct, performance, monitoring, auditing, recording, analyses, and reporting of clinical trials that provides assurance that the data and reported results are credible and accurate, and that the rights, integrity, and confidentiality of trial subjects are protected." This definition accurately captures the whole of GCP, both data integrity and subject protection, and specifies areas of trial implementation that directly affect GCP. In a clinical study there are pre study, during study and end of the study activities. These activities have been shown in the study flow chart.

Protocol

In a clinical study protocol, CRF, IB and ICD are important documents. Some of the main information about Protocol and CRF is mentioned below.

Protocol is a document, which states the background, objectives, rationale, design, methodology (including the methods for dealing with AEs, withdrawals, etc.) and statistical considerations of the study. It also states the conditions under which the study shall be performed and managed. The content and format of the protocol should take into consideration the adopted SOPs, the regulatory requirements and the guiding principles of GCP.

In the conduct of the study, if all the aspects as mentioned in the protocol are not followed thoroughly, there may be deviations. The failure to adhere to protocol may be accidental or due to negligence and in either case, the protocol deviation should be documented.

Case Record Form (CRF)

This is a document designed in consonance with the protocol, to record data and other information on each study subject. The Case Record Form is designed in such a format that allows accurate input, presentation, verification, audit and inspection of the recorded data. A CRF may be in printed or electronic format. Instructions to fill the CRF are part of the CRF.

Prior to Commencing the Study (Pre-study Site Visit)

Before the start of the study the sponsors should visit the principal investigator to verify that the site, staff and facilities for the study comply with the requirements of the protocol and sponsor SOPs. The sponsor's staff may accompany the monitor during this visit.

Laboratories participating in the study should be checked by the monitor to ensure that they are accredited by an appropriate accreditation organization like CAP (College of American Pathologist) and NABL (National Accreditation Board For Testing and Calibration) and have adequate quality assurance.

Start-up activities for a new study cover the activities that occur between the time a site is chosen to participate in a study and the time that the first participant is enrolled in the study.

Site Initiation Visit

Before the patient enrollment starts, it is important to have a meeting with patient site(s) personnel with the purpose to acquaint them with the relevant aspects of the study. This involves the review/discussion of the protocol, case report form completion, missed visits, IRB/IEC reporting requirements, adverse event reporting, etc.

This site initiation visit is scheduled once all regulatory documents and approvals are received, during this visit; the sponsors are required to discuss the following with the principal investigator and his/her staff as appropriate:

- Study objectives and obligations
- Investigator brochure
- Protocol procedures (particularly inclusion/exclusion criteria, enrollment goals, adverse events, primary efficacy variables and GCP compliance)
- Informed consent procedure
- Randomization procedure
- AE/SAE reporting
- CRF completion and error correction/need for adequate source documentation
- Maintenance of the investigator binder and site visit log
- Laboratory sample handling procedures and results reporting procedures
- Clinical supply dispensation, accountability and storage procedures
- Any other issue as deemed important to the conduct of the study
- After visit a report is to be prepared based on the SOP.

Techniques to Avoid Bias

a. Randomization: Randomization alleviates the treatment assignment bias. It introduces a deliberate element of chance into the assignment of treatment to subjects in a clinical trial. During subsequent analysis of the trial data, it provides a sound statistical basis for the quantitative evaluation of the evidence relating to treatment effects. It also tends to produce treatment groups in which the distributions of prognostic factors, known and unknown are similar. In combination with blinding, randomization helps to avoid possible bias in the selection of subjects arising from the predictability of treatment assignments. Although unrestricted randomization is an acceptable approach, some advantages can generally be gained by randomizing subjects in blocks. This helps to increase the comparability of the treatment groups, particularly when subject characteristics may change over time, as a result, for example, of changes in recruitment policy. In multicenter trials the randomization procedures should be organized centrally. It is advisable to have a separate random scheme for each center, i.e. to stratify by center or to allocate several whole blocks to each center. More generally stratification by important prognostic factors measured at baseline may sometime be valuable in order to promote balanced allocation within strata; this has greater potential benefit in small trials. The use of more than two or three stratification factors is rarely necessary, is less successful at achieving balance and is logistically troublesome.

b. Blinding: Blinding is done to limit the occurrence of conscious and unconscious bias in the conduct and interpretation of a clinical trial administered which may come with the knowledge of treatment administered. This bias may occur in patient care, the attitudes of patients to the treatments, the assessment of end-points, the handling of withdrawals, the exclusion of data from analysis, and so on. The main objective is to prevent identification of the treatments until all such opportunities for bias have passed. In a single-blind trial the investigator and or his staff are aware of the treatment but the subject is not or vice versa. In open-label everybody knows the identity of the treatment. A double-blind trial is one in which neither the subject nor any of the investigator or sponsor staff who are involved in the treatment or clinical evaluation of the subjects are aware of the treatment received. This level of blinding is maintained throughout the conduct of trial, and only when the data are cleaned to an acceptable level of quality will appropriate person be unblinded. Blinding, during the conduct of the study, should not be broken unless it is essential for patient's physician to know the drug for the management of adverse event etc.

c. Monitoring: Monitoring is an act of overseeing the progress of a clinical trial, and of ensuring that it is conducted, recorded, and reported in accordance with the protocol, Standard Operating Procedures (SOPs), Good Clinical Practice (GCP), and the applicable regulatory requirement(s).

The purpose of trial monitoring is to verify that:

i. The rights and well being of human subjects are protected and the patient has given written informed consent.
ii. The reported trial data are accurate, complete, and verifiable from source documents.
iii. The conduct of the trial is in compliance with the currently approved protocol/ amendment(s), with GCP, and with the applicable regulatory requirement.

d. Source Document . The source document are original documents, data, and records (e.g., hospital records, clinical and office charts, laboratory notes, memoranda, participant diaries or evaluation checklists, pharmacy dispensing records, recorded data from automated instruments, copies or transcriptions certified after verification as being accurate and complete, microfiches, photographic negatives, microfilm or magnetic media, X-rays, participant files, and records kept at the pharmacy, at the laboratories, and at medico-technical departments involved in the clinical trial.

e. *Source Data Verification (SDV):* Source data verification is done to conformity of the data presented in case report forms (CRFs) with source data. In this process, information reported by an investigator is compared with the original records to ensure that it is complete, accurate and valid. The aim of SDV is to ensure that the data collected are reliable and allow reconstruction and evaluation of the study. Study monitor carries out source data verification when site visit is done.

f. Source Data Verification Vs Data Monitoring: In data monitoring (DM), the clinical trial monitor checks completed CRF pages to ensure that the data have been correctly entered and that all corrections have been dated and initialed. Data monitoring is essentially a review of the CRFs by the sponsor company to check for errors and inconsistencies. On the other hand, in SDV, the data collected in CRF is checked against source documents.

g. Clinical Data Management: Madision and Plaunt (2003) define Clinical Data Management (CDM) as the process of collecting and validating clinical information with the goal of converting it into an electronic format to answer research questions and to preserve it for future scientific investigations. CDM is an integral part of the clinical trials process, which ensures the validity, quality and integrity of data collected from trial subject to a database system. CDM delivers a clean and high-quality database for statistical analysis and consequently enables clinical scientists to draw conclusions regarding the effectiveness safety and clinical benefit/ risk of the drug product under investigations. An invalid and /or poor quality database may result in wrong and / or misleading conclusions regarding the drug product under investigation. Thus the objective of the CDM process in clinical trials is not only to capture the information that the intended clinical trials are designed to capture, but also to ensure the validity, quality and integrity of the collected data. In general the CDM process includes:

i. Case report form (CRF) development
ii. Database development and validation
iii. Data entry, query, and correction
iv. Data quality assurance and
v. Data lock, archive, and transfer.

The implementation of good data management practice (GDMP) is necessary. GDMP is a set of standards/procedures for assurance of the validity, quality and integrity of clinical data collected from trial subjects to a database system.

h. QC/QA Procedures: In order to ensure the integrity and accuracy of the study data, various Quality Control (QC) and Quality Assurance (QA) Procedures shall be applied at every step during the conduct of the study. These procedures shall be performed as per ICH- GCP and sponsor's applicable Standard Operating Procedures.

i. Quality Control (QC) : The internal operational techniques and activities undertaken within the quality assurance system to verify that the requirements for quality of trial related activities have been fulfilled, i.e. data and form checks, monitoring by study staff, routine reports, and correction procedures.
j. Quality Assurance (QA): The externally planned and systematic actions that are established to ensure that the trial is performed and the data are generated, documented (recorded), and reported in compliance with GCP and the applicable regulatory requirement(s), i.e. site or center audits, external monitoring, etc.

RECENT ADVANCES

Drug discovery, lead candidate selection and preclinical development are undergoing rapid changes, driven in part by scientific advances in areas such as combinatorial chemistry, molecular and cell biology and high throughput technology and also by the fierce competition and economic forces.

Pharmacogenomics and Drug Development

Pharmacogenomics information is anticipated to have large impact on drug development and to facilitate individualized drug treatment.

Different patients respond in different ways to the same medication. These differences are often greater among members of a population than they are within the same person at different times. The existence of large population differences with small intra-patient variability is consistent with inheritance as a determinant of drug response. It is estimated that genetics can account for 20 to 95 percent of variability in drug disposition and effects.

Pharmacogenomics is a rapidly evolving science with the potential to revolutionize drug discovery and development. FDA had published a draft guidance in November 2003 regarding the submission of pharmacogenomic data to investigational new drug applications (INDs), and new drug applications (NDAs).

Pharmacogenomics involves the use of genome-wide analyses to identify genes with altered expression or activation as a result of exposure to a drug. Pharmacogenomics can identify markers to aid drug development. Markers of exposure can determine whether the desired target tissues of a subject have been exposed to a drug at physiological concentrations. Markers of efficacy can provide molecular evidence above and beyond traditional clinical endpoints. Stratification markers can identify a subset of patients who may uniquely benefit from a given therapy. Finally, toxicity markers can predict and prevent adverse events.

Integrated Drug Development

In order to accelerate the drug development process, pharmaceutical companies are going for integrated drug development plan which help them to optimize the resources and timelines and carry out development faster thereby saving cost and bringing in the drug faster for the patients.

CONCLUSIONS

Drug development is a complex, time and money intensive process. The role of scientists, clinical pharmacologists, investigators, regulatory agencies and other development partners is very important. The scientific framework in which development of a drug proceeds is dynamic and new approaches are required to be developed.

With the dynamic character of scientific and regulatory framework and also that the process involves many constituents like pharmaceutical industry, the scientific and health care communities, the government, and society at large—a potential synergism exists in which involved constituents could work collaboratively to improve methods and procedures for development of innovative, life-saving, safe medications for fighting various diseases and sufferings of the mankind.

SUGGESTED READING

1. DiMasi JA, Hasnsen RW, Grabowski HG, Lasagna L. Research and development costs for new drugs by therapeutic category: a study of US pharmaceutical industry. Pharmacoeconomics 1975; 7: 152-69.
2. Guo Y, Shafer S, Weller P, Usuka J, Petlz G. Pharmacogenomics and drug development pharmacogenomics 2005 (8); 857-64.
3. Good Clinical Practices: Guidelines for clinical trials on Pharmaceutical Products in India, Central Drugs Standard Control Organization, Directorate General of Health Services, Ministry of Health and Family Welfare, Government of India, New Delhi, 2001.
4. International Conference on Harmonization, Good Clinical Practices: Consolidated Guidelines E6 (R1, Section 5); Federal Register, 1997.
5. Madison T, Plaunt M. Clinical Data Management. In By Chow, S C Dekker (Eds): Encyclopedia of Biopharmaceutical Statistics (2nd ed) New York. 2003;181-8.
6. Schedule Y (Amended Version 2005) Under Drugs and Cosmetics Rules 1945, by CDSCO, Ministry of Health, Government of India.

3

Designing Clinical Trials

MUR Naidu, P Usha Rani

INTRODUCTION

Clinical trial, which is properly planned and executed, is a very powerful experimental technique for assessing the effectiveness of intervention. Careful planning is required before the collection of data begins for conducting successful clinical research projects. Some investigators know the planning process; others must learn how to plan clinical research by observing their mentors and reading books on research designs. It is important that the investigator should recognize the difficulty encountered in studies with human subjects and planning any clinical trial and attempt to estimate the magnitude of participant's failure to protocol compliance. Ideal clinical trial is one, which is randomized and double blind. In most of the clinical trials, drawbacks are unavoidable, but these deficiencies can be prevented by adhering to fundamental features of clinical trial design, conduct and proper analysis.

HISTORY OF CLINICAL TRIAL

The earliest evidence of the clinical trial dates back to 20th May 1747, where in his classical study James Lind evaluated six treatments in 12 patients of scurvy. One of the two patients who were given lemons and oranges quickly recovered from signs and symptoms of scurvy and were fit for their duty after 6 days. Earliest experiments involved arbitrary, non-systematic schemes for patients, assigned to various therapeutics as that described by Lind. The concept of process of randomization in clinical trials was first introduced by Fisher. In year 1926, Fisher applied randomized in an agriculture research. The study by Amberson et al in 1931 was the first clinical trial that used a form of random assignment of subject to study group. In this study a flip of coin determined which group of 12 subjects would receive Sanocrysin, a gold compound for pulmonary tuberculosis versus control. British Medical Research Council in year 1948 for the first time used a properly randomized control for

Streptomycin in the treatment of pulmonary tuberculosis study. The principle of blindness was also introduced in clinical trials by Amberson. In 1938 Deichi et al gave saline solution to the subjects in the control placebo group in a cold vaccine trial.

The clinical trial has evolved into standard procedure in the evaluation of new drugs after World War II, which included use of control groups, random allocation of patients to control and experimental groups and use of blind or masked assessment. It is only in the past few decades that clinical trials have emerged as the preferred method in the evaluation of medical intervention. Subsequently, several other comparative studies were conducted. Some of them are given in Tables 3.1 and 3.2.

Table 3.1: A selective history of clinical research

Authors	*Periods*	*Events*
Frederick II	1200 CE	Effects of exercise on digestion
Van Helmont	17th century	Effects of bloodletting on fever
Billroth	Late 1800s	Value of simple mastectomy in treatment of breast cancer
Various Frei	1940's –50s	Tuberculosis trials6-MP and childhood ALL
Doll Wynder	1950	Link between smoking and lung cancer

Table 3.2: Historical events in the development of clinical research

Periods	*Authors*	*Events*
1747	James Lind	Experiment with untreated control group (Lind, 1743)
1799	Haygarth	Use of sham procedure (Haygarth, 1800)
1800	Waterhouse	US Based small pox trial (Waterhouse, 1800, 1802)
1863	Gull	Use of placebo treatment (Sutton, 1965)
1923	Fisher	Application of randomization to experimentation (Fisher and Mackenzie)
1923	MRC Britain	Special committee on clinical trial created by the Medical Research Council of Great Britain (Medical Research Council, 1931)
1931	Amberson	Random allocation of treatment to groups of patients (Amberson et al, 1931)
1937	NIH	Start of NIH grant support with creation of the National Cancer Institute (National Institute of Health, 1981b)
1944	PCTC	Publication of multicenter trial on treatment for common cold (Patulin Clinical Trials committee, 1944)
1962	Curran	Promulgation of Nuremburg Code for Human Experimentation (Curran and Shapiro, 1970)
1962	Hill	Publication of book on clinical trials (Hill, 1962)
1962	Kefaiver and Harris	Amendments to the Food, Drug and Cosmetic Act of 1938 (United `States Congress, 1962)
1966	US PHSR	Publication of US Public health service regulation leading to creation of Institutional Review Boards for research involving humans (Levine, 1981)
1967	Chalmers	Structure for separating the treamtment monitoring and treatment administration process
1979	SCT	Establishment of Society for Clinical Trials Society for Clinical Trials, Inc, 1980
1980		First issue of Controlled Clinical Trials

DEFINITION

Research is a systematic investigation (including development, testing and evaluation) designed to discover or contribute to a body of generalizable knowledge. Not all research involves human participants, but when they are involved, researchers and their teams are legally and ethically obligated to protect them. A clinical trial is defined as a systematic and prospective study aimed to compare the effect and values of interventions against a control group in human subjects.

It is a prospective rather than a retrospective study in which trial participants are followed forward in time. This is in contrast to case-control study, a type of retrospective study in which participants are selected on basis of presence or absence of clinical condition or events. By definition, this type of study is not a clinical trial, since the participants are not directly observed from the moment of study initiation.

A clinical trial can also be defined as - the controlled experiment having a clinical event as an outcome measure and done in a clinic or clinical setting and involving person having a specific disease or health condition (Meinert, 1996).

An experiment is a series of observations made under conditions controlled by the scientist; thus a clinical trial is an experiment testing medical treatment on human participant (Piantadosi 1997). The term clinical trial may be applied to any form of planned experiment, which involves patient and is designed to elucidate the most appropriate treatment of future patients with a given medical condition.

BASIC PRINCIPLES

A clinical trial must employ one or more intervention techniques like prophylactic, diagnostic, therapeutic devices, regimens and procedures etc. Without active intervention the study is observational because no experiment is being performed. To compare the intervention group a clinical trial must contain a control group. It is essential that the control group must be sufficiently homogenous with respect to intervention group at the start of clinical trial, so that the difference in outcome may reasonably be attributed to proposed intervention. New interventions most often should be compared with best current standard therapy. In clinical trials, the investigators cannot dictate individual participant to do as per their requirement unlike animal studies. Investigator can only encourage trial participant to withdraw or avoid certain medication or procedures, which can interfere with trial outcome.

The design and conduct of any type of clinical trial requires three important considerations.

1. Study must examine valuable and important biomedical research questions
2. It must be designed and based on a rigorous methodology that can answer a specific research question and
3. Must be based on a set of strong ethical principles to minimize the risk to trial participants.

The choice of an appropriate study design depends on the following factors and considerations

i. Ability of study design to answer the primary research question
ii. Whether the trial is studying a potential new treatment for a condition for which an established, effective treatment already exists
iii. Whether the disease for which new treatment is sought is severe or life threatening
iv. The probability and magnitude of risk to the participants
v. The probability and magnitude of likely benefit to the participant
vi. The population to be studied – its size, availability and accessibility.

Because the choice of study design for any particular trial will depend on these above mentioned factors and other considerations, no general outline can be offered for the design of clinical trial. Judgment about effectiveness of given intervention ultimately rests on an interpretation of the strength of evidence arising from the data collected. In general, the more controlled the trial stronger is the evidence. The study design of clinical trial can take several forms, most of which are based on an assumption of accessible sample population.

Whenever feasible, standard trial design must be used which contains adequate statistical power. Scientific research has a long history of using well-established, well-documented and validated methods for the design, conduct and analysis of clinical trial. An appropriate study design must include sufficient sample size, statistical power and proper control of bias to allow a meaningful interpretation of the trial results.

CLINICAL TRIAL

This is a schematic general flow chart format for conducting a clinical trial. The exact sequence of events may vary with any given situation. The sponsor, the site, the particular protocol and a host or other variables play a role in the exact flow of a clinical trial. In fact, no two protocols follow the exact same sequence. Flow chart 3.1 given below present the steps of what a "typical" clinical trial conducted commonly would look like.

Phase III trials are advanced stage clinical trials, designated to show conclusively, how well a new drug works. Phase III trials are usually larger, multi-institutional and typically involve from 100 – 1000 participants. They are comparative in nature in which participants are usually assigned by randomization to at least 2 arms, one of which serves as control, or a reference arm and one or more of which involve new intervention. Phase III trials generally measure whether a new intervention extends benefit or improves the health of participants.

Phase IV trials usually performed after a new drug or biological has been approved for use. These trials are post marketing surveillance studies aimed at obtaining additional information about the risks, benefits and optimal use of an intervention.

A much more inclusive and general approach that subsumes the 4 phases of clinical trial is suggested by Piantadosi 1979 and tabulated in Table 3.3 as:

Flow chart 3.1: Clinical research

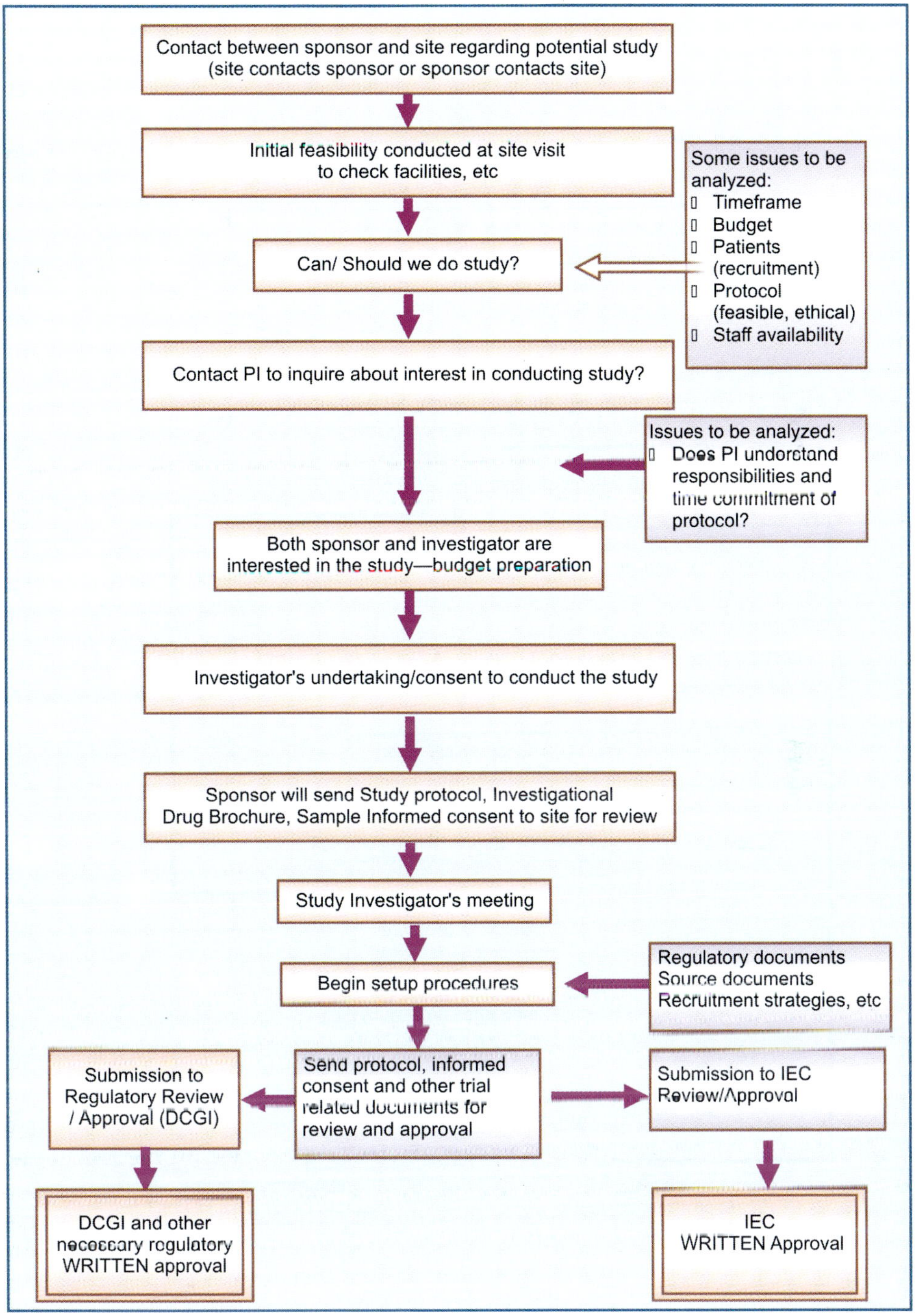

Contd...

Contd...

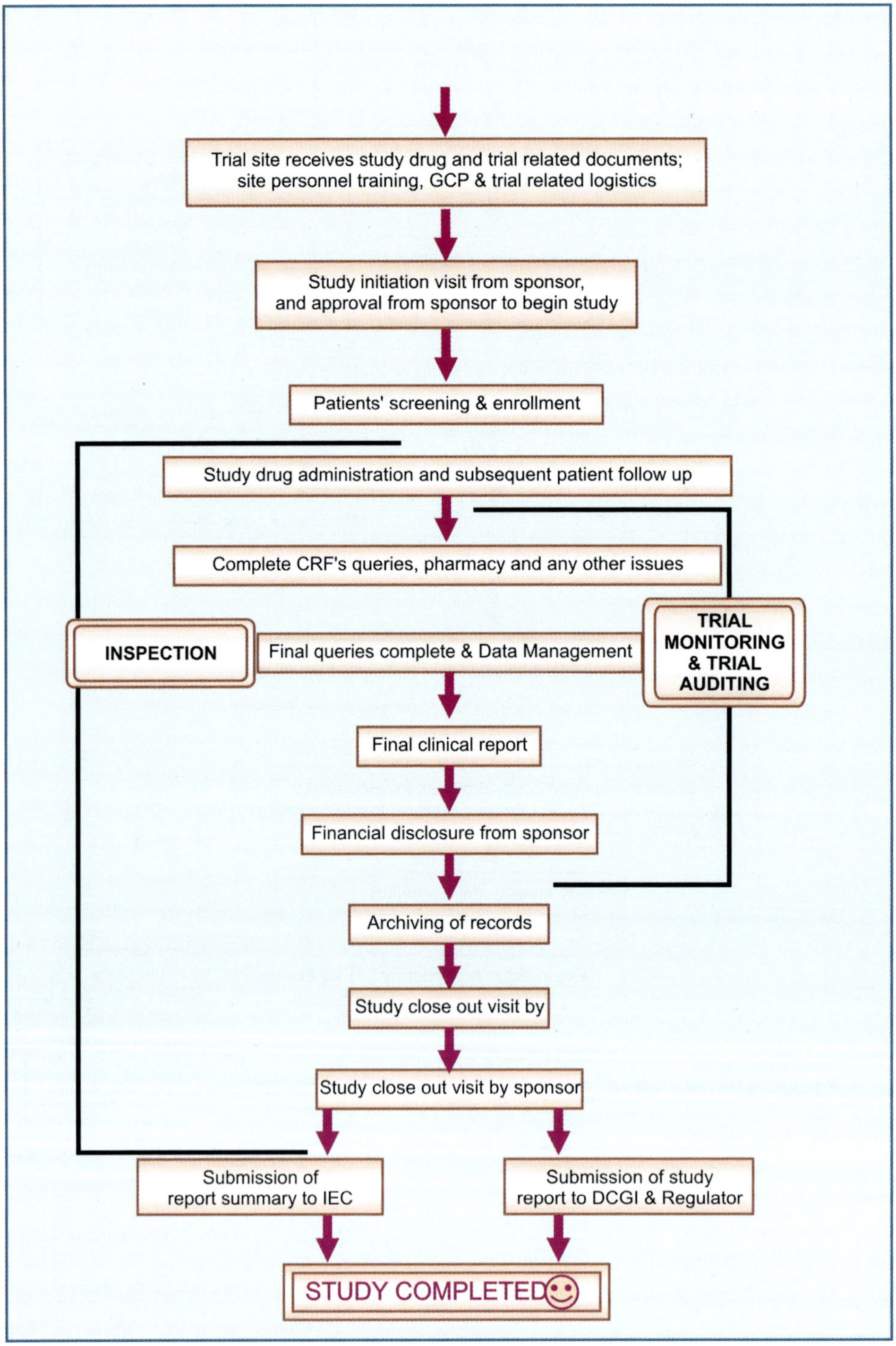
Trial site receives study drug and trial related documents; site personnel training, GCP & trial related logistics
Study initiation visit from sponsor, and approval from sponsor to begin study
Patients' screening & enrollment
Study drug administration and subsequent patient follow up
Complete CRF's queries, pharmacy and any other issues
INSPECTION
Final queries complete & Data Management
TRIAL MONITORING & TRIAL AUDITING
Final clinical report
Financial disclosure from sponsor
Archiving of records
Study close out visit by
Study close out visit by sponsor
Submission of report summary to IEC
Submission of study report to DCGI & Regulator
STUDY COMPLETED

i. Early development study - testing the treatment mechanism (proof of concept)
ii. Middle development studies – treatment tolerability
iii. Comparative – Pivotal confirmatory studies
iv. Late development studies

Table 3.3: Phases of clinical investigation

Phase of trial	*Number of subjects*	*Duration of study*	*Purpose*
Phase I	20 – 200	Several months	Safety pharmacokinetics
Phase II	Several hundred	1-3 years	Safety, efficacy, pharmacokinetics
Phase III	Several hundred to thousands	1-4 years	Safety, efficacy

DESIGNING CLINICAL TRIAL

Process of designing and carrying out clinical research can be divided mainly into two parts: The first part is to deal with processes required in planning the study before data collection begins and second part deals with the execution steps carried out in data collection, analysis, and publication. Ideally, the clinical investigator should be aware of and address all of these steps in the design phase to ensure the feasibility and success of the clinical trial project.

Planning Steps

Develop Hypothesis for Research

One of the most important steps in successful clinical research is to come up with an important idea to study. Developing good and important research hypothesis requires experience in the clinical field to be studied and interaction with other experienced investigators. With the help of other investigators or one's own experience; the investigator must ask, "*What is an important question that, if I could answer, would greatly advance the understanding or practice in my* field?" Approaches like attending national research meetings, seeking insights from experienced colleagues, and simply working in a field for a number of years, will provide the direction. One should not adopt only a research method or technique or an existing clinical database with the idea, to analyze and answer some important questions. Efforts that begin with methods or databases and proceed to questions rarely generate important conclusions. It is always better that one should determine the important questions in the field and design the methods and databases to answer them.

Once the hypothesis has been identified, the clinical investigator should review the scientific literature and discuss the idea with mentors and colleagues. These days, a complete scientific literature review can be conducted rapidly through use of the National Library of Medicine's MEDLINE database, which can be accessed by computer in any medical library and via personal computer and modem from home. After reading the titles and abstracts of articles indexed under appropriate keywords, the researcher should go to the library and read the articles most relevant to the research. This will determine whether others have attempted to address the subject, identify research approaches and methods used successfully or unsuccessfully by prior investigators, and provide additional contextual information of importance in designing the project. Armed with knowledge from the literature, one is then in the position to discuss the subject meaningfully with others. The discussion process helps the investigator refine the idea and think through complex issues or impediments to the research. The researcher must realistically assess the idea and narrow its scope to something that can be accomplished with the time and resources that might realistically be obtained.

Define the Objectives and Establish Priorities

Early in the planning process, the researcher must make a list of all the objectives that are to be accomplished. When the objectives are not formally written, often there is an unrecognized confusion over how many objectives are there and exactly what they are. They can only be clarified by writing them down in formal word statements. Usually you may find, when writing down the objective of the study, that there were really two or three somewhat different objectives being interchangeably discussed when the original research idea was being formulated.

Once all of the objectives are identified, they must be rewritten in order of priority and relative importance. A common fault in study design is to have too many objectives in a single study. Objective must be clearly and concisely stated. If a study has more than one objective, they should be listed in order of priority. The fewer the questions to be answered in one study, the greater the likelihood that they will be answered conclusively. In some instances, the competition among objectives is so extreme that two or more objectives can simply not be addressed in the same study. It is better to avoid studies with several objectives, which will otherwise require additional study resources, sample size, financial resources, and personal time. It is therefore important to set the priorities among objectives before going further in the design. The key to successful study design is simplicity.

Define the Variables Needed

Once the objectives are formally written, the investigator develops a plan to accomplish the objectives. Generally, the first decision in developing the plan is to enumerate the variables that will have to be measured to answer the questions. After enumerating all the variables, later steps will deal with defining the variables in greater detail, anticipating problems in measuring and comparing the variables, and formulating a study design in which the measurements can be used for drawing casual inferences. In any clinical study, there are mainly three types of different variables. They may serve as dependent variables, independent variables, or extraneous variables.

The *dependent variables* are the measures of the outcomes of the study. They are often referred to as outcome variables, response variables, disease variables, or effect variables. They constitute the effect in the cause-and-effect relationship.

The *independent variables* are the presumed casual variables in the cause-and-effect relationship. They are often referred to in different contexts as treatment variables, casual variables, classification variables, and factor variables. In epidemiological studies they are often referred to as risk factors. In experiments, the independent variable is assigned by the investigator and is under the investigator's control, where as in observational studies it is not.

The *extraneous variables* are additional variables not of direct interest to the investigator but that might be adversely affecting the study unless they are accounted for in the design or the analysis. They are often referred to as confounding variables, biasing variables, noise variables, co-variables, or effect modifiers.

As an example, in a clinical trial to determine the efficacy of an investigational drug for epilepsy, the group to which the patient was assigned (drug or placebo) would be the independent variable; whether the patient subsequently experienced epileptic attack (or the number of attacks) would be the dependent variable; and such measurements as the cause of the epilepsy (trauma versus infection and tumors), the extent and severity of epileptic attacks, and the number of previous epileptic attacks might be extraneous variables of interest. The investigator should make a list of all the variables of interest in the study. When the list has been narrowed down the best variables for each of these uses, the investigator should write a formal definition for each variable, including the valid codes, or values, with which the variable is coded in the data collection process. When studying diseases, the dependent variable is often a measure of whether or not a patient developed the disease, and the definition of this variable is called the *case definition*.

The wording of the variable definitions is extremely important and should be carefully formulated because these definitions will be applied literally in classifying patients in the data collection process. If the definitions are too broad or unclear, this may result in serious misclassifications that could bias the study results. Often the definitions will need to be discussed among collaborators or with a mentor to ensure that they are precisely and appropriately stated.

After they have been defined, a concise description of how each variable will be measured should also be written. For some variables, this will be a short statement, but for others it might require a several-page description of laboratory methods or equipment configurations.

In defining and describing the variables, the investigator must also anticipate the statistical analysis that will be applied at the end of the study. While many new investigators find it uncomfortable to think of analyzing the data before it is even collected, at least a broad outline of the analysis is essential before finalizing the definitions of the variables. Some investigators even go through the motions of writing out the methods and results sections of their scientific paper in mock fashion before data collection begins, imagining what they are predicting to find to ensure that the list of variables and codes is going to be adequate for their needs. Such advance scrutiny of the variables is important because the approach that can be used for the statistical analysis is determined to a large extent by the types of variables and their codes measured in the study.

Define the Study Population

While determining the variables to be measured, the investigator simultaneously defines the population to be studied. In clinical research, the population is generally a group of patients found in the hospital, admitted to a clinic, or simply identified in the population. In defining the population to be studied, however, it is frequently not sufficient to include simply a group of patients that can be conveniently assembled.

To guide the definition of the study population, one must ask "What is the *target population*?" or "What is the group of people to which the study's results are to be generalized at end of the study?" The investigator should write a description of the target population.

Any clinical trial design requires precision in the process by which participants are determined to be eligible for inclusion. The objective is to ensure that participants in clinical trial are representative of some future class of patients or individuals to whom the trial findings might be applied.

The four main types, or forms, of variables used in clinical research are:

- *Categorical, dichotomous:* The variable has only 2 categories, such as mortality ("yes"/"no") or gender ("male"/female").
- *Categorical, multicategoried, nominal:* The variable has more than 2 categories but they are naming (nominal) and intrinsically ordered such as color ("white"/ "black"/"green"/"red") or dept. ("Medicine"/ "Surgery"/ "Obstetrics"/ "Pediatrics").
- *Categorical, multicategoried, ordered:* The variable has more than 2 categories and they are intrinsically ordered (ordinal), such as titer ("non-reactive"/"1:8"/"1:32"/ "1:64") or Age groups ("18-34"/"35-49"/"50-74"/"75 and older").
- *Continuous (or interval):* The variable is measured on a continuous scale, such as blood pressure (in mm Hg), or has a large number of discrete, ordered values, such as age (in years); height (in cms); weight (in kgs/lbs).

Once the target population has been described, the investigator must decide whether to enroll all members of the target population into the study or to select a small sample of them. In most research, it is not feasible to study all members, and therefore samples of the target are almost always studied. In selected population of sample, the investigator must select the types of samples carefully to ensure that the final results can be generalized back to the large population.

There are three basic kinds of sample. A *statistical sample* is a sample of the target population selected by some process of random numbers. The advantage of a statistical sample is that the results obtained in the sample will be true of the large population within a range of error that can be calculated from the information in the sample. Its disadvantage is that it is often infeasible when the target population is ill defined or when there are no lists or other means for selecting a random sample.

The second type of sample is a *convenience sample*. It generally comprises a group of patients, nonrandomly selected, who could be conveniently enrolled in the study and who seem to make up a reasonably representative sample of the population. Since the samples were not selected by a true random sampling method, one will not have the same degree of assurance that the results can be generalized, as one would have with a random sample.

The third type of a sample is referred to as *chunk*. When random sampling is infeasible and there are no convenience samples to be had, an investigator may be forced to study a group of subjects who's similarly to the target population is unknown and possibly unknowable. When studying a chunk, the investigator must admit that the results might give a highly misleading picture of what is true in the target universe. On the other hand, there are many circumstances in which biological characteristics or effects are so universal in the population that the degree of similarity of the sample to the target universe is of no importance. In such instances, studying a chunk of patients gives quite satisfactory results and may prove far less expensive than either a convenience sample or a random sample.

Finalize the Objectives into Testable Hypothesis

Once the objectives have been written, the variables defined, and the study population determined, it is necessary to refine the written objects into a set of written, testable hypothesis. This must be done before the study design can be determined. Basically, a hypothesis is simply a prediction of how the variables will be found to be associated in the final statistical analysis. It differs from the written objective in that; it is stated in terms of the actual statistical associations that will be found among the precisely defined variables formulated in Step 3.

The hypothesis may be stated in one of two forms. Statisticians generally prefer what is called the null hypothesis. For example, in a study to test the efficacy of a new drug in treating bronchial asthma, the null hypothesis (abbreviated H_0:) might be stated as H_0: The mean FEV1 (Forced Expiratory Volume in one second) in the treated group will be *no different from* that in the untreated group, this statement of the null hypothesis is nondirectional, that is, the null hypothesis would be rejected (proved untrue) if the FEV1 in the treated group is found to be either higher or lower than that in the untreated group.

The corresponding alternative hypothesis would be - The mean FEV1 in the treated group will be *different* (either higher or lower) from that in the untreated group. For a nondirectional hypothesis like this, a two-tailed statistical test must be used in the analysis. In contrast, the null hypothesis may sometimes be expressed in a directional manner as, the mean FEV1 in the treated group will be *no higher than* that in the untreated group. The corresponding alternative hypothesis would be, the mean FEV1 in the treated group will be higher *than* that in the untreated group. For a directional hypothesis like this, a one-tailed statistical test must be used in the analysis. In some studies, however one may not know the direction in which the difference will go, thus necessitating a nondirectional null hypothesis and subsequently the use of less powerful, two-tailed significance tests. Often moreover, the way the hypothesis is expressed has important implications on the way the study is actually designed. This is why the hypothesis must be quantitatively stated before the study design can be determined.

A clinical trial is often formulated as a hypothesis as to whether an experimental therapy is effective. However, confidence intervals may provide a better indication of the level of uncertainty. In the clinical trial settings, the hypothesis test is natural because the goal is to determine whether an experimental therapy should be used.

Predict Error and Bias

All scientific studies are subject to error and bias, no matter how well designed or carried out. Poorly designed studies, however, are usually more seriously affected, and these distorting influences may invalidate the results and render a study useless and unpublishable. To minimize the occurrence of error or bias in a study, it is crucial to anticipate the types of error or bias or allow the investigator to control for them in the statistical analysis. Bias in clinical trials is the potential of any aspect of the design, conduct, analysis or interpretation of the result of a trial to lead to conclusion about the effects of an intervention that are systematically different from the truth. It is relatively easy to identify potential source of bias in clinical trial, but investigators have a limited ability to effectively remove the effects of bias. It is often difficult to even determine the net direction and effect of bias on study results. Randomization and blinding are the two techniques generally used to minimize the bias.

There are basically four types of bias in research studies. These are sampling error, selection bias, information bias, and confounding. Although there is a highly developed system for anticipating, avoiding, and testing for sampling error, the other types of bias are often more difficult to detect and control. Biases can lead to errors in the results that would cause one to conclude erroneously that there is an association (e.g., a difference between groups) when, in fact, there is not (a Type I error) or to conclude erroneously that there is not an association when in fact there is (a Type II error).

Sampling error is defined as a distortion in the estimate of an association between two variables, resulting from chance variation in the selection of the sample. It usually occurs when the study sample is too small and differences between the comparative groups result from purely random variation. After a study is completed, one can analyze the results to determine the probability that the findings were attributable to a sampling error.

If the study came out with a positive finding, a statistical significance test can be performed to obtain a p value that expresses the probability that the difference occurred by chance alone. On the other hand, if the study came out with a negative finding, a statistical test can be performed to calculate the beta probability, which expresses the probability that the failure to find a difference occurred by chance alone. In assessing sampling error, the p-value is used in a study with a positive outcome to estimate the probability that a Type I error occurred and the beta probability is used in a negative study to estimate the probability that a Type II error occurred.

Selection bias is defined as a distortion in the estimate of an association between two variables, resulting from the manner in which subjects were selected for the study sample. For example, if an investigator asked volunteers for a study on the causes of lung cancer, it is possible that smokers with longstanding cough who are concerned about lung cancer might be less likely to volunteer for that study than smokers without symptoms. If the smokers who volunteered are compared with nonsmoker volunteers, it is likely that the risk due to smoking will be underestimated because of a selection bias. This would be known if the investigator anticipated this possibility and included in the project a pilot study to compare the smoker volunteers with smokers in the general population. Unless this is anticipated, the selection bias would lead to an erroneous conclusion.

Sampling error is a distortion in the estimate of an association between two variables, resulting from chance variation in the selection of the sample. It usually occurs when the study sample is too small.

Information bias is defined as a distortion in the estimate of an association between two variables, resulting from measurement error or misclassification of the subjects, when the error or misclassification is different in the comparative groups. For example, in a study of the dietary risk factors for coronary artery disease, patients with the disease might be more likely to be concerned about the fat content of their diets and might therefore more likely to record the consumption of fatty foods than would patients without the disease. This might result in an exaggerated estimate of the effect of dietary fat on coronary artery disease due to an error in the way the information was collected. As with selection bias, the potential for information bias must be anticipated and, if a likely possibility, it must be controlled for, if possible, in the analysis of the study.

Confounding is defined as misleading (spurious) association that results when the casual effect of an independent variable on a dependent variable is inflated (or deflated) in a particular set of data by the presence of a third casual variable that is co linked with both the independent variable and the dependent variable. For example, several early studies found that people who drank more than four cups of coffee per day had a higher rate of myocardial infarctions than did people who did not drink coffee. Upon further study, however it was found that coffee drinking and cigarette smoking were closely linked and coffee drinkers are more likely to smoke, than are people who do not drink coffee. Since smoking is known to be a casual factor in outcomes of coronary artery disease) and is also associated with coffee drinking, it was identified as a potential confounding variable in the analysis. When the analysis was repeated controlling for cigarette smoking, coffee drinking was found not to be associated with myocardial infarction either in smokers or in nonsmokers.

Note that confounding is different from sampling error, selection bias, and information bias; like the latter two; however, it can only be identified by the anticipation of one who is familiar with these facts. Therefore, before finalizing the study design, the investigator must think deeply about the types of error and bias that are likely to be encountered in the design and analysis.

Selection of Appropriate Study Design

It is often tempting to decide on the study design earlier in the planning process, but this should be avoided. In practice, however, it is common to start with a tentative study design, but the design must not be finalized until the above-mentioned first six steps are completed.

a. *The Purposes of Studies:* It is important to identify consciously the purpose of the study to develop the most appropriate design for a study. The objective of the study often determines the most useful study design. The purpose of studies is divided into descriptive, hypothesis generating, and hypothesis-testing. In descriptive studies the aim is simply to describe the frequency or magnitude of some events or disease. These studies utilize a survey design, almost always utilizing a statistical or convenient sample, most often a cohort or case-control design. For the more definitive hypothesis-testing purpose, experimental studies or observational studies are used, and must employ extensive design features to avoid or control bias.

b. *Important Study Designs:* Study designs can be divided into three main types: surveys, experiments and observational (epidemiological, quasi-experimental) studies. The survey study design is usually used for studies with descriptive purposes. It involves measuring a set of parameters in one pass through a population or sample of subjects. It is usually performed with a carefully developed and pre-tested questionnaire. This type of study design is most effective for estimating the frequency or magnitude of parameters. It may also be used for measuring associations between variables, although it is usually less satisfactory than other study designs for this purpose.

Most often, surveys are performed in samples of a target population using one of the many well-described statistical sampling techniques, for example, a simple random sample, a stratified random sample, or a cluster sample.

The experimental study designs provide a powerful means of testing causal hypothesis in circumstances where treatments or risk factors can be assigned to patients or experimental animals by the investigator. The feature that distinguishes an experimental design from surveys and observational studies is that the treatment or risk factor is assigned by the investigator. Usually, the assignment is randomly determined using a system of random numbers, and ideally both the investigator and the subjects are unaware of which groups the subjects were assigned to (the so-called "double-blind design"). Three of most commonly used experimental designs – the simple experiment, the repeated measures design, and the repeated measures with crossover design.

Most commonly, experimental subjects are randomly assigned to treatment and control (or placebo) groups. The treatment is administered to those in the treatment group, and no treatment (or placebo) is administered to the control group. This basic experimental design, referred to as a simple experiment, is often varied according to the circumstances of the study.

If the investigator expects a great deal of baseline variation in the outcome measurement, a repeated measures design is often used. In this design, two (or more) measurements are performed in all subjects in both the experimental and the control groups, one before the intervention with the treatment or placebo and the second after the intervention has had time to exert its effect. It is important to note that the simple experiment and the repeated measures required different approaches to the statistical analysis.

For populations involving extreme variation in the outcome event among the subjects, a crossover component can be added to the repeated measures design. Under this plan, after completing the repeated measures study, the experiment is repeated in the same experimental and control subjects except that the groups are switched; the treatment is now administered to the control subjects and the placebo to the experimental subjects, and the outcome is measured again after the treatment has had time to work.

Observational study designs, also called epidemiological studies or quasi-experiments, are useful in circumstances where experiments are either infeasible or unethical. In observational studies, subject who receives the treatment or risk factor is not under the control of the investigator. Instead, the investigator measures and analyzes the natural occurrence of independent and dependent variables and performs statistical analyses to obtain the most powerful casual inference possible from the experience.

Observational studies are usually performed in one of two designs: Cohort studies or case-control studies In a cohort study the subjects are selected on the basis of whether they are exposed to the risk factor (or treatment) and are then followed to determine which ones get the disease. This design is also called a follow-up study. In a case-control study, sometimes referred to as a "backward study," the design proceeds in the opposite direction from that of a cohort study. The subjects are selected on the basis of whether they have the disease and are then studied to determine which ones had been exposed to the risk factor (or treatment). An uncommon but sometimes useful hybrid of the cohort and case-control designs is a nested case-control study. The data are initially collected as a typical cohort study (subjects selected on the basis of exposure to the risk factors), but later the investigator selects from the cohort those patients with the disease and a group of controls (with or without matching) for analysis of risk factors, like a case-control study. This can reduce computing costs by reducing the number of patients in the analysis or hold down the costs of recontacting the patients to collect additional risk factor information.

Determination of Sample Size

Determination of the optimal sample size for a study is a critical feature of the design. If too few subjects are chosen, the study is likely to fall prey to sampling error, ending in either a Type I error or a Type II error (see Step 6 above). On the other hand, selecting too many subjects may increase the cost of the study beyond the financial resources available. To avoid either extreme, the investigator must predict the optimal number and use that in selecting the subjects for study.

To select the optimal sample size, the investigator must make an educated guess about the number of subjects who will be needed to obtain a valid test of the hypothesis under study. To do this, one must simply predict what numerical results will be obtained at the end of study and then work backward to the sample size needed to test for statistical significance. New investigators are often uncomfortable with determining the sample size on basis of an educated guess. What if the guess is wrong? Unfortunately there is no way of guaranteeing an adequate sample size. Instead, a great deal of effort must be put into making the best educated guess possible for determining the sample size. For instance, one may find data in published studies or perform pilot studies to obtain more reliable guesses of the parameters.

In most instances, new investigators should consult a qualified statistician to assist in estimating the required sample size, since the exact method depends on the type of study design selected (See Step 7). In general, though, for each type of study design, there are only a small number of parameters that must be measured, estimated, or guessed at to form the basis for estimating the optimal sample size. For example, in a simple survey for estimating the frequency of some clinical parameter in a population, one simply needs to know the estimated frequency (percentage) at which the parameter will be found in the population and then specify how far off the estimate can be from the true value due to sampling variation (e.g., the desired width of confidence intervals around the estimate) and the degree of assurance that the estimate will be made with a specified level of precision (the alpha and beta probabilities). By making a best guess at these parameters, the investigator provides all the information needed for the statistician to calculate the sample size for the study. With experience, one can often arrive at a satisfactory sample size estimate by entering the required parameter estimates into the sample size program of one of the standard statistical packages for personal computers.

Execution Steps

Data Collection Process

To ensure accuracy of the measurements of the independent variables, the dependent variables, and the extraneous variables, it is necessary to plan a proper method of data collection. Forms used to record the data should also be developed and, if appropriate, tested for accuracy and clarity in a pilot study ahead of the main data collection process.

Where a "gold standard" (an alternative method known to be highly accurate) exists, the new laboratory method should be compared with it in a pilot study to measure the validity of the new method. Measurements of validity result in estimating four parameters: sensitivity, specificity, the positive predictive value and the predictive value of a negative result. In general, the sensitivity and specificity are most useful when doing scientific studies, and the predictive value parameters are most useful when using a screening test in the care of an individual patient. When no "gold standard" method exists, one can at least measure the reproducibility, or reliability, of the new measurement method.

Data Entry and Management

Most importantly, the investigator must learn to distinguish between what is scientifically right and what is easy. Compromise often results in misclassification of subjects. If the misclassification is merely random, it reduces the chance of finding a significant difference. If it is systematic and related to the hypothesis under study, it constitutes a bias and will distort the study's results. Further, as data collection progresses, the investigator must continue to monitor the accuracy of the data to ensure that assistants do not become lax in the accuracy of their work.

Almost always the analysis of the research database is done with one of the many computerized statistical packages. At first the investigator should work closely with a statistician to ensure that the analyses are done correctly and completely. Since well-qualified statisticians often have preferred methods and approaches to analyses, it is wise to involve the statistician, who will assist with the analyses of the results, in the design phase of the project.

To choose the right statistical test in the majority of circumstances, the investigator must ask four simple questions:

i. First, one asks, "What are the variables being compared?" To answer this question, the investigator identifies the independent variable(s) and the outcome variable that are to be compared in the central hypothesis test at the end of the study.
ii. Second, when the variables are identified, the investigator asks, "What is the form of these variables?" and identifies what type of variable each is. Is each a categorical, dichotomous variable; a categorical, multicategoried, nominal variable; a categorical, multicategoried, ordered variable; or a continuous (or interval) variable?

iii. Third, if the outcome variable is continuous, the investigator asks, "Does it meet the normality assumption?" This question is answered by graphing the distribution of the outcome variable in the population to be studied.
iv. Finally, the investigator asks, "Are the comparison groups independent or paired?" In simple experiments, most cohort studies, and some case-control studies, the observations on the study subjects are independent of one another, and the answer to the question is "no". In repeated measures experimental designs and in matched case-control studies, the observations on the subjects are paired, in which case the answer to the question is "yes".

The final end product of all statistical tests is the ***p*** value. The *p* value is nothing more than the probability (measured from 0 to 1) that the observed difference is between the experimental and the control groups occurred by chance alone due to sampling error. When the *p* value is less than 0.05 it is generally conceded that sampling error has been ruled out as an explanation for the difference.

Publication

Finally, the end product of a successful study is the publication of an article in a scientific journal, for if a study is not published, it was never done. Successful writing for scientific journals is an art form that must be acquired through study and practice. It is different from other styles of writing. Author should always decide on a specific journal before starting to write a scientific article, consult the "INFORMATION OF AUTHORS" page that appears in most of journals, customize the article according to those instructions, and photocopy several articles from recent issues of the journal to serve as models.

Generally, a good scientific article presents no more than five or four main points that are key findings in the results section. These should be illustrated by tables and graphs in nearly final form before sitting down to write. The writing process goes much smoother if the tables and graphs are completely laid out and the results are written to describe and relate to them.

CONCLUSIONS

Modern clinical trials date back more than 40 years, and a wide variety of clinical trial designs have been developed and adopted over the past 25 years. To the extent possible, each of these designs uses the concepts of controlled and randomization to make comparison among group. Designing clinical research is a creative and rigorous process that requires attention to a large number of details, each of which can determine the success or failure of the project. For the planning and execution of clinical research to be successful, the investigator must be fully aware of the many aspects that must be planned so that all are addressed as early as possible in the research process. The steps outlined in this chapter provide a road map to give clinical investigators a framework and a checklist for the issues that they must address in planning their research projects.

ACKNOWLEDGEMENTS

The authors sincerely acknowledge the assistance and help rendered by Ms. Sridevi; Y. Sridhar and G.Venkata Ramana in preparation of this manuscript.

SUGGESTED READING

1. Altman LK. Probe into flawed cancer study prompts federal reforms, The New York Times,B6,Tuesday,April 26,1994.
2. Amberson Jb, Jr.McMahon Bt, Pinner M A Clinical trial of sanocrysin in Pulmonary tuberculosis, AmRev Tuberc 1931;24:401-35.
3. Armitage P. Controversies and achievements in clinical trials. Control Clinical Trial 1981; 5: 243-51.
4. Boissel JP. Impact of randomized clinical trials on medical practices, Controlled Clin.Trials 10:Suppl.1989;1208-348.
5. Burkhardt R, Kienle G. Controlled clinical trials and medical ethics, Lancet ii:1978;1356-9.
6. Doll R. Clinical trials:retrospect and prospect, Stat Med 1982;1:337-44.
7. Iber FL, Irley WA, Murray PJ. Conducting clinical trial. NewYork 1987; Plemun.
8. Lavi NW. Factors influencing clinical research success. In MJ Finkel, ed; Principle and Techniques of human research and Therapeutics; Vol 11; Mount Kisco, New York 1976; Futura; 133-42.
9. Lawrence M, Friedman, Curt D, Furberg, David L DeMets. Introduction to Clinical Trials. Lawrence M.Friedman, Curt D.Furberg, David L DeMets ed in Fundamentals of Clinical Trials, 3rd ed. New York: Springer 1998; pp 1-15.
10. Medical Research Council:Streptomycin treatment of pulmonary tuberculosis, Br.Med.J2"1948;769-82.
11. Meinert CL. Clinical trials: Design, conduct and analysis. NewYork 1986.Oxford University press.
12. Pocock SJ. Clinical trials: A practical approach. NewYork 1983: John Wiley and Sons.
13. Richard A.Guarino. Clinical Research Protocols. Richard A Gaurina ed in New Drug Approval Process.Third Edition.The Global Challenge. 3rd ed. New York: Marcel Dekker, Inc; 2000; pp 219 – 70.
14. Shapiro SH, Louis TA (Eds). Clinical trials: Issues and approaches. New York, 1983; Marcel Dekker.
15. Spilker B. Guide to clinical trials. New York 1991; Raven Press.
16. Spodick DH. The randomized controlled clinical trial:scientific and ethical basis, Am J Med 1982;73:420-5.
17. Spriet A, Dupin Spriet T, Simon P. Methodology of clinical trial. 2nd ed. Basel 1994; Karger.
18. Storer BE. Design and analysis of Phase I clinical trials, Biometrics 1989;45: 925-37.
19. Vere DW. Ethics of clinical trials. In Good CS ,ed: The Principles and practice of clinical trials, Edinburgh, Churchill Livingstone,1976.
20. William M.Troetel. The Investigational New Drug Application and the Investigator's Brochure. Richard A Gaurina ed in New Drug Approval Process (3rd ed). New York: Marcel Dekker, Inc; 2000; pp 55-92.

4 Ethical Issues in Clinical Research

Urmila Thatte

Research has been called a good business, a necessity, a gamble, a game. It is none of these; It is a state of the mind.
—*Martin H Fischer.*

INTRODUCTION

Clinical Research is defined as a systematic investigation in human beings designed to discover or contribute to a body of generalisable knowledge. As clinical research involves human participants, researchers and their teams are legally and ethically obligated to protect them. In clinical practice a physician would be expected to use interventions that have a reasonable expectation of success and are designed solely to enhance the well-being of an individual patient. As against this, clinical research is designed to test a hypothesis, permit conclusions to be drawn; and thereby develop or contribute to generalisable knowledge – here the participant, therefore may not get the best known treatment and, therefore the obligations on the researcher are more. Thus, the key principle of ethics in Biomedical Research attempts to protect the right of every human subject to understand the nature of research, the risks and benefits involved and then choose to agree or disagree to participate.

This chapter reviews some ethical aspects that arise while designing and conducting clinical research. After discussing some historical milestones, I shall cover some of the key issues elaborated in some of the codes, declarations, and other documents that govern the ethical conduct of human subject research; define and discuss the basic principles of ethical research, review the critical elements of informed consent; explore controversial issues relating to clinical research especially in developing countries; and finally review the roles and responsibilities of Ethics Committees.

HISTORICAL ASPECTS

The *Charaka Samhita* and the Hippocratic Oath both describe the ethics that govern medical practice. However, they did not cover research. In the 18th century, clinical investigations were exemplified by self-experimentation. The work of Edward Jenner

(1749-1823) is illustrative as he tested his ideas of the smallpox vaccine on his own son and other neighborhood children! Another scientist, Johann Jorg (1779-1856) swallowed several drugs in various doses to record their properties. To the extent that Celcius is on record for saying, "It is not cruel to inflict on a few, criminal sufferings which may benefit multitudes of innocent people through all centuries"!

In the absence of codes, guidelines, rules or laws there was much scope for what we recognize today as exploitation. Due to implicit faith in the treating physicians, and no recognition of the vulnerable sections of society, it required major mishaps that have punctuated history to push the medical fraternity into developing ethical guidelines and codes for research. The 20th Century has been carved in stone for the experiments conducted by Nazi physicians during World War II because they were unprecedented in their scope and the degree of suffering and harm they caused to human beings. Horrific studies such as injecting people with gasoline and live viruses, immersing people in ice water, and forcing people to ingest poisons dot the pages of history. The end point of these experiments was often death of the participant. At the end of the Second World War, in December 1946, 23 physicians and administrators were indicted before the War Crimes Tribunal at Nuremberg for their willing participation in such experiments. Sixteen of them were found guilty and imprisoned, while 7 were sentenced to death. In the August 1947 verdict, the judges included a section called "Permissible Medical Experiments" and this section became known as the Nuremberg Code, which formed the basis for ethics codes internationally.

Unfortunately, the Nuremberg Code was not honored by some researchers and the Willowbrook Study conducted from 1963-1966 is a good example illustrating the point. Children admitted to the Willowbrook State School (an institution for mentally defective children) were deliberately infected with the hepatitis virus (by being fed stools from infected persons or later by being injecting with purified virus preparations) to observe the natural history of this disease and then to test the effects of γ-globulin in preventing or ameliorating the disease. Researchers defended the deliberate infection of these children by stating that the majority of them acquired the infection anyway while at Willowbrook, and perhaps it would be better for them to be infected under controlled research conditions! What was worse was that during the course of these studies, new inmates were admitted only if they agreed to participate in the hepatitis program! There was obviously no full disclosure and clearly coercion and undue pressure was used to enroll vulnerable (children and mentally challenged) subjects.

At the other end of life's spectrum, came the Jewish Chronic Disease Hospital Study where live cancer cells were injected into chronically ill and debilitated patients who had been told that they were receiving a skin test. The patients were provided oral information about the test but no consent was documented.

The Declaration of Helsinki published first in 1964 sought to address ethical aspects of clinical research and is a milestone in bioethics of research.

The most notorious example of prolonged and knowing violations of the rights of a vulnerable group of research participants was the long-term study of black males conducted at Tuskegee by the United States Public Health Service. Initiated in the 1930s to examine the natural history of untreated syphilis, continuing until 1972, this study recruited more than 400 black men suffering from syphilis. These participants were recruited without informed consent and, were misinformed that some of the procedures done in the interest of research (e.g. spinal taps) were actually "special free treatment." Although along the way antibiotics became available, these were not given to the patients and the study resulted in 28 deaths, 100 cases of disability, and 19 cases of congenital syphilis. The Belmont Report published by the National Commission for the Protection of Human Subjects of Biomedical and Behavioral Research on April 18, 1979 was one of the outcomes of the public outcry that resulted when the story of the Tuskegee study broke.

CODES, DECLARATIONS AND GUIDELINES (TABLES 4.1 AND 4.2)

The Nuremberg Code (available at http://ohsr.od.nih.gov/guidelines/nuremberg.html) is the first international standard laid down for the conduct of research and contains ten clear principles to be followed by researchers while conducting human experiments. For the first time this code mandated the need to obtain "voluntary consent of the human subject" before recruiting him/her as a participant in research. The emphasis on safety is clear in that the Code specifies the need for animal experimentation to precede human experimentation and that unnecessary physical and mental suffering and injury should be avoided. The Code also specifies that the degree of risk to participants should never exceed the expected benefit to either the participant or to society at large. The issue of minimizing risks is also addressed further specifying that participants should always be at liberty to withdraw from experiments.

The Declaration of Helsinki (available at http://www.wma.net/e/policy/b3.htm) first accepted by the 18th World Medical Assembly in 1964 has been revised 5 times and the latest version was published in 2000 at the 52nd WMA, Edinburgh, Scotland. Subsequently two notes of clarification on Paragraph 29 and 30 were added by the WMA General Assembly, at Washington in 2002 and Tokyo in 2004. It contains 32 principles and has made informed consent a central requirement for ethical research while allowing for surrogate consent when the research participant is incompetent, physically or mentally incapable of giving consent, or a minor. There are several key aspects of the Declaration worth noting. For example, it states that research in vulnerable groups should be conducted only when the research is necessary to promote the health of that population and when this research cannot be performed on legally competent persons. It further emphasizes the importance of obtaining assent (where possible) of the participant in addition to legal consent. An important feature of the Declaration is the statement "The benefits, risks, burdens and effectiveness of a new method should be tested against those of the best current

Table 4.1: Guidelines for ethical conduct of research in human subjects

1. Nuremberg Code 1947 (http://ohsr.od.nih.gov/guidelines/nuremberg.html)
2. Declaration of Helsinki, 1964 (http://www.wma.net/e/policy/b3.htm)
3. The Belmont Report, 1979 (http://ohsr.od.nih.gov/guidelines/belmont.htm)
4. International Ethical Guidelines for Biomedical Research Involving Human Subjects, 1982, 1993, 2002 (http://www.cioms.ch/frame_guidelines_nov_2002.htm)
5. The Ethics of Research related to Healthcare in Developing Countries, Nuffield Council, 2002 (http://www.nuffieldbioethics.org/go/screen/ourwork/developingcountries/publication_309.html)
6. Indian Council for Medical Research Ethical Guidelines for Biomedical Research on Human subjects (http://icmr.nic.in/ethical.pdf).

prophylactic, diagnostic, and therapeutic methods." The Declaration of Helsinki clearly mandates that "all protocols must be submitted to an Ethics Committee for review, which must be independent of the investigator, the sponsor or any other kind of undue influence".

Following the revelation of the Tuskegee Study, US Congress established the National Commission for the Protection of Human Subjects of Biomedical and Behavioral Research to make recommendations for the conduct of research involving humans. In 1979, the National Commission wrote the Belmont Report, *"Ethical Principles and Guidelines for the Protection of Human Subjects"* (available at http://www.wma.net/e/policy/b3.htm), which specified the fundamental Principles of Ethical Research, namely:

i. Respect for persons
ii. Beneficence
iii. Justice

The Belmont Report also defines how these principles must be applied in clinical research in the informed consent process, assessment of risks and benefits and the equitable selection of patients.

Table 4.2: Indian guidelines for ethical conduct of research in human subjects

1. Policy Statement for Biomedical Research involving Human subjects-1980
2. Ethical Guidelines for Biomedical Research involving Human subjects- 2000 http://icmr.nic.in/ethical.pdf)
3. Ethical Guidelines for Social Science Research in Health in 2000by CEHAT http://www.cehat.org/initiatives1.html
4. Ethical Guidelines for Stem Cell Research, DBT. http://dbtindia.nic.in/publication/publicmain.html
5. ICMR Draft Guidelines
6. Guidelines for ethical practices in studies involving animals, ICMR (http://icmr.nic.in/bioethics/Guidelines_medicalcollege.pdf) INSA, (http://icmr.nic.in/bioethics/INSA_Guidelines.pdf)
7. Guidelines for Vaccine trials, DBT http://dbtindia.nic.in/publication/publicmain.html
8. Guidelines for Genetics and Genomics by DBT http://dbtindia.nic.in/publication/publicmain.html

The Council for International Organizations of Medical Sciences (CIOMS), an international organization established jointly by WHO and UNESCO in 1949, published the *International Ethical Guidelines for Biomedical Research Involving Human Subjects (fifteen in all)* in 1993 (available at http://www.cioms.ch). The CIOMS guidelines are particularly relevant for research planned in developing countries.

The Indian Council for Medical Research (ICMR) ICMR Policy Statement on Ethical Considerations involved in Research on Human Subjects was promulgated in 1980 where several ethical issues were addressed including the role of Ethics Committees, informed consent, research on Traditional Medicine and Publications related issues. By the mid nineties, a need was felt for revision of this statement as critical issues in the area of biogenetic research were emerging and it was becoming mandatory for clinical trials to be conducted for new drugs. Hence, the Central Ethics Committee for Human Research (CECHR) comprising of 27 members was set up under the chairmanship of Justice Hon'ble MN Venkatachaliah in August 1996. Five sub-committees of experts were set up for drawing up the guidelines in respective areas, namely:

i. Clinical evaluation of drug/devices/ diagnostics/vaccines/herbal remedies
ii. Epidemiological research
iii. Human genetic research
iv. Transplantation research including fetal tissue transplantation
v. Assisted reproductive technologies

A draft consultative document was prepared in December 1997, which was given nation wide circulation January 1998. Regional public debates were held between 1998 and 1999 and meetings of the sub-committees for special issues were held in 1999 and the document (Indian Council for Medical Research Ethical Guidelines for Biomedical Research on Human subjects available at http://icmr.nic.in/ethical.pdf) was published in 2000.

Currently, it is expected that all institutions in India, which carry out any form of biomedical research involving human beings, should follow these guidelines in letter and spirit to protect safety and well-being of all individuals. The guidelines have been submitted for legislation.

The Indian GCP guidelines were published in late 2001 (www.cdsco.nic.in) and the current Schedule Y (www.cdsco.nic.in) dated 20th January 2005 gives timely legal support to these GCP guidelines. It is the investigator's responsibility to ensure GCP compliance of the approving Ethics Committee. An important feature of the current Schedule Y is that Investigators may now start trials after they obtain approval from EC of another site or an independent ethics committee in case they do not have access to a Schedule Y compliant EC. However, he/she is expected to allow oversight of the trial by the approving EC. The Schedule Y also specifies the composition and quorum of Ethics Committees, and prescribes that SOPs are mandatory. Ethics Committees are expected to review agreements, insurance and subject compensation details and the approval format is prescribed. It is expected that there will be improvements in the quality of clinical trials with this notification.

BASIC PRINCIPLES OF CLINICAL RESEARCH

The Belmont Report described the basic principles of ethical clinical research. The first is to have respect for individuals participating in research. It is necessary to treat individuals as autonomous human beings and not use them as a means to an end. They must be allowed to choose to participate or not in the research for themselves. It is also a basic principle to provide extra protection to those with limited autonomy. The elements of autonomy (self determination) include mental capacity and voluntariness and the application of this principle is in the requirement to obtain informed consent, respect privacy of research subjects and protect vulnerable subjects.

Beneficence is the second principle governing ethical clinical research. It is expected that the researcher will minimize harms and maximize benefits. The application of this principle is the over-riding responsibility of investigator and applies to physical, mental and social well being of the research participant. This principle is applied by using the best possible research design to minimize harms and maximize benefits, making sure the researchers are able to perform procedures and handle the risks and prohibit research without a favorable risk-benefit ratio, all ensured by appropriate ethical review of the proposal.

The third basic principle is justice. This principle requires that all people are treated fairly. Hence, research has to be so designed that its burdens and benefits are shared equitably. This principle is applied practically by ensuring that selection of subjects is done equitably (i.e. distribute risks and benefits) taking special care to avoid exploitation of vulnerable populations.

The two important pillars that support the application of these basic principles of clinical research include review by ethics committees and informed consent process. One of the common questions raised is "which studies require the use of these patient protection methods". To answer this it is necessary to define "Who is a research participant". The human participant is a living individual about whom a researcher obtains data through intervention or interaction with the individual or identifiable private information. Thus, protection of participants covers a wide range of research, including that which involves tissue specimens, medical records, genetic material, behavioral and/or biomedical assessments, and treatments. Further, research involving residual diagnostic specimens, including specimens obtained for routine patient care that would have been discarded if not used for research, private information, such as medical data that can be readily identified with individuals, even if the information was not specifically collected for the study in question also requires safeguards. Research on cell lines or DNA samples, that can be associated with individuals, falls into this category.

INFORMED CONSENT

Informed consent is defined as consent given by a competent individual who has received the necessary information, has understood the information and having understood the information has arrived at a decision about participation without having been under any coercion, undue influence or inducement or intimidation. It is necessary to document this consent as a written, informed consent and has to be given voluntarily. It must be obtained from every subject before any study related procedure and documented on a form approved by the Ethics Committee. Generally, the informed consent document has to adhere to GCP and is based on the Declaration of Helsinki.

The informed consent process is based on the principle that competent individuals are entitled to choose freely whether to participate in research or not. This process protects the individual's freedom of choice and respects the individual's autonomy. It is a shared process and protects the subjects' rights.

It is preferably the research participant who gives consent, always. If the subject is unable to give consent (e.g. minor, dementia, unconscious) then the subject's legally acceptable representative (LAR) is expected to consent. However, the subject should be informed to the extent compatible with his/her understanding and assent to participate should be sought and documented.

It is at all times the investigator's responsibility to obtain consent. Either the Principal Investigator or his delegate (who must be qualified to administer consent) should discuss all pertinent aspects of the study including the informed consent form, answer any queries/doubts, request consent and if given, documented on the ethics committee approved form. The consent should be signed and dated by the subject or the subject's legally acceptable representative, the person conducting the informed consent discussion and if the subject or subject's legally acceptable representative is illiterate, an impartial witness. It is important to ensure that no coercion/undue influence is used and the subject is given ample time for decision, and adequate opportunity to discuss issues. If a subject does not understand English a vernacular consent form (approved by the ethics committee) must be administered in the language he understands. In the case of an illiterate individual, consent is administered in the presence of an impartial witness. The subject can give a thumb impression in the place of the signature. It is important to document the method of obtaining consent in all these cases. A signed and dated copy of the consent form must be provided to the subject or his legally acceptable representative

In the case of older children, Schedule Y now mandates obtaining an assent as well as the consent of the parents.

The contents of a consent form have to be approved by the ethics committee and should never imply waiving of any legal rights of subject. It is necessary before requesting an individual's consent to participate in research that the investigator provides the individual with information in the language he or she is able to understand which should not only be scientifically accurate but should also be sensitive to their social and cultural context. The Schedule Y (Appendix XI) specifies the content of the Informed consent document and these are the minimum elements that must be part of this, including the fact that the trial involves research and that his participation is strictly voluntary. The purpose of the study including the interventions and procedures, risks, benefits, and alternative treatments must be mentioned. Compensation or treatment for injury is an important part of the consent form. The subject's responsibilities must be delineated and if any payment is to be made this should be clarified. How the confidentiality of the patient will be protected must be specified, as well as whom to contact for study related information including the ethics committee details must be mentioned.

If important new information is obtained during study the informed consent form must be revised, Ethics Committee approval obtained before use and the subject or subject's legally accepted representative informed in timely manner and consent obtained to continue in the study.

An informed consent is, therefore, not a piece of paper or a signature. It is a process by which we ensure that our subject's right to be informed and right to consent to research, is protected and document our efforts to protect the subject's rights to the satisfaction of independent observers.

SPECIAL ISSUES

Participant Selection

As has been mentioned researchers are responsible for ensuring that selection of participants is equitable. While selecting participants, the researcher must consider the population from which the sample is drawn, the feasibility of acquiring the number of participants needed and the recruitment procedures that ensure an equitable distribution across the population.

Patients may be susceptible to real or imaginary pressure to participate, for example, if a researcher also serves as a patient's primary physician, the patient may feel obliged to participate in the research out of a desire to please or out of fear that failure to do so will result in hostility or abandonment. This type of coercion must be avoided.

Vulnerable Populations

Persons who are relatively or absolutely incapable of protecting their own interests are termed as vulnerable research participants. When such individuals are to participate in research, special responsibility falls on all stakeholders of that research, including (and especially) the research team. They should, thus, be cognizant of the special problems of research involving such patients. The very poor, illiterate patients, children, individuals with questionable capacity to consent (including psychiatric patients), prisoners, foetuses and pregnant women, the terminally ill, students or employees, comatose patients, tribals, and the elderly are examples of the vulnerable populations.

Special justification is needed for including these populations in research, and the protocol must include additional safeguards for their safety and welfare. Risk benefit analysis has to be made carefully.

When children are to be included in research, the whole family has to be considered while devising the protocol as well as while obtaining informed consent from the parents or guardians. If the research is based in schools, appropriate involvement and permission must be obtained from the school authorities. Adequate measures must be developed to protect children's privacy and to ensure that their participation does not stigmatize them in the present or future. Further in children and others who have diminished ability to give legal consent, all efforts must be made to ensure that the potential participant agrees to participate (gives assent).

Because prisoners are a special population that is confined and readily available in large numbers, they may appear an attractive population in whom to conduct certain type of research. However, they are a vulnerable population because they are under the strict control of their wardens whom they feel they must please and to whom they must appear cooperative if they are to earn their release. Hence, these potential participants may believe, probably as a result of their dependent situation, that their agreement to participate in research will be viewed positively by their wardens.

Often it is useful to include as a member of the Ethics Committee a representative of the vulnerable population that is to be researched upon while reviewing the protocol to further ensure no exploitation.

Stigmatization as a Result of Participation in Research

An issue that needs consideration is whether participants will suffer stigmatization as a result of their participation in research. When research is conducted on behaviors, lifestyles, or conduct that is unpopular or even illegal, the mere act of being included in a study may cause an individual to be labeled in a negative manner.

Payment to Research Participants

A dilemma that is faced by investigators and ethics committee members is that of payment to participants. What would be "adequate compensation" *vs.* "inducement"? The line is often fine especially when the potential participant is a poor, illiterate patient attending tertiary care institute in India. There is no agreement about whether it is right to pay research subjects at all. If payment for participation is to made, then there are no clear rules or standards for payment other than a general prohibition against coercion or the exercise of undue influence, and hence, each research organization must create and document its own rules.

Developing Countries

Economic disparity, an authoritative or corrupt political system, lack of human rights protection, lack of individual autonomy (especially when this applies only to certain sectors), lack of infrastructure for scientific/ ethical review and low education or literacy of participants create special situations in developing countries that need to be addressed. The Nuffield Council Report on "The ethics of research related to healthcare in developing countries" (available at http://www.nuffieldbioethics.org/go/print/ourwork/developingcountries/publication_309.html) has identified four major concerns: informed consent issues, standards of care, post-trial access and ethics review mechanisms in developing countries.

In developing countries, participants often consent to research because they believe it is their only means of receiving healthcare or other benefits. Social and cultural environment is such that the Doctor is considered next to god and therefore, anything recommended by the doctor is accepted (and therefore, negating the concept of free choice). The Nuffield Council has recommended that if relevant, it may be appropriate to obtain agreement from the particular community or assent from a senior family member, before any prospective participant in research is approached.

Standard of care for the control arm is an issue that worries many ethics committees. Should it be the best current treatment available anywhere in the world or treatment based on an alternative standard (locally available) of care or placebo? Clearly, the appropriate answer to this question is that patients should be offered a universal standard of care for the disease being studied. However, where it is impossible to offer such a standard, the minimum that should be offered is the best intervention currently available as part of the national public health system. In any case, the final approval would rest with local ethics committees which would be aware of local scenario.

An important issue that needs attention in developing countries is what happens to the patient when the trial is complete? It is clearly unacceptable that research should begin without having a policy in place for making available the trial treatment (if found effective) after the trial.

The most crucial issue in developing countries is that of ethics review processes and this is discussed below.

ROLES AND RESPONSIBILITIES OF IRBS

The Declaration of Helsinki and the ICMR guidelines have mandated that all proposals on biomedical research involving human subjects undergo ethical review. This activity is generally performed by an Ethics Committee, which is needed to protect the study subjects' well being, rights and confidentiality, to meet the mandate of the Declaration of Helsinki as well as to make clinical research socially respectable and acceptable to regulatory authorities and journal editors.

Ethics Committees could be either institutional or independent. The Ethics Committee (EC) is made up of a reasonable number of members, who collectively have the qualifications and experience to review and evaluate the science, medical aspects, and ethics of the proposed trial. Generally, members should be aware of local, social and cultural norms, and this is why approval of local ECs is required even if central or international ECs have already approved the proposal.

The ICH-GCP guidelines (available at http://www.ich.org) recommend that an EC may contain an odd number of members (at least 5 members familiar with GCP), including at least one member whose primary area of interest is not science, and one member independent of the institution. The ICMR guidelines suggest, while the Schedule Y mandates that the Chairperson should be from outside the Institution and not the head of the same institution to maintain the independence of the Committee. The Member Secretary, however, belongs to the same institution to facilitate administration of the EC. The Schedule Y (2005 Amendment) specifies in Appendix VIII that the EC should have at least 7 members, being a mix of medical/ non-medical, scientific and non-scientific persons, including layperson. The quorum for an EC meeting has been specified as at least 5 members consisting of a basic medical scientist (preferably one pharmacologist), a clinician, a legal expert, a social scientist/representative of non-governmental voluntary agency/philosopher/ ethicist/theologian or a similar person and a lay person from the community.

An investigator can be an EC member although he/she cannot opine or vote on a proposal in which he is the investigator. The EC can invite *ad hoc* subject experts for a meeting if they feel a lack of expertise within themselves. However, these experts can only offer expert advice or opinion on a scientific, legal or such other issue and they cannot vote on a proposal. They must be named, their participation justified in writing, and their opinion or advice recorded.

It is necessary for an EC to function according to written standard operating procedures (SOP) which define the composition of the EC and the authority under which it is established, the scheduling of, notifying its members of, and conducting its meetings, as well as the process of conducting initial and continuing review of trials. A list of members and their signed and dated CVs must always be available for audit or inspection.

The chief investigator, not the sponsor always communicates with the EC although the sponsor can help the investigator to respond to the issues raised by the EC, supply additional information required and amend the study plan if necessary as well as comply with the ECs other requirements.

The ECs responsibilities extend from before start of research, including review and approval of the proposal, while research is in progress to monitor the study and review SAEs to after completion of research including publication and archiving.

Table 4.3 enlists the documents the Ethics Committee is expected to review (per ICMR guidelines and Schedule Y) before taking a decision on a proposal.

The ECs must provide independent, competent, and timely review of the science, ethics and medical aspects of the proposed studies according to an established review procedure.

The elements of review have been well described in the WHO's Operational Guidelines for Ethics Committees that Review Biomedical Research (available at http://www.who.int/tdr/publications/publications/pdf/ethics.pdf).

Table 4.3: Documents an ethics committee must review

- Trial protocol(s)/amendment(s), with date and version
- Written informed consent form(s) and consent form updates that the investigator proposes for use in the trial
- Subject recruitment procedures (e.g. advertisements)
- Written Information to be provided to the subjects (Patient Information Sheet and Informed Consent Form (including updates if any) in English and/or vernacular language
- Investigator's Brochure(IB), available safety information
- Information about payments and compensation available to subjects
- Investigator's current curriculum vitae and/or other documentation evidencing qualifications
- Any other documents that the EC may require to fulfill its responsibilities
- May request more information be given to subjects when, in the judgment of EC, the additional information would add meaningfully to the protection of the rights, safety and/or well being of the subjects
- Insurance policy/compensation for participation and for serious adverse events occurring during the study participation
- Investigator's agreement with the sponsor.
- Investigator's undertaking (Appendix VII of Schedule Y).

The scientific design and conduct of the study has to be reviewed at the outset as poor science is poor ethics. The appropriateness of the study design in relation to the objectives of the study, the statistical methodology (including sample size calculation), and the potential for reaching sound conclusions with the smallest number of research participants has to be assessed. There must be a justification for the predictable risks and inconveniences weighed against the anticipated benefits for the research participants and the concerned communities. The justification for the use of control arms, criteria for prematurely withdrawing research participants and for suspending or terminating the research as a whole may be assessed. The EC should also review the policies for monitoring and auditing conduct of research, including the constitution of a data safety monitoring board (DSMB).

The adequacy of the site, including the qualifications of the Principal Investigator and supporting staff, available facilities, and emergency procedures are also assessed by the EC before approving a study. Recruitment of research participants is a central aspect to be reviewed by the EC. The characteristics of the population from which the research participants will be drawn, the means by which recruitment is to be conducted, and how will full information be given to the potential research participants must be reviewed.

Any plans in the protocol to withdraw or withhold standard therapies for the purpose of the research, and the justification for such action needs careful review. What medical care will be provided to research participants during and after the course of the research is another important facet to be assessed, including adequacy of medical supervision and psycho-social support for the research participants. Plans for post-trial access to the study product must be evaluated. It is crucial to assess the description of any financial costs to research participants, rewards and compensations for research participants (including money, services, and/or gifts) as well as provisions made for compensation/treatment in the case of the injury/disability/death of a research participant attributable to participation in the research (including insurance and indemnity arrangements).

Maintaining confidentiality of the patient is important in the study, and the EC must review the plans to protect this.

The informed consent process has to be studied in detail, including the identification of those responsible for obtaining consent. The adequacy, completeness, and understandability (including vernacular forms) of information to be given to the research participants must be reviewed. The EC must be satisfied regarding the justification to use a vulnerable population and special attention paid to the process of informed consent and assent should be clarified.

The EC may evaluate the impact and relevance of the research on the local community, and study where relevant, proposed community consultation during the course of the research. The manner in which the results of the research will be made available to the research participants and the concerned communities may also be addressed.

When reviewing proposals, the EC must assess whether the anticipated benefit of the research (could be new knowledge or improved health for the research participant) justifies undertaking the risks. The EC should not approve research in which the risks are believed unreasonable in relation to the anticipated benefits.

Risks can be physical, psychological, social, legal, and economic and can be graded as minimal or greater than minimal risk. The EC must ensure that risks to participants are minimized. ECs should assess the degree of therapeutic misconception that may occur in a protocol.

The EC must review proposals within a reasonable time, document its views in writing, clearly identifying the trial, documents reviewed, and the dates for approval/favorable opinion, modifications required prior to its approval/favorable opinion, disapproval/negative opinion or termination/suspension of any prior approval/favorable opinion.

An expedited review may be conducted if the research proposal involves minimal risk to the study subjects, or involves a minor amendment to a study already approved by the IEC.

A written approval containing the date of the meeting, documents reviewed (versions and dates), list of members present indicating that quorum was complete should be given. It is mandated that no clinical study can be started without EC permission and no deviations or changes initiated without prior written EC approval except when necessary to eliminate immediate hazards to the subjects.

During a trial the PI must submit updated documentation, written summaries of the trial status annually or more frequently if requested, serious adverse events within 7 working days (and provide additional information as requested), a summary of the trial's outcome upon completion as well as amendments to the protocol or informed consent document.

Some Issues with Ethics Review

The most common problem the EC faces is that of scientific and ethical review. Investigators do not appreciate scientific review and ethics committee members often lack training in ethics review. Often investigators submit incomplete protocols, level of evidence generated using the design is very low and many of the planned studies are of a "me-too" variety. Efficacy and failure end points are also often not specified. In practical terms it is often useful to have a checklist for members related to major scientific and ethical aspects while reviewing a proposal so that major issues are covered.

As new members are recruited into any EC, it becomes necessary for training in the review process as well as to inculcate within them an understanding of their roles and responsibilities so that the committee becomes compliant with relevant guidelines in letter and spirit. Further, as guidelines and laws change it becomes necessary to have continued training of members.

Ethics committees are also often overburdened. Increasing number of projects per meeting and the "size" of each proposal leads to superficial review. The time available for discussions is also limited leading to inadequate review.

An aspect that is never addressed and there are no guidelines about is the one related to compensating ethics committee members for their expertise and time.

ECs usually perform preliminary review of the proposal – and then no further monitoring is performed. Investigators submit SAEs (often not in prescribed formats, and with very incomplete data) and the EC often only acknowledges that these SAEs have been received. But there is rarely further follow-up action. Naturally, again, the question of time, expertise and funds is crucial to this aspect.

The EC must have an independent office with open communication lines. The role of the Chairperson cannot be emphasized enough – this individual has to knit together a number of (very busy and often senior) individuals from diverse backgrounds and ensure compliance to GCP guidelines. The Secretary and Secretariat also have a very important role. The Secretary acts as a liaison between the investigator and the committee and therefore, needs to ensure appropriate communication between them.

It is necessary to increase communication between ethics committees to prevent the phenomenon of "EC shopping" where sponsors may change investigators because of rejection by EC of a proposal at one site. There is also a strong need for national audits of Ethics Committees and a functional accreditation system. It would also be useful to create awareness and train apart from researchers and Ethics Committee members, sponsors, administrators and policy makers in this area.

I end with a quote by Valdemar W Setzer who says "Ethics is not definable, is not implementable, because it is not conscious; it involves not only our thinking, but also our feeling".

SUGGESTED READING

1. http://ohsr.od.nih.gov/guidelines/nuremberg.html
2. http://www.wma.net/e/policy/b3.htm
3. http://www.cioms.ch/
4. http://icmr.nic.in/ethical.pdf
5. http://ohsr.od.nih.gov/guidelines/belmont.htm
6. http://www.cioms.ch/frame_guidelines_nov_2002.htm
7. http://www.nuffieldbioethics.org/go/screen/ourwork/developingcountries/publication_309.html
8. www.cdsco.nic.in
9. http://www.cehat. org/initiatives1.html
10. http://dbtindia.nic.in/publication/publicmain. html
11. http://icmr.nic.in/bioethics/ Guidelines_medicalcollege.pdf
12. http://icmr.nic.in/bioethics/INSA_Guidelines.pdf
13. http://www.ich.org
14. http://www.who.int/tdr/publications/publications/pdf/ethics.pdf.

5

ICH-GCP Guidelines

Sonal Vora, Sunita Nair

INTRODUCTION

A paradigm shift has occurred in the way clinical research is being conducted today. Times are changing fast and research has become more prevalent globally. There is a more intense search for expanding research sites beyond US/Europe to countries that are called "emerging" countries. Thus, an increasing number of trials are being conducted in multicultural and multinational environments. Various trends facilitate this, including increasing industry pressures on clinical development and improved infrastructure and medical expertise in these emerging countries. India is such an "emerging" market and the various opportunities that lie here are by now well acknowledged worldwide.[1] In the same breath, it is important to realize the challenges that clinical researchers face here before, during and after conducting clinical studies – most (if not all) would be prevalent in various degrees in other (more developed) countries, too.[2]

Amongst all the challenges that have been described in various publications, it is somewhat ironical that, while the concept of globalization of clinical trials is gaining momentum, the main challenge across all countries worldwide still appears to be protecting human subjects and ensuring that trials are conducted according to good clinical practices ([GCP], Fig. 5.1). Certainly, we have many universal standards and ethical principles or codes guiding clinical trials – the Nuremberg Code, Council for International Organizations of Medical Services (CIOMS), the Declaration of Helsinki, National Institutes of Health (NIH) Policy, the National Research Act, the Belmont Report and the International Conference on Harmonization (ICH) – GCP Guidelines. However, a major issue remains the training of all clinical researchers in GCP. It is very important to ensure, not only the satisfactory knowledge of GCP, but also the willingness to comply with the above-mentioned principles/ codes. This will provide assurance that the rights, safety and well being of subjects are protected and that the trials data are credible. This chapter attempts to give a broad outline of perhaps the most widely accepted ethical code, the ICH-GCP guidelines. While the entire ICH guidelines are available[3], the scope of this chapter includes only the salient features of the guidelines as an outline.

The introduction of ICH Guidelines for GCP in 1966 defines GCP as "an international ethical and scientific quality standard for designing, conducting, recording and reporting trials that involve the participation of human subjects". Thus, we can see that ICH places primary importance on both the ethics and science of clinical research.

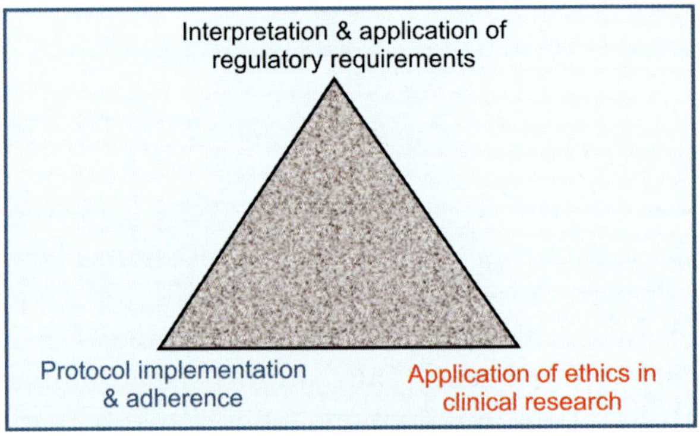

Fig. 5.1: Cornerstones of GCP

HISTORY OF ICH

Several historical events led to the realization that it was important to have an independent evaluation of medicinal products, before they were allowed to reach the market. In the US, it was a tragic mistake in the formulation of a children's syrup in the 1930s, which sparked the setting up of product authorization, while in many countries in Europe, the trigger was the thucalidomide tragedy of the 1960s. In Japan, government regulations for the registration of medicinal products started in the 1950s. But it was not until the 1960s and 1970s, that a number of laws, regulations and guidelines for reporting and evaluating data on safety, quality and efficacy of new medicinal products, were enforced.[3]

Box 5.1: ICH: Objectives

Thus, the ICH was established as a joint regulatory/industry project to improve, through harmonization, the efficiency of the process for developing and registering new medicines in Europe, Japan and United States, so that these products can be provided to patients with minimum of delay.

Interestingly, while the industry was moving towards globalization, each country had to register its own medicines at a national level. While the objective of each and every regulatory system was the same, i.e. to evaluate the safety, quality and efficacy of new products, there emerged divergent technical requirements by different regulatory systems in various countries, leading to duplication of many time-consuming and costly testing procedures for marketing new products globally. In lieu of the rising costs of health care and research and development coupled with the need to minimize any delays in making new medicines available to needy patients, there was an urgent need felt to rationalize and harmonize regulation.

These issues were taken up in a joint European Community Mission to Japan in 1988, which comprised of representatives from the European Commission (EC). The industry was represented by the European Federation of Pharmaceutical Industries' Association (EFPIA). It was at this meet that a project on harmonization of regulatory requirements was conceived, which finally came into force in October 1989.[4] The success of the harmonization project in Europe paved the way for similar initiatives in Japan and the US. A Steering Committee comprising of representatives from EC, US Food and Drug Administration (FDA), Koseisho (Japanese Ministry of Health, Labor and Welfare), International Federation of Pharmaceutical Manufacturers Association (IFPMA), EFPIA, Pharmaceutical Research and Manufacturers of America (PhRMA), Japan Pharmaceutical Manufacturers Association (JPMA) and observers from WHO, Canada and Switzerland, was formed. A number of working groups of experts under the Steering Committee came into being. A specific plan of action was formulated at the WHO Conference of Drug Regulatory Authorities (ICDRA) in Paris, in 1989. This was followed by discussions between the ICDRA and IFPMA to formulate a joint regulatory-industry initiative on international harmonization, which led to the birth of ICH (Box 5.1). This is how the ICH process (the International Conference on Harmonization of the Technical Requirements for Registration of Pharmaceuticals for Human Use) was initiated. The ICH Steering Committee was set up at a meeting in April 1990 in Brussels (hosted by European Federation of Pharmaceutical Industries Association) and has been meeting, ever since, at least twice a year, with the location altering between Europe, USA and Japan.

The ***Terms of Reference*** Topics selected for harmonization were divided into *Safety, Quality and Efficacy,* which reflect the basic criteria for approving and authorizing new medicinal products (Box 5.2).

Box 5.2: Basic principles guiding the ICH process

- Development of scientific consensus through discussions between regulatory and industry experts
- Wide consultation of the draft consensus documents, through normal regulatory channels, before a harmonized text is adopted
- Commitment by regulatory parties to implement the ICH harmonized texts

During the same meeting, it was also agreed that six-party Expert Working Groups (EWGs) should be set up, through whom scientific and technical aspects of each harmonization topic could be discussed. The EWGs would meet in the same week as the Steering Committee and give a report of their progress to this Committee.

Initial Topics Selected for Harmonization

During the first Steering Committee meeting of ICH, the Terms of Reference were agreed. The topics that were selected for discussion at the three EWG workshops at ICH 1, especially those for Quality and Safety were very broad in their scope. Despite the success of ICH 1 conference, it was obvious that the harmonization topics would have to be more focused, with a clearly defined and realistic objective. This was the basis of the sub-division of most of the eleven ICH 1 Topics and also of ICH Codes (which are identified as simply as "Quality T1-T3", "safety T1-T4" and "Efficacy T1-T4).

Since ICH 1, at least one Topic has come "full circle". The single Quality Topic on "Specifications" was first divided into two topics – Analytical Validation (Q2) and Impurities (Q3). These were further sub-divided and developed into harmonized guidelines. After the completion of these tasks, it was agreed that work should recommence on a consolidated guidance for setting specifications for new drugs and products (Q6) at ICH 3.

In addition, the broad Safety Topic from ICH 1 – Toxicity Testing Program was also broken down into various elements, which resulted in harmonized guidelines. Other Topics such as Safety Testing for Biotechnology Products and the Timing of Toxicity Studies in Relation to Clinical Trials were put "on hold" but were re-visited subsequently.

ICH—STRUCTURE

The ICH is broadly an initiative that has been jointly undertaken by both regulators and the pharmaceutical industry, wherein both are equal participants in scientific and technical discussions of the testing procedures required to ensure and assess the safety, quality and efficacy of medicines. Technical requirements for developing new drugs have been the focus of ICH. Hence, the scope of ICH is mainly confined to Western Europe, the US and Japan, where the bulk of new drugs are developed.

The ICH is administered by the ICH Steering Committee, which is supported by the *ICH Secretariat*. The ICH Secretariat is, in turn, supported by the *International Federation of Pharmaceutical Manufacturers Association (IFPMA).*

ICH Participants

Founder Members

The ICH comprises of *six founder members* representing the regulatory bodies and the research-based industry in the EU, Japan and the US (Fig. 5.2). These groups are directly involved in the decision making process.

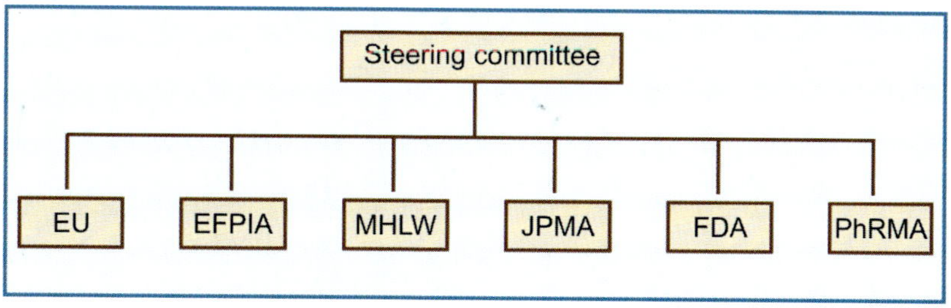

Fig. 5.2: Founder members of ICH

European Commission – European Union

The EC represents 25 members of the EU. The Commission is using harmonization of technical requirements and procedures to achieve a single pharmaceuticals market in the EU, which would allow free movement of products among the member countries. The Commission has set up the European Medicines Agency (EMEA) and the Committee for Medicinal Products for Human Use (CHMP) of the EMEA provides technical and scientific support for all ICH activities. EMEA is situated in London.

European Federation of Pharmaceutical Industries and Associations (EFPIA)

The EFPIA is situated in Brussels and comprises of 25 national pharmaceutical industry associations, including six associations with liaison status, and 43 leading pharmaceutical companies involved in research, development and manufacturing of medicinal products in Europe, for human use. The Federation works in lieu with the activities of EMEA.

Ministry of Health, Labor and Welfare, Japan (MHLW)

The approval and administrative responsibilities of drugs, medical devices and cosmetics in Japan fall under the auspices of the MHLW. All technical and scientific support for ICH-related activities are provided by the Pharmaceuticals and Medical Devices Agency (PMDA), the National Institute of Health Sciences (NIHS) and other expert academic bodies.

Japan Pharmaceutical Manufacturers Association (JPMA)

JPMA is a consortium of 90 major research-based pharmaceutical manufacturers in Japan. ICH work is coordinated through specialized committees of industry experts who also participate in the expert working groups.

US Food and Drug Administration (FDA)

The US FDA, which is the largest regulatory agency in the world, is responsible for the approval of all drug products used in the US. Two centers namely, the Center for Drug Evaluation and Research and the Center for Biologics Evaluation and Research give technical advice for ICH work.

Pharmaceutical Research and Manufacturers of America (PhRMA)

The research-based industry in the US is represented by PhRMA, which has 67 member companies and 24 research affiliates involved in the discovery, development and manufacture of prescription medicines. The PhRMA, previously known as the US Pharmaceutical Manufacturers Association, coordinates its technical input to ICH through its Scientific and Regulatory Section.

Observers

In addition to the expert groups, the ICH has observers to act as a link with non-ICH countries and regions. The observers are the World Health Organization (WHO), the European Free Trade Area (EFTA), which is represented at ICH by Swissmedic, Switzerland and Canada represented by Health Canada.

ICH Coordinators

Each of the six groups has a designated Coordinator who acts as the main point of contact with the ICH Secretariat. Each party also has an established Contact Network of experts within their own region to ensure that they reflect the views and policies of the co-sponsor they represent in various discussions.

ICH Secretariat

The ICH Secretariat is supported by the IFPMA and operates from its offices in Geneva. The Secretariat is mainly concerned with:

i. Preparations for, and documentation of, meetings of the Steering Committee
ii. Coordination of preparations for meetings of the Expert Working Groups and six-party drafting groups
iii. Technical documentation and for liaison with the speakers for the ICH Conferences, when they are scheduled. The industry and regulatory parties in the country where the Conference is taking place look after the organizational aspects of the same.

International Federation of Pharmaceutical Manufacturer's Association (IFPMA)

The IFPMA is a Federation of Member Associations, which represents the research-based pharmaceutical industry and other manufacturers of prescription medicines in 56 countries worldwide. The IFPMA has been in close association with ICH right from the beginning, with an objective of ensuring contact with the research-based industry, outside the ICH regions. The IFPMA runs the ICH Secretariat.

ICH CONFERENCES AND WORKSHOPS

One of the objectives of the ICH when it was first established was to organize an International Conference on Harmonization – therefore, this was the name given to the initiative.

Over the years, the name ICH is now somehow more linked with the harmonization process than the actual Conferences, though the latter played a very important role towards ensuring that the harmonization process was carried out in a transparent manner and that there was an open forum in which to present and discuss the various recommendations of the ICH.

The various conferences that were held are summarized in Box 5.3.

Box 5.3: Chronicles of ICH conferences

First Conference	Brussels	1991
Second Conference	Orlando	1993
Third Conference	Yokohama	1995
Fourth Conference	Brussels	1997
Fifth Conference	San Diego	2000
Sixth Conference	Osaka	2003

Sometimes, Regional Workshops have been organized by ICH parties on the implementation and use of the ICH Guidelines. These have been conducted at the time of a Steering Committee meeting in the region, so that the presence of Steering Committee members and ICH Experts could be benefited from. These types of workshops will continue in the future and will provide an opportunity for interaction with all the "users' of the guidelines.

ICH Harmonization – Brussels 1997

The Fourth International Conference on Harmonization (ICH 4) was held in Brussels on 16-18 July 1997. This marked the completion of the first phase of ICH activities, wherein significant progress, in reducing duplication in the process for developing new medicinal products and submitting technical data for registration, was made.

Statement by the ICH Steering Committee

Continuation of Harmonization Activities: At this meeting, it was decided that the six-party structure would continue as the operational basis for harmonizing technical requirements for new medicine development and registration of products containing new drug substances. It was decided to have a second phase of harmonization activities to ensure that:

i. There is a mechanism to harmonize new technical requirements resulting from scientific progress and developments in innovative drug research;

ii. There is a process for updating and supplementing the current ICH guidelines, when necessary and monitoring their use, so that the benefits of harmonization achieved so far are not lost;

iii. Future disharmony is prevented through early collaboration and exchange of information on newly emerging issues, originating in one of the regions.

Scientific Consensus: Since some of the topics selected for harmonization had implications for regulatory agencies and sectors of industry not represented by the six parties to ICH, observers from WHO, EFTA and Canada were selected and participation in the Expert Working Groups was extended on the basis of the topic selected. Despite the wider participation in technical discussions, the inception and implementation of new, updated or extended harmonized ICH guidelines will continue to be the responsibility of the regulators in the three ICH regions, taking into account the results of the regulatory consultative process, within each region.

Conferences and Workshops: It was decided that ICH would continue to organize periodic conferences and workshops, which serve as channels of communication and discussion of harmonization issues. The biennial International Conferences on Harmonization have been conducted to disseminate information on ICH and to ensure that harmonization is conducted in an open and transparent manner.

Globalization of the Benefits of Harmonization: The widespread dissemination and understanding of the objectives and outcomes of ICH need to be realized. This challenge would be met by the six parties of ICH, WHO and through IFPMA in conjunction with other concerned parties. The long-term benefits of international harmonization, in terms of quicker access to new medicines to patients throughout the world, would receive a boost with active participation from the WHO.

Second Phase of International Harmonization: It was decided that in the second phase of international harmonization, ICH would continue to work with the same zeal as in the early phase to ensure that good quality; safe and effective medicines are developed quickly and at competitive prices. The scope of these activities would be to safeguard patient, consumer and public health by preventing unwarranted duplication of clinical trials in humans and to minimize the use of animal testing without compromising the regulatory obligations of safety and effectiveness.

Revised ICH Terms of Reference:

i. To maintain a forum for a constructive dialogue between regulatory authorities and the pharmaceutical industry on the real and perceived differences in the technical requirements for product registration in the EU, USA and Japan in order to ensure a more timely introduction of new medicinal products and their availability to patients;

ii. To monitor and update harmonized technical requirements leading to a greater mutual acceptance of research and development data;

iii. To avoid divergent future requirements through harmonization of selected topics needed as a result of therapeutic advances and the development of new technologies for the production of medicinal products;

iv. To facilitate the adoption of new or improved technical research and development approaches, which update or replace current practices, where these permit a more economical use of human, animal and material resources, without compromising safety;

v. To facilitate the dissemination and communication of information on harmonized guidelines and their use such as to encourage the implementation and integration of common standards.

ICH PROCESS FOR HARMONIZATION OF GUIDELINES

The development of the ICH process for harmonizing guidelines on technical issues was one of the critical factors in the success of the ICH. The commitment to ICH was set out in a Steering Committee Statement from the meeting in Tokyo, October 1990 (Box 5.4).

Box 5.4: Statement by the ICH steering committee

- The Parties co-sponsoring this Conference, represented at the 2nd Steering Committee Meeting in Tokyo, 23-24 October, 1990 re-affirmed their commitment to increased international harmonization, aimed at ensuing that quality, safe and effective medicines are developed and registered in the most efficient and cost-effective manner. These activities are pursued in the interest of the consumer and public health, to prevent unnecessary duplication of clinical trials in humans and to minimize the use of animal testing without compromising the regulatory obligations of safety and effectiveness.
- This Conference will provide a unique opportunity for regulators and industry to reach consensus on the steps needed to achieve this objective through greater harmonization of technical requirements and to set out practical and realistic targets for harmonizing requirements where significant obstacles to drug development and the regulatory process have been identified
- Recognizing the substantial progress which has already been made in achieving this harmonization within Europe and through bilateral contacts between Europe, Japan, USA and other regions, the Conference will seek to make further progress through a trilateral approach, with clearly defined priorities, methods of work and recommendations to both industry and regulatory authorities.
- Whilst the Conference will be an important step forward, it is not seen as an end in itself, but as a stage in a developing process, at a high level, between regulators and industry.

Contd...

Contd...

- The Conference, its preparations and follow-up activities will be conducted in an open and transparent manner and the presence of observers from other regulatory authorities and WHO is welcomed as a means of ensuring that the benefits of progress towards harmonization can be utilized worldwide.
- The Conference will not only look at existing issues but will, based on past experience, seek to minimize future divergence of new registration requirements, as a consequence of technical progress.

It was in March 1992 at the Steering Committee meeting in Washington that the ICH process was first drawn up. It was further amended in Tokyo, September 1992. The process that was laid down comprised of five steps with "decision points" at Step 2 and Step 4, which permitted the monitoring of the progress of the topics selected for harmonization by the Steering Committee.

This "five-step approach" is also what is described as the "full" ICH process. It proved extremely successful for the first phase of ICH activities.

Apart from this "five-step" approach or the "full" ICH process, there is yet another process that is sometimes adopted which is called as the "Maintenance" process or the Abbreviated Process for Maintenance of ICH Agreements. This process is used when minor changes and revisions to existing ICH Guidelines are required to be made.

Before discussing the details of both these processes, it is necessary to understand how the basic ICH Harmonization is initiated.

Initiation of ICH Harmonization Action

This can be described under the following headings:

i. How proposals are made for harmonization action
ii. The preparation of a short summary of the proposal through a Concept Paper
iii. Selection of a procedure depending on the nature of the proposal.

Proposals for Harmonization Action

There could be various fora at which some suggestions for new harmonization activities are triggered. Some of these fora include ICH Regional Guideline Workshops; other regional and international conferences, workshops and symposia dealing with R and D and regulatory affairs; recognized Associations, Federations and Societies, which represent scientific and technical professionals who are concerned with the development, testing and registration of medicines.

However, it is necessary that formal proposals for ICH action be channeled through one of the six ICH parties or one of the Observers on the Steering Committee.

Any proposal for harmonization action may fall into one of the following groups:

i. **New types of medicinal products:** Under this, proposals for guidelines to cover new products that result due to advances in technology and techniques for producing medicines are covered such as products arising from gene therapy and other developments in biotechnical and genomic research.

ii. **Lack of harmonization in current technical requirements:** This group includes proposals for further harmonization of existing requirements such as a result of work on the Common Technical Document.

iii. **Transition to technically improved testing procedures:** In this group are included proposals for action to facilitate the replacement of currently established testing procedures to more efficient and economical methods where these provide equal or better assurance of the safety and/or quality of new drugs.

iv. **Review of an existing ICH Guideline:** Proposals for significant changes to the technical aspects of an ICH Guideline or proposals for a major addition to the guideline are included here.

v. **Maintenance of an existing guideline:** This group includes proposals for relatively minor modification, updating clarification or review of ICH agreements to take account of problems with implementation, new information or new scientific knowledge.

Preparation of a Concept Paper

Whoever proposes a new harmonization action (i.e. the ICH party or Observer) has to present the issue in the form of a Concept Paper, which provides a short summary of the proposal (maximum 2 pages) while giving the following information:

i. **Type of harmonization action proposed:** e.g. a new tripartite harmonized guideline /recommendation, or an amendment/update of an existing guideline.

ii. **Statement of the perceived problem:** i.e. a brief description giving an indication of the extent of problems that are currently caused by a lack of harmonization, or – in the case of new scientific developments – anticipated if harmonization action is not taken.

iii. **Issues to be resolved:** a summary of the main technical and scientific issues, which require harmonization.

iv. **Background to the proposal:** further relevant information such as the origin of the proposal, references to publications, references to the publications, discussions in other fora

v. **Type of Expert working Group:** if an EWG is needed, a recommendation on whether it should be a six-party group (for topics related to the R and D of new drug substances and products) or an extended EWG (for topics with implications beyond new drug research).

Note: A formal EWG is not required for actions designated as "maintenance" of existing guidelines.

Further documentation and reports may be annexed to the Concept paper.

Selection of Procedure

Proposals that are in the following groups will automatically be subject to the full ICH Process ("five-step approach"): *New types of medicinal product, lack of harmonization in current technical requirements, transition to technically improved testing procedures and review of an existing ICH Guideline.* These are groups a-d as mentioned above.

The proposal and Concept paper should be sent to members of the Steering Committee, Observers and ICH Coordinators and the copy to the ICH Secretariat should ask for the item to be included on the agenda for the next Steering Committee meeting.

Proposals for maintenance of existing guidelines (i.e. of group e above) – where the sponsor feels that an abbreviated process is appropriate, should be sent to the ICH Secretariat with a request that the Maintenance Process (which is described below) be initiated.

Some revisions in the ICH procedures

Subsequent to ICH 4 in 1997 and ICH 5 in 2000, the ICH Steering Committee agreed upon certain working procedures upon to ensure that the objectives that were laid down could be met.

Towards this, harmonization initiatives would be designated as "Major" and "Minor". A major topic would include proposals for new guidelines and changes to existing guidelines, which involve interpretations of statutory or regulatory requirements, changes in interpretation or policy that are more than a minor nature, usually complex scientific issues. Other changes are considered as "minor".

Because of this modification, major topics will be handled under the full ICH Process as described above ("five-step approach"). Proposals for "Minor" changes to existing tripartite harmonized guidelines will be handled through the abbreviated Maintenance Process (described below).

Another important point to note is that in the first phase of ICH activities, the main focus was on the technical requirements for developing and registering products containing new substances in the EU, Japan and the USA. Also, the Expert Working Groups, which worked on more than 40 guidelines for new products were made up of scientists from six ICH parties – the regulatory agencies and the research-based industry in the three regions.

Now with the revised ICH procedures, however, the second phase of activities may cover a wider range of topics and issues, which have implications for parties outside the six ICH parties.

It must be remembered, though, that the basic principles guiding the ICH process as described in Figure 5.1, which have been the cornerstone of ICH work, remain unchanged.

Full ICH Process for Major Harmonization Topics

Topic selection

An item on *Proposals for New Topics* is routinely included as an item in the agenda of the Steering Committee. The sponsoring party, or Observer will have circulated the Concept Paper to Coordinators and the Secretariat in advance and the Concept Paper and any comments will have submitted to the Steering Committee. A preliminary assessment is made as to whether the topic is of sufficient interest to all parties and whether it can be accommodated within the ICH work program.

As noted, the Concept Paper will indicate the type of EWG that is appropriate for the topic (i.e. whether it should be a six-party membership only, or with membership extended to other interested parties). In the event of requiring an extension of membership to other interested parties, the Steering Committee will invite, as appropriate, those additional parties to discussions on the topic just prior to its acceptance by them (the Steering Committee) as an ICH topic.

Steering Committee Action

Once a topic is adopted for harmonization action, the Steering Committee will:

i. Confirm the *Objectives and Expected Outcome* of the harmonization action
ii. Confirm the composition of the *EWG* appointed to discuss the technical issues
iii. Set a *Timetable and Action Plan* for the EWG

The Concept Paper will be revised and updated to reflect these decisions.

Expert Working Groups

Each of the six ICH parties will be asked to designate a Topic Leader for the new topic. These leaders will participate in the EWG meetings and be the point of contact for any consultations that are carried out between meetings (by correspondence, fax, e-mail etc. A Deputy Topic leader may also be designated. The Observers to the ICH will also be invited to nominate an expert to the EWG.

In case of EWGs with extended membership, the Secretariat will invite the designated organizations to nominate an expert to participate in the EWG and act as the contact point for receipt of documents on technical issues

Organizations that have never participated in ICH EWGs before should be informed that ICH does not cover the cost of travel or accommodation for EWG participants and that their participation is at their own cost – it is possible to make a request for a contribution to the expenses of holding the meetings, though.

Also, if one of the non-ICH parties is absent from EWG meeting, it will not prevent the meeting from taking place

EWG Reports to the Steering Committee: Other interested parties and their experts will be present and able to express their views to the Steering Committee when topics in which they have a particular interest are discussed. The agenda for the Steering Committee will be accordingly arranged.

For managing the likely numbers of attendees from interested parties during the discussion of these topics, attendance will be limited to one representative in addition to their expert.

Timetable and Action Plan: The Steering Committee will agree to a "target" timetable for development of scientific consensus in the EWG for each new harmonization topic. This would not generally exceed 2 years.

One of the six ICH parties will be designated to nominate the R*apporteur* and all involved parties will be asked to nominate their respective experts within a fixed time limit.

Steps in the ICH process (Box 5.5)

Step 1: Consensus Building: It is the duty of the Rapporteur to prepare an initial draft of the guideline or recommendation based on the objectives set out in the Concept Paper (in consultation with experts designated to EWG) and circulate it for comments within a defined timeline. Since formal meetings are usually held along with the biannual Steering Committee meetings, communication is usually by fax and e-mail. Additional, formal meetings of the ICH EWG need to be agreed, in advance, by the Steering Committee.

Interim reports are made to each meeting of the ICH Steering Committee. If there is consensus on the interim report within the defined timelines, it is submitted to the Steering Committee with EWG signatures for Step 2 adoption.

If no consensus can be reached within stipulated timelines, a report regarding the exact extent of agreement is submitted to the Steering Committee. Experts from all

Box 5.5: Steps in the ICH process

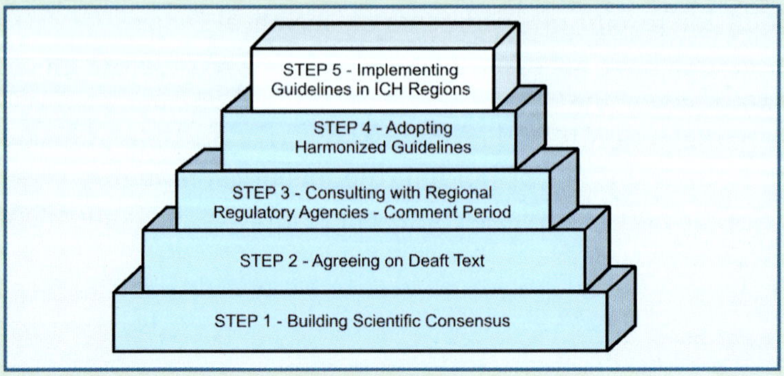

parties represented on the EWG will have the opportunity to explain their position to the Steering Committee who may then either allow an extension of timelines, or decide to suspend/abandon the harmonization project or decide to proceed to Step 2.

Sign-off by EWG Members: When consensus is reached on the technical issues, all parties represented on an EWG would be invited to sign the document to indicate their agreement to the consensus text, which is submitted to the Steering Committee. If all other parties are not present or able to sign the consensus text, the Steering Committee will have to decide whether to proceed to Step 2.

Step 2: Start of Regulatory Action: At this stage, there is an agreement by the Steering Committee for proceeding to the next stage of regulatory consultation. The Steering Committee Members confirm this agreement for each of the six signing parties signing their assent.

Step 3: Regulatory Consultation: The guideline now leaves the ICH process and is the subject of regulatory consultation in the three regions. The guideline is subsequently published as a draft CPMP guideline in the EU and as draft guidance in the Federal register. The MHLW translates and issues it in Japan for internal and external consultation. After exchanging information amongst themselves and at times taking inputs from various industry associations and regulatory authorities in non-ICH regions, the three regulatory parties form a single harmonized text.

A designated *Regulatory Rapporteur* obtains agreement on the final document.

Step 4: Adoption of a Tripartite Harmonized Text: At this stage, the *Regulatory Rapporteur* submits the report to the Steering Committee who adopts the text in the event of both industry and regulatory parties being satisfied that the consensus at Step 2 is not significantly altered further to the consultation. However, if one or more parties representing industry object to the adoption of the guideline, or introduce new issues, the regulatory parties may suggest that a revised version of the text be submitted after further consultation.

Step 5: Implementation: This is the final stage, which is carried out in accordance with the national/regional procedures that apply to other regulatory guidelines and requirements in the EU, USA and in Japan. Details on the type of regulatory action taken and dates of implementation are reported back to the Steering Committee and published by the Secretariat.

Abbreviated Maintenance Process (Abbreviated Process for Maintenance of ICH Agreements)

The objective of the Abbreviated Maintenance Process is to provide a rapid and flexible way of making minor changes and revisions to existing ICH Guidelines, using the minimum of resources consistent with the achievement of a scientifically valid result. It is necessary that as far as possible, maintenance work be completed via a written procedure. Meetings should be held only in exceptional cases.

The Abbreviated Maintenance Process is summarized below:

Contact Network for Maintenance of Guidelines

A network of experts is established by each of the six ICH parties for dealing with maintenance issues. In addition, they should also identify one Maintenance Contact for each Step 5 ICH guideline or implemented agreement, which work in close association with their respective ICH coordinators (who are the first point of contact) to deal with all maintenance issues concerning their respective guidelines. These coordinators should provide the ICH Secretariat with details of the Maintenance Contacts for each guideline.

Procedure: Maintenance Network

After the identification of a maintenance issue, a *Concept Paper,* which is as specific as possible is prepared and then sent to the ICH Secretariat and the Coordinators. If the Coordinators are in agreement regarding the proposal being a "minor" change, the maintenance process is initiated.

Further to this, there is a *review and sign-off process*:

i. The secretariat registers the maintenance proposal, designates a code

ii. Number and prepares a draft sign-off sheet identifying the proposed

iii. Changes to the guideline which is attached to the concept paper and sent

iv. To the maintenance network via the ich coordinators.

v. The steering committee members and observers are informed about the proposal.

vi. The maintenance contact from the sponsoring party (which provided the concept paper) acts as a *topic coordinator whose* responsibility is to circulate comments and further proposals as necessary.

vii Subsequent to regional/internal consultation, each of the *Maintenance Contacts* indicates whether he or she agrees with the proposal made. Minor changes may be proposed to the wording.

viii In the event of an agreement not being reached, the matter will be referred to the next Steering Committee for a decision on establishing an Expert working Group and initiating the full ICH process (as described above)

ix. If all experts agree, the completed sign-off sheet is returned to the ICH Secretariat who circulates the signed-off proposal to the Steering Committee, requesting a response within a month.

Procedure: Steering Committee

i. The Steering Committee now has to opine as to whether:

ii. The proposal is accepted and can be implemented immediately (without further consultation). An example of this might be the changes to the residual solvent lists in the impurity guideline.

iii. **Secretariat Action:** The text of the ICH Guideline is updated and circulated to the Steering Committee and Maintenance Contacts. The revised text is announced and published.
iv. The proposal is accepted but requires wider consultation. The proposal should then be treated as a Step 2 document for formal regulatory consultation, in accordance with the procedures set out in the "full" harmonization process.
v. **Secretariat Action:** Signatures for all six parties will be required on the Step 2 consultation document, after which the consultation will be announced following normal procedures.
vi. There are further issues to be resolved and the matter needs to be discussed at the next Steering Committee meeting.
vii. **Secretariat Action:** The Maintenance Contacts will be informed and the item will be included on the agenda for the next ICH Steering Committee meeting.

ICH GUIDELINES

The ICH topics are basically divided into four broad and major categories:

A. Quality
B. Safety
C. Efficacy and
D. Multidisciplinary

The ICH topic codes are assigned according to these categories. These categories have been introduced in *Section 2* and details on each are mentioned below.

Quality

Quality topics are those relating to chemical and pharmaceutical quality assurance. These comprise of:
Q1-stability testing, Q3- impurity testing, Q5- quality of biotechnological products and Q7- good manufacturing practices.

Safety

These are topics related to *in vitro* and *in vivo* pre-clinical studies, for example, S1-carcinogenicity testing, S2-genotoxicity testing, S5-reproductive toxicology, and S7-pharmacology studies.

Efficacy

These include topics relating to clinical studies in human subjects. For example, E4-dose response studies, carcinogenicity testing, E5-ethnic factors, E6-good clinical practices, and E7-clinical trials.

Multidisciplinary

Multidisciplinary topics ("M") are those that do not fit uniquely into one of the above categories. The multidisciplinary topics considered by ICH are M1 – medical terminology, M2 – electronic standards for transmission of regulatory information (ESTRI), M3 – timing of pre-clinical studies in relation to clinical trials, and M4 – the common technical document.

The ESTRI project includes the verification of procedures for consistent, accurate transfer of information; the evaluation of encryption technologies and key certification procedures for the transfer of regulatory information. The working group has undertaken test projects to define logical electronic communication standards to ensure the integrity of information and data exchange between pharmaceutical companies and authorities. Tests have also been conducted which involves transferring encrypted and non-encrypted files between a limited numbers of international centers.

FUTURE OF ICH — STATEMENT OF ICH STEERING COMMITTEE[1]

The Fifth International Conference on Harmonization (ICH 5) held in San Diego in November 2000, marked the end of a decade of harmonization for the ICH. This meeting provided a scope for evaluating the results achieved during the past years and for identifying future activities in the area of international harmonization.

This Conference was preceded by a meeting of the ICH Steering Committee and Expert Working Groups during which the Common Technical Document (CTD) – a harmonized format for regulatory submissions - was completed.

Success of ICH

The success of the ICH process was attributed to the scientific consensus developed between industry and regulatory experts and also to the commitment of regulatory bodies to implement the ICH tripartite, harmonized guidelines and recommendations.

If the ICH is to continue being successful it will have to ensure that it addresses current issues for harmonization in an increasingly dynamic international environment. To facilitate this, it will be necessary to focus more on the implementation and monitoring of ICH commitments, especially the Common Technical Document (CTD), in which the creation of implementation groups or task forces will be of prime importance (Box 5.6).

Future Topics for Harmonization – The "Way Forward"

The Steering Committee agreed to continue with the work of harmonization after ICH 5 and select new topics in a systematic and focused manner. It was felt that an

Box 5.6: ICH activities in future

In the future, the ICH intends to focus its activities on:
- Implementing and maintaining existing guidelines
- Preventing disharmony
- Encouraging scientific dialogue and harmonization in new areas
- Undertaking efforts towards global co-operation with non-ICH regions /countries

even more careful advance examination of a potential topic for future harmonization is essential, in order to ensure that the projects are feasible, implemented within timelines and add value for all ICH partners. ICH is expected to undertake new activities in areas where there are new technological advances and innovative medicines. It was decided that a feasibility study and/or scientific pre-screening should precede topic selection, wherever necessary. Post-marketing areas have been identified as a major area to focus on too, in future.

Structure and Participation of Steering Committee

It was felt that the existing Steering Committee structure was appropriate. If any topic were of interest to any other parties, however, they would be welcome to participate in a flexible and ad hoc manner.

Dissemination of Information

The Steering Committee felt that it was necessary to disseminate information and communicate with non-ICH parties, too. Regular large conferences would facilitate communicating results of harmonization activities to wide audiences, as would the increased involvement of WHO through its regional centers. These were a part of the recent emphasis on *global co-operation* actions by ICH.

Modern techniques such as video-conferencing and electronic communication could be considered to increase the communication between parties of ICH as well as with other parties.

Revised ICH Terms of Reference

i. To maintain a forum for a constructive dialogue between regulatory authorities and the pharmaceutical industry on the real and perceived differences in the technical requirements for product registration in the EU, USA and Japan in order to ensure a more timely introduction of new medicinal products, and their availability to patients.
ii. To contribute to the protection of public health from an international perspective
iii. To monitor and update harmonized technical requirements leading to a greater acceptance of research and development data.

iv. To avoid divergent future requirements through harmonization of selected topics needed as a result of therapeutic advances and the development of new technologies for the production of medicinal products.
v. To facilitate the adoption of new or improved technical research and development approaches which update or replace current practices.

CONCLUSIONS

With the ICH harmonization process, it is possible to bring new medicinal products to the market place in a shorter and streamlined manner, with coordinated and integrated efforts between various research-based industries and regulatory authorities across the world. Sharing common objectives and thought processes through harmonization have further facilitated aligning these efforts in a single direction in order to ensure that through the endeavors of any country participating in global clinical research, the data generated is of good quality and of a standard that can be accepted by any regulatory authority worldwide.

Individual country efforts at releasing their own local guidelines are, by far and large, in accordance to ICH-GCP guidelines while highlighting some local issues of importance that need special attention.

The continuous revisions of the ICH process further to its introduction highlight the efforts to ensure that current topics pertaining to strengthening globalization of clinical trials always remain under focus.

With the road ahead clearly mapped out as can be seen in various statements made in the 2000 revision (ICH 5, San Diego), it is quite evident that the success of ICH in the past will not only continue, but increase in leaps and bounds, while providing a common link between regulatory authorities and research-based industries worldwide.

For countries like India, continuous success in global clinical research requires training for all clinical research professionals in ICH-GCP. Ensuring the same standard of knowledge and understanding of ICH-GCP amongst all clinical research stakeholders (especially entire study teams representing the sponsor and investigator) is of equal importance – well before conducting any clinical research activity.

REFERENCES

1. Nermeen Varawalla. Conducting clinical trials in Asia. Applied Clinical Trials 2006. Available at: http://www.actmagazine.com/applied-clinicaltrials/content/printContent Popup.jsp?id = 334577.
2. Isal JP. India: Have we made progress? Applied Clinical Trials 2006.
3. History and Future of ICH. Available at: Accessed July 17, 2006. http://www.ich.org/cache/compo/276-254-1.html
4. Korteweg M. Standardizing quality in international studies. In: Hamrell MR, ed. The Clinical Audit in Pharmaceutical Development. Vol 104. Chpt 5. Marcel Dekker, Inc., New York 2000;63-97.

6

Informed Consent Process: Protecting Subjects' Rights

Surinder Kher

INTRODUCTION

The oath that the physicians have been taking for more than two thousand years clearly articulates that the physician knows what is best for his or her patient. For over two millennia, the culture has put the physician in an almost God like position in terms of his or her wisdom to practice in the patient's best interest. However, the last fifty years have been different than the past history. The concept that the physicians should prefer to protect their patients from information about their diseases or treatment options has totally changed and we have seen a trend towards patient rights. That has included the right to know what the physician intends to do and why. This is the essence of informed consent.

Ensuring that study subjects are engaging voluntarily, without coercion and in the knowledge they can withdraw at any time, is a fundamental ethical principle of research. With the current changing research environment and the various regulations governing biomedical research, the informed consent process should also assure subjects that the information they give will be securely stored with complete confidentiality and used responsibly by the various parties involved in the research.

THE HISTORY OF INFORMED CONSENT AND THE SYSTEM OF SUBJECT PROTECTION

The last fifty years have seen the international and US medical communities taking various steps to protect people who take part in clinical research.

A comprehensive movement towards informed consent began after World War II with the 1947 Nuremberg trials. In these war trials, physicians conducted medical experiments on concentration camp prisoners. This research included human experimentation with germ warfare, freezing individuals to learn what temperature can kill individuals most effectively, and similar other horrifying research trials.

Between 1930 and 1945 Japan conducted human experiments in biological warfare, including physical responses to infection and trauma, which lead to deaths of thousands of people. As a result of these unethical trials the Nuremberg Code was defined in 1947. It was the first major international document to provide guidelines on research ethics. It made voluntary consent a requirement in clinical research studies, emphasizing that consent can be voluntary only if:

- Subjects are able to consent
- They are free from coercion (i.e., outside pressure)
- They comprehend the risks and benefits involved.

The Code also states that investigators should minimize risk and harm, make sure that risks do not significantly outweigh potential benefits, use appropriate study designs, and guarantee subjects' freedom to withdraw at any time. The Nuremberg Code was adopted by the United Nations General Assembly in 1948. With this, the modern era of ethics within biomedical research emerged with particular emphasis on the patient's rights expressed by the practice of informed consent.

In the year 1962, the Kefauver-Harris Bill was passed to ensure greater drug safety in the United States after Thalidomide was found to have caused birth defects in thousands of babies born in Western Europe. At the 18th World Medical Assembly in Helsinki, Finland in 1964, the World Medical Association adopted 12 principles to guide physicians on ethical considerations related to biomedical research. This was the landmark declaration known as the Declaration of Helsinki laid the foundation of current ethical guidelines on biomedical research. It emphasized the distinction between medical care that directly benefits the patient and research that may or may not provide direct benefit.

It was in 1972 that the term "informed consent" first received wide awareness and prominence in public health research, as well as in the practice of medicine. There was a public outcry regarding unethical practices in the Tuskegee trials. In 1932 the US Public Health Service initiated a study that examined the effects of untreated syphilis among rural black men in Tuskegee, Alabama. Thousands of men were kept in total ignorance of the experiment, their infection, and the seriousness of syphilis. They were kept away from receiving effective treatment so the United States government could monitor how the disease progressed, its many serious side effects, and its rate of fatality. Following this public outcry the National Commission for the Protection of Human Subjects of Biomedical and Behavioral Research was established. The US Congress passed the National Research Act in 1974. This Act prompted the establishment of Institutional Review Boards (IRB) at the local level and required IRB review and approval of all federally funded research involving human subjects.

After four years of work, the National Commission for the Protection of Human Subjects of Biomedical and Behavioral Research in 1979 issued "The Belmont Report: Ethical Principles and Guidelines for the Protection of Human Subjects of Research." The report set forth three principles underlying the ethical conduct of research:

- *Respect for persons:* Recognizing the autonomy and dignity of individuals, and the need to protect those with diminished autonomy (i.e. impaired decision-making skills), such as children, the aged, and the disabled;
- *Beneficence:* An obligation to protect persons from harm by maximizing benefits and minimizing risks;
- *Justice:* Fair distribution of the benefits and burdens of research.

The Belmont Report explains how these apply to research practices; for example, it identifies informed consent as a process that is essential to the principle of respect. In response to the report, both the US Department of Health and Human Services and the US Food and Drug Administration revised their regulations on research studies that involve people.

On the basis of these ethical guidelines and regulations that evolved over the years the various regions and countries adopted these ethical principles for biomedical research.

In India the Indian Council of Medical Research (ICMR) also came out with the ethical guidelines for conducting biomedical research. The Declaration of Helsinki and the components of the Belmont Report also drive these guidelines.

BASIC PRINCIPLES

To differentiate the key components of informed consent, we need to understand the ethical issues of research involving human subjects. We need to understand the underlying principles that lay the foundation of the ethics of the informed consent process. These principles are autonomy, beneficence, and justice.

Autonomy

Autonomy means that each person should be given the respect, time, and opportunity necessary to make his or her own decisions. Prospective subjects must be given the information they will need to decide to enter a study or not to participate. There should not be pressure to participate. The principle of autonomy requires that protection be given to potentially vulnerable populations such as children, the elderly, the mentally ill, or prisoners. Individuals in these groups may be incapable of understanding information that would enable them to make an informed decision about study participation. They are considered potentially "vulnerable." Consequently, careful consideration of their situation and needs is required and extra care must be taken to protect them.

Beneficence

Beneficence obligates the investigator to secure the well being of all study subjects. It is the responsibility of the investigator to protect subjects from harm, as well as ensure that they experience the possible benefits of involvement. Balancing risks and benefits is an important consideration. The key is to "maximize possible benefits and minimize possible harms."

Justice

The principle of justice requires that the study subjects should not be selected on the basis of class, socioeconomic status, or race unless justified by the study objectives. The basis of including or not including a study subject in a study should be explained and justified by the investigator. For example, it should be explained why women are not included in a study population. Similarly investigator has to be careful about any bias that might arise due to relationships like an existing doctor-patient relationship or a teacher-student relationship. There is a possibility of influence or coercion in such situations. The informed consent process should reflect the precautions taken to balance the relationship and guard against even the perception of coercion.

The investigator is likely to be a valuable source of advice and information to the study subjects, but only the study subject should make the decision. Even medical experts cannot predict whether a treatment, screening, prevention, or supportive care method under evaluation in a trial will prove successful. The investigator is the central point of the informed consent process and is ethically and morally responsible to ensure that the basic principles of consent process are followed.

INFORMED CONSENT PROCESS

Informed consent is about people's understanding and willingness to participate in a study and not about signing a form. Study subjects must understand the purpose, the procedures, the potential risks and benefits of their involvement, and their alternatives to participation. While consent document that gives this information, and more, is a vital part of the process, the opportunity to discuss any questions or concerns with a knowledgeable research team member is also necessary. In addition, prospective subjects may need time to think about their decision and to discuss it if necessary, with family, friends, or religious or legal advisors. Investigators have to understand that the informed consent involves educating prospective subjects and not just disclosing information that is just a part of the process. The informed consent process should provide the study subject with ongoing explanations that will help him/her make educated decisions about whether to begin or continue participating in a trial. Investigator has to understand that a written document alone may not ensure that the study subjects fully understand what participation means. Therefore, before a study subject makes a decision, the research team should discuss with the study subject the trial's purpose, procedures, risks and potential benefits, and the rights as a subject. The research team should continue to update the study subjects on any new information that may potentially affect the continuation of the study subject. Before, during, and even after the trial, the study subjects should have the opportunity to ask questions and raise concerns. Thus, informed consent is an ongoing, interactive process, rather than a one-time information session.

Typically the informed consent document provides a summary of the clinical trial that includes its purpose, the treatment procedures and schedule, potential risks and benefits, alternatives to participation, etc. and explains the rights of the study subjects.

In all studies the investigators should follow all the essential steps for conducting informed consent. These include the following:

- Obtaining informed consent from each study subject
- Obtain the Informed consent before the start of the study
- The person receiving the information and giving consent (usually the study subject) must sign the consent form.
- In a situation where the study subject is incapable of providing informed consent (e.g. subject is unable to write or understand the consent document) or the study subject is in a 'vulnerable' population (e.g. children, elderly), the informed consent document should be signed by the study subject's legally acceptable representative.
- The person who provides the information and obtains consent (usually the investigator) must sign the consent form. This person must be qualified enough to inform the study subjects of all the aspects of the study and should be in complete knowledge of the protocol that is indicated through his/her on the protocol. If other personnel (e.g. study coordinator) assist in providing information or obtaining consent, he/she should also sign the consent form, clearly describing his/her role in the consent process. The signatories (study subject, investigator and any other person involved in the consent process) should personally date the informed consent document.
- Subjects who cannot understand (read, write or comprehend) the local language may not be eligible for studies that require subjective interpretation (e.g. studies requiring filling of quality of life forms).
- If a subject is unable to read or if a legally acceptable representative is unable to read, an impartial witness should be present during the entire informed consent discussion. The witness will ensure that there was no coercion in the obtaining the informed consent and that the study subject was given adequate time to consider participation in the study. The witness must be able to confirm that the consent procedure was adequate and must have no vested interest in clinical study. The witness should be independent of the study. The relationship of the witness to the study subject and to the investigator or the study should be documented. After the written informed consent form and any other written information to be provided to subjects is read and explained to the subject or the subject's legally acceptable representative, and after the subject or the subject's legally acceptable representative has orally consented to the subject's participation in the trial, and, if capable of doing so, has signed and personally dated the informed consent form, the witness should sign and personally date the consent form. By signing the consent form, the witness attests that the information in the

consent form and any other written information was accurately explained to, and apparently understood by, the subject or the subject's legally acceptable representative, and that informed consent was freely given by the subject or the subject's legally acceptable representative.

The following steps may be followed while preparing obtaining consent:

- Obtain approval of the informed consent from the IRB
- Present the prospective subject with the consent document
- Explain significant points about the research or participation to the study subject
- Prompt the subject to ask questions and answer all/any questions. Make sure to discuss risks, benefits, and alternative therapies in addition to purposes and procedures. It is advisable to read the consent document together with the subject/ the legally acceptable representative
- Give the prospective subject a copy of the consent document
- Allow the subject time to discuss participation, if desired, with family, friends, family physician, etc
- Meet with the subject again and ask open-ended questions about the nature of the study and participation. This helps in assessing that the study subject understands the process correctly
- If the subject is willing, have him or her sign the consent document.

Preparing the Informed Consent Document

During the clinical trial pre-study activities the task of drafting the proposed information sheet and consent form is undertaken as soon as the protocol is final. The protocol and the standard operating procedures should state the need for informed consent. Once the information sheet and the consent document are drafted the investigator should be invited to comment prior to finalization, taking into account knowledge of the local IRB requirements. During the study site assessment visits the sponsor should ensure if there are any standardized forms or formats required by specific study sites, which might necessitate further revision of the information sheet and consent form. Before releasing the information sheet and the consent form to the IRBs and regulatory authorities, these documents must be reviewed and approved internally by the sponsor. Following external review by the IRBs and/or the regulatory authority, if changes are suggested to these documents the proposed changes must be reviewed and approved prior to the enrollment of study subjects.

As the study progresses there might be changes to the protocol or there might be significant events (e.g. serious adverse events). The impact of such changes or events on the informed consent should be evaluated to determine if amendments to the information sheet and/or the consent form are required. If the consent form and/or information sheet are amended, this information must be submitted to the IRB and/ or the local regulatory authority, if applicable. These changes may mandate the need to inform the study subjects and obtain their consent again to continue participation in the study. Information sheets and consent forms should typically include the items in Checklist below.

Checklist

Information about the Consent Procedure

- Consent will be given by the study subject's free will
- Adequate time will be provided to allow the study subject to decide on participation in the study
- Reasonable amount of time will be given to ask questions
- Statement that participation is entirely voluntary
- Statement that refusal to participate in the study will not lead to loss of usual medical benefits
- Description of the situations under which participation would be terminated
- That the subject has right to withdraw at any time without prejudice or consequences.
- That a signed copy of the information sheet and consent form will be provided to the study subject.

Information about the Study Drug /Devices

- Name of sponsor and/or the clinical research organization
- Explaining that the study is a research procedure
- Description of study type and research objectives and purpose of the study
- Description of procedures to be followed
- Description of study medications/devices
- Instructions on use and storage of study medication /device, if relevant
- Description about comparator or other treatments that will be used in the study
- Randomization procedures that will be followed in the study
- Statement explaining the method and reason for selecting the subjects: an explanation of why the subject had been approached for study participation might give the subject a better understanding of the study
- Approximate number of other study subjects participating in the study: it might be helpful for the subjects to understand that they are one of many others rather than the first person participating in the study
- Statement about the expected duration of participation in the study
- The number of times the subject will need to visit the clinic.

Information about the Risks/ Benefits

- Description of the known therapeutic benefits of the study drug/device. Never overemphasize the benefits
- Explanation of the foreseeable risks, inconvenience, discomfort, and any other side effects as a result of participation in the study

- Description of the available and accessible alternative therapies
- Statement explaining that any new findings, that become available during the course of the study that could affect the safety of the study subject will be disclosed to study subjects
- Description about the measures that will be taken for any adverse events or therapeutic failure
- Detailed explanation of the assurance of compensation for treatment-induced injury with specific reference to local laws and guidelines
- Explanation of the financial remuneration, if any for incidentals such as travel cost, lost of work or fee for participation. The anticipated prorated payment, if any, to the subject for participating in the trial
- Explanation of any expenses that may result from participation.

Other Elements

- IRB approval obtained
- Name of IRB with details of contact person on the IRB (if applicable by local requirements)
- Name, address and telephone number (24-hour availability) or contact person at study site for information or in the event of an emergency
- Need to disclose details of current and past medical history, any habits of smoking and alcohol intake
- Medical records will clearly identify study participation
- Explanation that participation is confidential, but records and data will be reviewed by authorized representatives of the sponsors and also may be disclosed to a regulatory authority and the purpose of such disclosure
- The duration for which the data will be stored and the measures that will be taken to ensure physical security of data
- Statement that the family physician or referring physician will be informed of study participation and any significant problems arising during the study. (This sometimes becomes extremely important to confirm vital medical history from this physician)
- Explanation about all conditions that apply to women of childbearing potential
- For genetic studies an explanation that the samples will be used for genetic research with description of the ownership of the sample, the duration for which the samples will be retained, secondary use of these samples and the accessibility of the test results.

Ensuring Readability of the Information Sheet and the Consent Form

The informed consent process can only be effective if subjects understand the study information presented to them. Thus, readability of the consent document is very important. The information provided should be in a very simple and non-technical language so that the subjects can understand and interpret it. A good way to achieve this is to ask a layperson to read and explain the document after it has been drafted. So while writing the document, ensure the following few points are taken care of:

- Write the document consistently in second person (You, Your)
- Print the documents appropriately and ensure that the font size used for typing is appropriate
- Use simple, straightforward sentences
- Use commonly recognizable terms and measurement amounts
- Direct it at an eighth-grade reading level
- Avoid technical language and jargon
- Offer explanation for terms that may be difficult to understand. Remember that study subjects cannot be excluded based on language barriers. If subjects do not understand the language of the consent document, a translated consent document in the language that the subjects can understand should be used. Sometimes qualified interpreters can be used to translate the explanation and questions from the subject. The consent form thus should be simple and straightforward without compromising the content. This helps all the parties involved in the process-investigators in explaining to study subjects, study subjects to understand and thus, participate in research and the reviewers (IRB) in reviewing the documents. It should be borne in mind that if the document is not understandable, a claim could be made that the subject did not understand what was signed.

Some Special Considerations

While conducting research in special population groups (children, incapacitated or challenged individuals) one will need to have special considerations for the informed consent process.

Informed Consent in Children

While considering children in a study specific benefits for participation must be described. At the same time the discomforts that the child may have should be described and explained. A parental consent should be sought for all such children. One or both parents have to give consent for the child based on the extent of risk involved in the study. If the study involves more than minimal risk without any benefit, both the parents should consented. Besides the parental consent the child should give an "assent" for participation in the study provided that the child can comprehend the aspects of research. Typically children who are more than 7years of age are assumed to be fit to give "assent". This is done through a separate assent form. Assent means, simply, that the child who is the potential subject affirmatively agrees to participate in the research.

Informed Consent in Incompetent Individuals

A lot of times investigators will come across people who are not competent enough to give consent (mentally challenged or elderly people with difficulties of vision and hearing). In such situations the investigator should seek the consent of a proxy (legally acceptable representative). The proxy should discuss the decision with family members and/or the medical staff caring for the person and it must be ensured that the decision taken by the proxy would have been in line with the decision made by subject if he/she were competent. The point to remember here is that the person should be considered competent to refuse even if he/she has been considered incompetent.

Oral Consent

Though not recognized by most investigators as a practical and an appropriate approach of obtaining informed consent, an oral "short form" written consent can be obtained from the subjects. This "short form" written consent form states that the elements of the informed consent have been presented to the subject or subjects' legally acceptable representative. For an oral consent it is necessary that

- There is a witness to the oral presentation
- The IRB must approve a written summary of what will be said to the subject/representative
- Subject/representative, the witness and the person administering the consent should sign the short form
- Copies of the summary and the short form should be given to the subject/representative.

Informed Consent in Emergency Situations

There is a provision within the regulations for an emergency use of an investigational product. If the investigator has determined that there is insufficient time to obtain informed consent from the subject /legally authorized representative, the investigator should have the determination reviewed by another physician who is not a part of the study. The investigator should obtain a written certification of the following before the use of the product:

- That the subject is facing a life threatening situation, hence necessitating the use of the investigational product
- That informed consent cannot be obtained due to inability to communicate with the subject or obtain a legally effective consent from the subject
- That there is insufficient time to obtain consent from the legally acceptable representative of the subject
- That there is no alternative method of approved or generally recognized therapy that could provide at least an equal likelihood of saving the subject's life. In a

situation where the investigator is unable to seek the review of the independent physician prior to administering the investigational product, the investigator must have the determination of the use reviewed, evaluated and submitted to the IRB within 5 working days of the use of the investigational product.

Revisions and Continuing Review

The written informed consent form and any other written information to be provided to subjects should be revised whenever important new information that is relevant to the subject's consent becomes available. The IRB should approve revisions to the informed consent form. The subject/legally acceptable representative should be informed in a timely manner if new information becomes available that may be relevant to the subject's willingness to continue participation in the study. The communication of this information should be documented. As the study progresses the investigator should continually review the study and be able to analyze the anticipated risk benefit profile- whether these are reflected in the actual experience of the subjects or not. Investigators should ensure that they are involved in the study on a continued basis and are evaluating the risks and the benefits experienced by the study subjects.

COMMON AUDITING AND INSPECTIONAL FINDINGS OF INFORMED CONSENT PROCESS

Informed consent related issues are amongst the most common findings cited by the regulatory inspectors / auditors. These findings typically include the deficiencies in the content of the informed consent and also deficiencies in the administration of the informed consent. The frequently raised findings include

i. Inadequate or incomplete content of the information sheet and/ or the consent form
ii. Non-inclusion of all the basic elements of the informed consent as required by the regulations
iii. Approval of the consent or the revision of the consent by the IRB not obtained
iv. Improper administration of the informed consent to the subject/legally acceptable representative
v. Study subjects/legally acceptable representatives not reconsented with amended consents

To reduce or prevent inspectional findings it is important to have a proactive approach and get auditor reviews of the consent before submitting to the IRB for approval. Inadequacy regarding content results generally due to use of technical rather than the layperson language, readability that is above eighth-grade level and contents that may not be consistent linguistically or culturally. These aspects are frequently overlooked. It is important to ensure that the study subjects are provided with the most recent version of the IRB approved informed consent it is recommended that the informed consents contain the version number, date and the page number on each page of the consent form that has been signed or initialed and dated. Once compliance issues related to informed consent document have been satisfied, it is important to document the comprehension and the administrative procedures regarding the informed consent process.

CONCLUSIONS

Informed consent process must be conducted according to the standards that have been formalized in national and international guidelines and regulations. The ultimate aim is to protect the rights of the study subjects. Having said that research involving humans poses complex ethical issues. It requires careful thought and consideration especially from the investigator's perspective. The key lies in the effectiveness of the information given to the subject. As time progresses informed consent will continue to evolve in response to continued advances in medical treatment and new avenues of biomedical research. The right of a subject to understand any medical treatment, procedure, or participation in research will still continue to be the primary focus of the informed consent.

SUGGESTED READING

1. A Bhan, M Majd and A Adejumo. Informed Consent in International Research: Perspectives from India, Iran and Nigeria. Medical Ethics 2006;3, No.1.
2. Annas, George J, and Michael Grodin. The Nazi Doctors and the Nuremberg Code. New York: Oxford University Press, 1992.
3. Beauchamp, Tom L, and James F Childress. Principles of Biomedical Ethics. Oxford: Oxford University Press, 1994.
4. Code of Federal regulations and ICHGuidelines GCP Reference Guide, 2006.
5. Griffin JM, Struve JK, Collins D, Liu A, Nelson DB, Bloomfield HE. Long term clinical trials: How much information do subjects retain from the informed consent process? Contemp Clin Trials, 2006 May 12.
6. Hanssen, Michael. "Balancing the Quality of Consent." Journal of Medical Ethics 24, no. 3 (1998):182-87.
7. Indian Council of Medical Research Ethical Guidelines for Biomedical Research on Human Subjects, 2000.
8. Richard A Guarino. New Drug Approval Process: The Global Challenge. Marcel Dekker Inc, 2000.
9. Wendy Boyachuk and Graham Ball. Conducting GCP Compliant Clinical Research. John Willey and Sons, 1999.

7

Role of CRC and CRA in Clinical Trials

Sauren Das

INTRODUCTION

Over the years, it has become more and more necessary to have a multidisciplinary specialist approach in planning and conducting clinical trials. The team conducting the clinical trial usually consists of the principal investigators, the co-investigators, the Clinical Research Associates (CRAs), the Clinical Research Coordinators (CRCs), the data management team and the statisticians. Each person in the research team has a key role to play in the smooth and accurate conduct of the clinical trial. In this chapter, we shall discuss about the key roles and responsibilities of the CRAs and the CRCs.

Several guidelines like the FDA regulations and the international guidelines for Good Clinical Practice (GCP) have very clearly defined the roles and responsibilities of the investigators, sponsors and monitors. Very little formal description is, however, available about the importance of CRAs and CRCs and their roles and responsibilities. The CRC and the CRA are like the 'two pillars' of any clinical trial and they are the key members who ensure that the data is obtained faster and is clean.

THE CLINICAL RESEARCH COORDINATOR (CRC)

The clinical research coordinator (CRC) is a vital link between the trial subjects and their family, the investigator and other team members at the site, central laboratory personnel, the courier service personnel, the contract research organization (CRO), the site management organization (SMO), the sponsor and other players involved in the trial. The concept of a CRC is a relatively new addition to the trial team at the site. No matter what these individuals are called or designated, they act like the 'Central Hub' of the wheel of clinical trial at a site. The CRC is a specialized research professional who works with and under the guidance of the clinical investigator at the trial site. It is seen that many sponsor companies do not place a trial at a site that does not have a CRC working alongside the investigator.

The increase in the number of clinical trials and the advent of complicated and data intensive clinical trials further demands the vital role and contribution of a CRC.

THE CLINICAL RESEARCH ASSOCIATE (CRA)

The CRA is usually from the Sponsor or the CRO who is responsible for the overall monitoring of the clinical trial at the site. The responsibilities begin from the identification of the site, initiation and monitoring of the trial, validation of the (Case record form) CRF data and ensuring that the trial has been conducted in conformation to the protocol, ICH GCP guidelines and the applicable SOP. Such responsibilities do vary from organization to organization. The nature of responsibilities also varies according to the phase of the trial, the therapeutic area as well as the trial medication/device.

So how is the CRA any different from the CRC? We shall discuss this as the chapter progresses. For now, let us just understand that the CRC is present at the site and monitors the day-to-day conduct of the clinical trial at the site. The CRA is not present and at the site but visits the sites from time to time in order to monitor the trial. The CRC preferably manages just one site, whereas the CRA has to monitor the study at a number of sites.

WHO CAN BE A CRC/CRA?

Most CRCs and CRAs are nurses, physician assistants, medical graduates or other medical professionals. Such a requirement is, however, not mandatory. Whenever a CRC/CRA is from a medical background, it is seen that he or she is usually better prepared for the post. A medical personnel taking up the responsibilities of a CRC/CRA is more familiar with the prevalent system at the sites where clinical trials are conducted and, therefore more effective within that system.

Non-medical people who become CRCs or CRAs can also obtain training for an efficient functioning. CRCs/CRAs can obtain training from various sources. Such training is mostly informal, provided by another CRC/CRA who is more experienced in the field. Sponsor companies may also provide formal training in the form of workshops. When a sponsor provides the training, it is usually specific to the study to be conducted or the protocol used. Books and other relevant materials are also available as guides for CRCs and CRAs. Certain organizations also provide formal training courses as well as certificate programs for CRCs and CRAs. Such organizations include the Association of Clinical Research Professionals (ACRP), the Society for Clinical Research Associates (SoCRA) and the Drug Information Association (DIA).

THE SITES WHERE CRC/CRA WORKS

A CRC has to work at the clinical trial site–which can be a state-of-the-art Corporate/Private Hospital or a Government Hospital. He/she must be prepared mentally to work at all varieties of set ups. The true skills of a good CRC can be assessed within the confines of a huge Government hospital—the administrative hiccups, the huge patient load and the lack of adequate documentation.

A CRA also works at similar sites. But they visit these sites at regular intervals to ensure the compliance of the trial to the protocol and are not posted at those sites.

RESPONSIBILITIES OF THE CRC AND CRA

The roles and responsibilities of a CRA and a CRC are similar in many aspects but there are critical differences in key functional areas that shall be dealt with later in the chapter.

A CRC/CRA usually has multiple responsibilities to handle and needs to keep juggling around. The art of 'Multi-tasking' must be practiced and adhered to right throughout his/her career. The responsibilities of a CRC/CRA may vary depending on the specific requirements of a particular trial.

The responsibilities are broadly divided into:

General Responsibilities

1. Capacity building
2. Training new CRCs and CRAs

Trial Specific Responsibilities

1. Site identification
2. Pretrial documentation
3. IRB
4. Regulatory
5. Financial
6. Administrative
7. Training of the site staff
8. Informed consent form
9. Site initiation visits
10. Investigator's meeting
11. ICF, screening and recruitment/enrollment
12. Scheduling of visits
13. Research Pharmacy and Drug Accountability
14. Laboratory
15. Amendments
16. Monitoring.

General Responsibilities

Capacity Building

This is done by the CRC/CRA to ensure that the pool of potential investigators and sites keeps increasing. The CRC and the CRA in all major organizations are on the constant lookout for new sites with Investigators who are novice to the clinical trial arena. Sometimes, this is an exercise on its own, with the CRC and CRA visiting new sites and evaluating their capability to participate in global clinical trials. They run an in-depth survey to assess:

i. Manpower presence and competence
ii. Support staff and constant support
iii. Infrastructure
iv. Presence of a functional ethics committee
v. Compatible management
vi. Major diseases–incidence and prevalence rates.

The data obtained is analyzed and shared with the Business Development teams of the organizations to leverage their sales calls. This crisp and specific information helps in sealing off more clinical trial projects. This also helps in determining the total number of sites required to be undertaken for a particular trial and to have the RIGHT MIX of sites ensuring the timely fulfillment of target.

Training New CRCs and CRAs

The pool of research professionals in the form of CRC and CRA must also increase to keep abreast with the influx of additional clinical trials. The best method to train the newcomers into the field of clinical research is to hand-hold them and the best person to conduct such training are the existing CRC and CRA. Each CRC and CRA takes the responsibility of hand-holding one new comer and ensuring that they learn the tricks-of-the-trade. The training can be imparted in every field of the trial — from the document design to feasibility to site set up to conduct of the trial and to the close out. Such training programs can also be extended to the allied field of data management and report writing and electronic data capture areas.

Trial-related Responsibilities

The Pre-trial period is very critical and a proper planning at this stage ensures the smooth functioning of the entire trial. If the CRC/CRA conducts his/her responsibilities during this period sincerely and accurately, it is "rewarding' later. This phase involves a lot of planning and co-ordination by the CRC/CRA and by the team assigned to the trial.

Site Identification

One of the key responsibilities of the CRC/CRA before the initiation of a trial is the identification of the 'RIGHT' site at the right time fulfilling all the criteria set forth by the clinical trial guidelines and the protocol. The CRC/CRA, with his/her own past experience of having worked at a site, is the best judge to identify the site for another trial. He/she has worked at the site for over an year and knows the nook and corner of the site and also knows the needs, expectations and the potential. He/she knows which 'nut' to tighten and which 'bolt' to oil.

In circumstances when the CRC/CRA has to identify a site where he/she has no prior experience, it involves a more in-depth scrutiny before finalizing the site. A discussion with colleagues helps in the identification of the right site. Depending on the sample size mentioned in the trial protocol, the CRC/CRA along with the project manager decides on the number of patients to be enrolled and the number of clinical trial sites to be identified for the particular trial.

The factors involved in site identification are listed in the Table 7.1 below. In a particular clinical trial, any one of these factors or a combination may be given a priority when choosing a potential site.

- The CRC/CRA's responsibility includes the selection of an appropriate clinical investigator for the trial. For this, he/she needs to judge the reputation of the investigator in his/her field of expertise. This information can be collected based on peer views, references, publications, previous experience in clinical trials and other such factors.
- If previous clinical trials have been conducted at the particular site, many of the initial hiccups of initiation of a trial have already been dealt with. The time taken to finalize such a site is often much less. Thus, a site where trials have been conducted in the past is usually a preferred site for future trials.
- The CRC/CRA should consider the infrastructure available at the site before identifying it as suitable for conduct of the trial. He/she should assess the availability of space, equipment, manpower trained to handle particular equipment, ancillary facilities such as laboratories, pharmacy, etc. and communication facilities including high speed Internet to facilitate Interactive Voice Recognition System (IVRS) and real time transmission of critical trial related reports and other essential data (Table 7.1).
- The type of the healthcare setup must also be considered when identifying a suitable site. A site may be a multi-specialty hospital, a teaching institution, a

Table 7.1: Factors involved in site identification
1. Reputation of the investigator in his/her field of expertise
2. Previous clinical trials conducted at the site
3. Site infrastructure
4. Type of organization
5. Presence of a suitable Ethics Committee/Institutional Review Board
6. Access to the patient population needed for the trial
7. Access to the sponsor
8. Anticipated time required for trial initiation
9. Anticipated time required for trial completion
10. Patient turnover
11. Cost of the trial
12. Geographical location of the site

stand-alone clinic or a private nursing home. Each particular site has its own set of standard operating procedures (SOPs) for administration and patient management.

- The CRC/CRA should ensure the presence of a functional Ethics Committee/ Institutional Review Board (IRB) that conforms to the ICH GCP and other specific guidelines. He/she should assess the ability of the Ethics Committee/IRB to conduct a fair and timely processing of protocols.
- Based on the trial protocol, the CRC/CRA should determine whether a particular site is accessible to the patient population essential for the particular trial. He/she should assess the patient turnover at the site and whether patient enrollment for the trial can be completed within the time specified in the protocol.
- The site should be suitably located with access to proper transport and communication. Such a site provides ease of accessibility to the sponsor, the auditor and the trial inspector who may need to conduct site visits during the trial.

Pretrial Documentation

The CRC/CRA ensures that all the documents to be collected from the site staff are done accurately and within the specified timelines. They collect the updated and signed CV of the site team and ensure that the following documents are completed:

- Form 1572
- Financial disclosure
- Undertaking from the Investigator
- Confidentiality Disclosure Agreement
- Any other document specifically required for the concerned trial.

IRB

The CRC/CRA collects the relevant information about the IRB at the clinical trial site. They collect the following information from the IRB:

- Presence of written SOP
- Membership list
- Submission requirements
- Reporting timelines for safety reports and interim reports
- Financial requirements for submission.

The CRC being present at the site on a continuous manner is able to ensure the timely submission of the IRB package. He/She can also actively follow up through the site team with the IRB for faster approval. The CRC also undertakes the responsibility of the timely submission of all the safety reports and the amendments to the trial documents. The CRC also ensures that he/she obtains the acknowledgment letters from the IRB. In contrast, the CRA has to rely on the site team to complete the submissions on time and obtain the acknowledgment letters.

Regulatory

The CRC/CRA is also responsible for preparing the regulatory package and ensures that the package contains all the requisite documents as specified for submission by the regulatory body. They ensure the receipt of the favorable approval from the regulatory authorities and the proper filing of the same at the site and dispatch to the concerned personnel of the Sponsor. The CRC also undertakes the responsibility of the timely submission of all the safety reports and any amendments to the trial documents. The CRC also ensures that he/she obtains the acknowledgment letters from the regulatory authorities. In contrast, the CRA has to rely on the site team to complete the submissions on time and obtain the acknowledgment letters.

Financial

The responsibility of discussing the finance is usually with the project manager of the organization. In certain cases, senior CRC/CRA may also be empowered to discuss the financial terms and conditions with the site staff. He/she negotiates the trial budget at the site, which includes the budget for the following:

- Investigator fees
- IRB Fees
- Site administrative fees, if applicable
- Lab cost, if lab tests are done in-house at the site
- Study subject travel and other reimbursements
- Any other trial specific budget.

The CRC posted at the site also tracks the trial on a routine basis and informs the concerned personnel on reaching the milestones. All milestone-related payments are followed up by the CRC.

Administrative

The CRC/CRA helps in the pre study set up of the clinical trial sites. The CRC has a significant advantage over the CRA under this responsibility. He/She can actively follow up with the concerned personnel to help in a faster site set up.

Training of the Site Staff

All CRCs/CRAs must be ready to undertake the training of the site staff on a regular basis throughout the period of the trial. A periodic session must be taken to ensure that the entire site team is aware of the protocol and they comply with the protocol. The CRC can undertake frequent training sessions with the site team on:

- Inclusion and exclusion criteria
- Schedule of visit, window period and visit specific activity
- Safety guidelines as per protocol, safety reporting timelines and importance of timely reporting of serious adverse events.

This will enable the site team to enroll the right study subjects, enhance compliance to the protocol and ensure the ethical and scientific conduct of the trial.

Informed Consent Forms

The CRC/CRA ensures that the informed consent form (ICF) and the Patient Information Sheet are translated and back translated into the local/vernacular languages as deemed necessary by the respective sites. The Principal Investigator decides on the required languages for his/her site. The CRC/CRA ensures that all certificates of translations are in place.

Site Initiation Visit

The CRA visits the site on a Site Initiation Visit and ensures that the site is compliant and ready for the trial. The CRA schedules the visit well in advance ensuring that the site team is present and all required facilities are in order. During the visit, they discuss the entire protocol and other essential trial documents. The most critical activity to be done at this stage by the CRA is discussion on the CRF filling guidelines. A good and experienced CRA will demonstrate to the site staff or to the CRC, the CRF filling so that the chances of errors become negligible.

The CRC on the other hand, is present during the entire site visit to ensure that the process is done as per the Clinical trial protocol and the Sponsor's SOP. He/she ensures that all necessary requirements are in place for the trial to begin.

The CRA ensures that the clinical trial materials reach the site before the SIV and are in proper condition. He/she does the accountability during the SIV and briefs the site staff on the process of dispensing, drug accountability, requesting for replenishments and drug return. The CRC takes the responsibility of ensuring that the clinical trial materials are stored at a safe and secure place, have limited accessibility and are stored under the appropriate environmental conditions.

Investigators Meeting

The CRC/CRA is also in charge of conducting the entire Investigators' meet for the clinical trial they are assigned. A well-trained and experienced CRC/CRA may also present at these meetings and discuss various aspects of the trial. Such meetings help in disseminating the common information to all participating investigators and ensuring that all of them are in sync with the trial protocol and other specific requirements.

ICF, Screening and Recruitment /Enrollment

The CRC and CRA constantly follow up with the site team to enroll faster and complete the enrollment within the timelines. The CRC present at the site also helps in devising innovative methods to enhance enrollment and keeps the CRA updated on the enrollment status. The CRC present at the site during the enrollment process ensures that:

- The ICF conforms to the ICH GCP guidelines
- ICF is read out to the study subject or to his/her legally acceptable representative as applicable
- The study subject is given adequate time and opportunity to put forth his/her queries
- All the queries are clarified upto his/her satisfaction
- All discussions during the administration of the ICF are captured in the source document
- The ICF is signed, dated and timed as per the sponsors' specific SOP/guidelines
- A copy of the signed ICF is handed over to the study subject
- The site copy of the ICF is filed in the appropriate section of the Trial Master File or a separate file, as deemed apt by the sponsor.

Scheduling of Visits

This is an activity undertaken by the CRC and not by the CRA by virtue of his/her presence at the site. A committed CRC ensures that the enrolled study subjects are informed about their schedule of visits well in advance and that they do not miss their visits. The CRC at the site perform the following activity to enhance subject compliance and minimize dropouts or missed visits:

- Prepare protocol specific visit calendars
- User friendly formats of the visit calendars
- Make study subjects aware of the window periods if applicable for the trial
- Brief subjects on the importance of completing the entire trial and prevent any missed visits
- Follow up with subjects prior to the scheduled visits to ensure that they make the visits on date and time
- Pick up subjects from residence in case of emergency
- Manage study subject reimbursements if applicable.

Research Pharmacy and Drug Accountability

The CRC at the site manages the entire drug accountability and the central pharmacy. At the initiation of the trial, he/she takes the responsibility of the stock and ensures that the entire materials are in good condition and in appropriate quantity. He/she is responsible for the following:

- Store the materials in the appropriate place at the site
- Ensure that the safety and security is maintained for the entire duration of the trial
- Restrict accessibility to the storage room to only the authorized personnel related to the trial

- Ensure that the storage conditions are maintained as per the specifications mentioned in the protocol
- Ensure that the daily recording of the temperature, humidity, etc. are maintained and recorded on a daily basis or as specified by the sponsor
- Keep track of the stock on a regular basis to avoid any short supply
- Request sponsor for replenishments as and when required
- Maintain regular updates of the stock to ensure that there is proper reconciliation between the amount dispensed, returned and balance at the site
- Instruct and sometimes, educate study subjects on the proper handling of the trial medications, return of all unused medications and empty containers.

On the other hand, the CRA visiting the site at regular intervals checks the drug accountability records to ensure that there is no discrepancy and the storage conditions are appropriate and befitting to the sponsors' requirements.

Laboratory

The CRC/CRA evaluates the capability of the Laboratory at the trial site. They may also identify the central laboratory if the protocol requires it. A visit to the laboratory is done to assess:

- Availability of trained technical manpower
- Provision to conduct the protocol specified range of tests
- Pre analytical requirements and timelines
- Facilities for timely pick up of samples from the sites
- Turn around time for the different tests
- Accreditation and certification and their respective validity
- Collection and filing of all essential documents
  - CV of Lab Director and other key members
  - Normal values for the protocol specific range of tests
  - Samples of requisition and report docs
  - Lab manual
  - Collection centers and contact details
  - List of holidays and 'No-pick up' days
- Negotiate on the lab rates
- Mode of reporting–paper or electronic
- Storage and archival of samples and records.

Amendments

In case of any amendments to the study documents, the CRC/CRA is responsible for undertaking the appropriate actions:

- For all protocol amendments – the CRC/CRA follow up with the sponsor for the amended versions. The new versions are submitted to the IRB for approval before implementation.

- For all ICF amendments – the CRC/CRA follow up with the sponsor for the amended versions. They ensure the timely translations of the amended versions. The new versions are submitted to the IRB for approval before implementation. The CRC at the sites ensures that all the previous versions are packed and kept out of reach to avoid any misuse and chance use of older versions.
- The CRC at the site has a very significant role to play in case of amendments to the ICF during the course of the trial. In case the amendments are done during the enrollment phase the CRC has to ensure the following:
  - All completed subjects must be informed, especially in cases of new safety issues observed and mentioned in the amended versions
  - All continuing subjects are to be informed too, but they need to be reconsented with the new version of the ICF
  - All future subjects to be enrolled need to be consented with the amended versions
- All CRCs ensure that the amended versions are not implemented at the site before the favorable written approval by the IRB.

Monitoring

This is an activity undertaken by the CRA only and not by the CRC. On successful identification of the site(s), the CRAs are assigned one or more sites. They have the schedule prepared for each trial and start planning for the next round of visits to these sites. The number of visits to each site may change during the course of the trial depending upon various factors:

- Enrollment rate
- Number of safety events
- Quality and ethical conduct of trial.

Monitoring visits are conducted to ensure that the site is compliant to the protocol and other guidelines governing the ethical conduct of a clinical trial. The CRA ensures that the rights, well being and safety of the trial subjects are well protected during the entire duration of the trial. Each monitoring visit by the CRA comprises of a pre-visit phase, a visit-phase and a post-visit phase.

The pre visit phase is a preparatory phase, wherein the CRA plans the visit. He/she ensures the following:

- Schedule the visit in consultation with the site staff
- Send confirmation letter to site
- Prepare the agenda
- Prepare the check list for the activities during the visit
- Compile list of queries from previous visit, if applicable.

During the monitoring visit, the CRA checks for the following:

- Enrollment status–whether the site is enrolling as per the plan and the target, device strategies with the site team for faster enrollment
- Informed consent form administration

- Compliance to the protocol–ensure that the inclusion and exclusion criteria are met, randomization and blinding are done, dosing regimen and schedules are maintained
- Safety reporting is on time
- Trial Master File is kept current and tidy
- Complete review of the CRF and source document verification. Ensure that the CRF data reconciles with that of the source document.
- CTM accountability–ensure that the storage conditions match to the requirements set in the protocol, the physical; stock matches with the CTM accountability log
- Communications between all the players involved in the trial are done and filed at the appropriate place
- Track the site payouts
- Generate queries on the CRF and resolve queries generated by the site team
- Ensure that the site team is constant and will continue in a similar manner till the end of the trial
- Summary meeting with the site team to discuss the issues and the apt methods to tackle them.

  Following the successful completion of the visit, the CRA will compile the monitoring report and follow up with the site team for any queries.

SKILLS OF BEING A GOOD CRC OR CRA

The job of the CRCs and the CRAs involves a wide range of responsibilities. In order to fulfill these responsibilities, they need to possess certain skill sets. The CRC/CRA needs to have a good knowledge of the ICH GCP Guidelines and the prescribed protocol for the particular trial. Beyond these prescribed guidelines, the CRC/CRA needs to have good communication and managerial skills. He/she acts as a communication bridge between the Sponsors and the site and also manages the day-to-day activities of the clinical trial at a particular site. He/she interacts with a multitude of personnel with varying mindset, characteristics and personality. Hence, the CRC and CRA need to be highly flexible and loaded with tons of patience to handle these loads of work pressure.

The communication skills of a CRC/CRA come into practice even much before the trial actually starts. It is the CRC/CRA who, during the capacity-building phase, meets the potential investigators and determines whether such investigators and the healthcare set up where they work are suitable for conduct of clinical trials. During his/her discussion with a potential investigator, the CRC/CRA should be able to ascertain his research interests, previous experience with trials, patient turnover, general motivation and enthusiasm for the proposed trial. CRCs/CRAs should have the requisite communication skills to be able to discuss with a potential investigator and give him a clear idea about the processes involved in the clinical trial. They should discuss the joint nature of the trial to be conducted and are responsible for giving the investigators a clear picture of the role of the sponsor, the regulatory authorities, the investigator and the site personnel.

During the trial, the main challenges that the CRCs/CRAs faces are those dealing with site personnel issues, the study conduct issues and the study subject issues.

Personnel issues are more frequent and are usually very delicate issues. Uncooperative or untrained site personnel can be hurdles to the smooth conduct of a trial. The managerial skills of the CRCs/CRAs come into play in such situations. They must be able to deal with such situations with patience and perseverance.

Issues related to the study conduct are usually more serious and may require strong actions. Sometimes there may be extreme issues such as fraud or negligence in the trial. In such situations, the CRCs/CRAs need to:

A. Watch
B. Listen
C. Document
D. Report.

Watch

A well-trained CRC should be watchful of what is happening at the trial site. He/she should always keep his/her eyes open for any loopholes in the study conduct and should be able to sense the problem much before it actually becomes a major issue. The CRC, being present at the site on a daily basis, needs to be more vigilant to the micro details of the trial process. A close watch enables the 'trained eyes' of the CRC to foresee the impending problems and to take preventive measures.

Listen

CRCs/CRAs should listen to what other research professionals at the site have to say. They may just confirm the CRCs/CRAs doubt or in certain cases, they may provide the lead for the CRCs/CRAs to be more vigilant of certain issues.

Document

The CRC/CRA must document everything concerning the study. All verbal communications with the site are documented in the form of a Telephone Contact Report (TCR) and sent to the discussing parties. They should be careful so that both they and their superiors have records to substantiate their claims whenever such issues are discussed.

Report

They should report and discuss such irregularities with the project coordinators, investigators and project managers. The CRC/CRA should avoid jumping to false conclusions in such cases. But if they have legitimate concerns, these should always be discussed in detail with their superiors so that the appropriate disciplinary action can be undertaken.

The clinical research coordinator always manages issues related to the subject. The CRC discusses with the subject and his/her attendant regarding the next visits. The CRC needs to have tons of patience and has to keep his/her cool to explain to the subject about the protocol and the visit specific activities. A continuous counseling of the study subjects by the CRC is essential to ensure cent percent compliance. The CRC starts building up the rapport and trust with the study subject right from the first day of the trial. In fact, it all starts with the initial discussion with the subject for the informed consent and this trust is gradually built up during each successive visit.

'IN-AIR AND OUT-OF-HOME' EXPERIENCE

The CRAs must be ready to travel and sometimes travel extensively. In fact, they must love this life 'in-air and 'out-of-home.' In some cases, it may also involve cross-country travel and they have to adjust to the different timelines, culture and language. It is a common sight to see dedicated CRAs completing the work in airports and hotel rooms.

The busy travel schedule of a CRA keeps him/her away from relatives and friends and this adds to the already existing stress in their lives. This does have an impact on the mental stress of these highly stressed individuals. Hence, each of these individuals must have the right 'shock-absorbers' to handle the high loads of pressure and stress.

The workspace for a CRC and the visiting CRA may vary from a plush room with all the amenities of luxury, to the remote little corner of a busy general hospital. The filling of a CRF by the CRC and the reviewing of the same by the CRA is a real tedious job requiring high degree of attention to detail. An excellent rapport with the site team is essential–the care and hospitality rendered by the site team is directly proportional to this relationship and rapport. The visits to the hospital canteen for a cup of coffee not only keeps the CRC/CRA active for the work, but are also the memorable events to store for posterity.

The CRC/CRA's life is not a 'bed of roses', it is a journey of immense commitment and dedication, all concentrated to the lone goal of getting a 'safe and effective' medicine to the market and to the gullet of innumerable patients across the globe. These people are the true 'life-line' of the clinical research path.

SUGGESTED READING

1. Department of Health and Human Service: Investigational New Drug Application. Responsibilities of Sponsors and Investigators, 21 Code of Federal Regulations 312.50–312.70. Revised as of April 1, 2003.
2. Rico-Villademoros et al. The role of the clinical research coordinator – data manager – in oncology clinical trials. BMC Med Res Methodol. 2004;4:6.
3. The European Agency for the Evaluation of Medicinal Products, ICH Topic E 6. Guideline for Good Clinical Practice. Note for Guidance on Good Clinical Practice (CPMP/ICH/135/95).
4. Vogelson. The art and science of monitoring. Modern Drug Discovery. 2001;4(3):25-26.

8 Protocol Designing

Anish Desai, Manish Garg

INTRODUCTION

This chapter outlines the main steps in designing a protocol for a research project. It is not our intention to be prescriptive in the outline; we are simply providing guidelines for the potential researcher who hopes to carry out a research project. The ideas in this chapter are a condensation of our experiences and those derived from several readily available sources. This chapter has been written to ensure that researchers have the necessary information to be able to write a protocol according to ICH Guidelines for Good Clinical Practice (ICH-GCP) standards for clinical trials.

PROTOCOL

A protocol is a document that explicitly states the reasoning behind and structure of a research project. Every well-designed clinical trial requires a protocol, which is the written mechanism that describes how the clinical trial design will be implemented. The study protocol can be viewed as a written agreement between the investigator, the participant and the scientific community. Protocol is also defined as a document that describes the background, rationale, objective(s), design, methodology, statistical considerations and organization of a trial. It also serves as a reference document that describes; why the trial is being conducted? How should it be executed and what is to be done in any eventuality?

Though there is no single approach in designing clinical trial protocols, there are a number of principles that are usually adhered to. A general approach is often followed although many variations are possible. One may begin to write a clinical protocol after many discussions with several experts. The initial draft/synopsis of a study protocol in the early stage of planning a trial may be a rather basic/incomplete document, which outlines the general scheme without detailed specifications. The initial draft helps to identify aspects of protocol, which are unspecified, confusing or contentious which may be resolved without delay. It will often require several redrafts of the study protocol until a final more extensive protocol is produced which contains full details of the trial's objectives and organization and is acceptable on scientific, organizational and ethical grounds.

The protocol should include the right amount of detail necessary for the reader to be able to understand exactly what is needed to conduct the study e.g. blood pressure measurement should be described in more details in a protocol for a hypertension study where it is a primary efficacy parameter than in a protocol for another disease area where BP is assessed as part of the general assessment/safety check.

PROTOCOL OUTLINE

A typical protocol has the following elements:

- Title page
- Signature page
- Background information and scientific rationale
- Objectives
- Study design
- Study population
- Study procedures
- Statistical considerations
- Subject confidentiality
- Informed consent process
- Literature references
- Supplements/appendices.

TITLE PAGE

Title page introduces the document, its title, precise number, sponsor and authors to the reader. It should contain:

1. Protocol title, protocol identifying number, and date. Any amendment(s) should also bear the amendment number(s) and date(s). Full title should include summary study design, medicinal product(s), nature of the treatment (e.g. treatment, prophylaxis, and diagnosis) comparator(s) and/or any placebo(s), indication, patient population and setting (e.g. in-patient, outpatient). e.g. Linezolid versus teicoplanin in the treatment of Gram-positive infections in the hospitalized critically ill: a randomized, double blind, and multiple studies.

   The protocol number must clearly indicate the version number, whether it is final or draft and the date of this version. Similarly amendments must be numbered and dated so it is clearly put in the chronological development of the protocol and trial.

2. Name and address of the sponsor and monitor (if other than the sponsor). Sponsor names and list of responsibilities with agreed allocations.
3. Name and title of the person(s) authorized to sign the protocol and the protocol amendment(s) for the sponsor. This would generally be the Chief Investigator for multicentre trials or the Principal Investigator for single centre trials.
4. Name, title, address and telephone number(s) of the sponsor's medical expert (or dentist when appropriate) for the trial.
5. Name and title of the investigator(s) who is (are) responsible for conducting the trial, and the address and telephone number(s) of the trial site(s). In the case of multicentre trials the Chief Investigator should be listed and the principal investigators for each of the participating centers.
6. Name, title, address, and telephone number(s) of the qualified physician (or dentist, if applicable), who is responsible for all trial-site related medical (or dental) decisions (if other than the investigator).
7. Name(s) and address (es) of the clinical laboratory (ies) and other medical and/ or technical department(s) and/or institutions involved in the trial.

SIGNATURE PAGE

Signature page of all healthcare professionals involved in the trial including contact details of participating site, sponsor and sponsor's medical advisor if not already given above. In the case of a multicentre trial this page can be tailored to each site, otherwise it can get very long. If site specific signature pages are used a signed copy for each site must be held in the Trial Master File, in addition to the site master file.

CONTENTS PAGE

This helps navigation through the document by a large number of different people that will be needed throughout the life of the trial.

LIST OF ABBREVIATIONS

All abbreviations used should be listed and defined. Accepted international medical abbreviations should be used. Project specific abbreviations should be standardized within each project.

COMPLIANCE STATEMENT

The protocol should include a statement that the trial will be conducted in compliance with the protocol, GCP and the applicable regulatory requirements.

PROTOCOL SUMMARY/SYNOPSIS

This summary should be only one to two pages long. It should give the reader sufficient information to understand the rationale for the trial, its objectives and the methods that will be used to achieve these objectives. It should contain title; phase of study; sample size; gender; age; general health status; geographic location of subject population being studied; inclusion and exclusion criteria; number of sites; study duration and duration per subject; primary and secondary outcome measures and methods by which these outcomes will be determined and study design.

BACKGROUND INFORMATION

A description of the background and general aims of the trial is a useful preliminary, which helps to explain why the trial is considered scientifically worthwhile and how it builds on experience gained from previous research. A detailed literature search provides clinical, epidemiological data on the disease under study; helps to select studies that have potential significance to the proposed study and also helps to identify deficiencies in the literature and ways to address them. The literature review should be of sufficient depth to identify potential confounders and effect modifiers and to determine areas where new knowledge is needed. This data should be described in a concise form to form the background information. In short the data in this background information should be able to justify the need for this study.

STUDY OBJECTIVES/AIMS, END-POINTS AND RATIONALE

Study Objectives/Aims

Clinical study objectives are concise statements of the major and minor questions that the trial is designed to answer. The author should reflect on the objectives and confirm that they represent valid and proper questions, or series of questions, to propose. The objectives of a clinical trial are the questions a clinical trial asks and tries to answer. In all areas of research, asking the right question is perhaps the most important part of the research. How the research problem is stated determines the trial design used, the data collected, the analyses conducted, and the conclusions that can be drawn. It is therefore essential that the objective(s) be clearly, completely and concisely expressed.

If too many objectives are defined in one protocol then it can lead to many methodological and statistical problems. A clinical trial often has both primary and secondary objectives, and these should be identified as such in the protocol. Ideally, no more than 1 or 2 of each should be included in a clinical trial.

Study End-points

In choosing efficacy parameters to evaluate in a clinical study it is especially beneficial if the parameters chosen can demonstrate end-points related to: reduced progression or even reversal of the disease process; improved quality of life; reduced mortality; improved symptomatology of the patient etc. The protocol should include a specific statement of the primary endpoints and the secondary end-points, if any to be measured during the trial. Methodologies for measuring these end points should be available and need to be well defined.

Study Rationale

The study rationale defines the need for conducting the study and how the results obtained from the study will help to advance the needs of the scientific community and add to the current understanding of the problem.

STUDY DESIGN

The scientific integrity of the trial and the credibility of the data from the trial depend substantially on the trial design. Study designs include, for example, double-blind, case-control, cohort, cross-sectional, nested case-control, double-dummy, or other hybrid designs. While choosing a study design one should consider issues such as choice of a control group, method of treatment allocation procedures for implementing blindness, and explanation of a crossover design if it is relevant and financial resources available. Resources and technology should be available to implement the study design. The rationale for the selection of the proposed design over others should be presented.

RANDOMIZATION

Randomization is a technique to ensure that statistical significance tests may be used in a valid manner. It is a process by which patients in a clinical trial are 'randomly' assigned to receive one of the treatments being evaluated. Randomization is used to reduce bias in assigning patients to treatment and is usually implemented through a randomization code that assigns patients to different treatments. The mode of randomization should be specified in the protocol.

INCLUSION AND EXCLUSION CRITERIA

Any clinical trial requires a precise definition of which patients are eligible for inclusion and exclusion. Inclusion criteria constitute the definition of patient characteristics required for entry into a clinical trial and may generally be used for patient exclusion as well as inclusion, since most criteria (e.g., age range of 18-50 years) establish both inclusion (18-50 years) and exclusion (lower than 18 or above 50 years) groupings. To identify specific inclusion and exclusion criteria for a study one needs to consider the narrow and broad limits as discussed below.

Narrow vs Broad Limits

If the limits for patient entry are set too broadly, then a heterogenous group of patients may be enrolled which may create a problem when the data generated are inadequate to address the clinical trial objectives. Under circumstances in which an excessively heterogenous group of patients is enrolled, the interpretation and relevance of the trial may be questioned. Conversely, if the limits of patient entry are set too narrowly, then it may be impossible to obtain an adequate number of patients to conduct the trial in addition, it may be difficult to compare data from such a population with data generated from a broader population (i.e., interpretation of the data may not be relevant for general clinical situations).

The advantage of using relatively 'tight' entry criteria is that the clinical trial will be conducted with a more homogenous population. This factor will often provide more meaningful data and interpretations, especially for Phase II controlled studies. The criteria used to determine patient inclusion can be divided into 4 groups:

Characteristics of Patients

Sex, age, weight, education, race and/or ethnic background, social and economic status, pregnancy and lactation, use of tobacco, ingestion of caffeine and/or alcohol, abuse of alcohol or drugs, diet and nutritional status, physiological limitations and genetic history, surgical or anatomical limitations, hypersensitivity to a clinical trial medicine or test, other medicine and nonmedicine allergies and emotional limitations.

Characteristics of the Disease and its Treatment

Disease being evaluated, concomitant medicines, previous medicine and nonmedicine treatments, history of other diseases, present clinical status, previous hospitalization, operations and procedures.

Environmental and Other Factors

Patient recruitment and cooperation, participation in another clinical trial/ participation in another part of this clinical trial or in any other clinical trial using this study medicine, institutional or environmental status, occupation, geographical location and litigation and disability.

Results of Screening Examinations

Laboratory and other investigations.

Choosing Criteria for Inclusion and Exclusion

In determining the criteria to be used for patient inclusion, it is important to exclude those patients for whom the clinical trial will create unacceptable clinical risks. If patients with a given disease, state, or attribute are to be excluded from a trial, then it is important to determine the procedures used to exclude these patients. For example, if all patients with a given disease are to be excluded from a trial, it may be sufficient for the investigator to question all prospective participants as to whether they presently have the given disease. An additional question that may be posed by the investigator is whether the patient has ever had the disease. A further step is to request that a laboratory or other test be performed to document that the patient does not have the disease. The degree of documentation required for patients to enter the clinical trial may be set at whatever standard is deemed appropriate to ensure that patients in the trial do not have the excluded disease.

The criteria established for inclusion and exclusion can be checked by patient history as detailed by the patient or as noted in medical records; findings observed by the investigator; findings documented by scores on tests or confirmed by other professionals using clinical judgement. It may be important for key tests to be performed by independent investigators, laboratories, or groups to prevent bias from entering into critical measurements that affect the patient inclusion. Inclusion criteria should be designed to eliminate (insofar as possible) hard-core nonresponders with the disease being evaluated. If this is not done, then no matter how well the clinical trial is designed and conducted in a large number of hard-core nonresponders, the data obtained may actually represent a false-negative result.

SCREENING

A screen is an evaluation of potential patients to determine their eligibility to enter a clinical trial. This evaluation may be entirely based on an interview or review of medical records, but in almost all prospective clinical trials, a series of tests (e.g., physical examination, laboratory evaluations) are conducted. Screens may also be conducted in stages so that only patients who pass an initial verbal screen are evaluated with more time-consuming and expensive tests. The tests for screening patients before enrollment in the trial should be elaborated in the protocol.

SAMPLE SIZE

The number of patients required for a clinical trial (sample size) refers to the number of patients who finish a trial rather than the number who enter. Thus, in planning a clinical trial the definition of a 'completed ' patient is important to establish, as is the expected rate of patient dropouts and discontinuers. An important result may fail to be detected if too few patients complete a trial.

Another problem that may occur if too few patients complete a clinical trial is that a false-positive result may occur. Although a false-positve result may occur in all trials, the chances of its happening are higher when fewer patients are enrolled than intended. Numerous biases and errors in a clinical trial may be minimized by increasing the number of patients entered until adequate power is obtained.

Often pilot studies with a small sample size, is conducted to obtain information, and work out the logistics and management, deemed necessary for further clinical trials.

STATISTICS

This section should include a description of the statistical methods to be employed, including timing of any planned interim analysis(ses); methods for statistical analyses for primary endpoints and secondary endpoints e.g. intention to treat; rules for any interim analysis or administrative look (e.g. in studies involving normally fatal indications). The level of significance to be used and how the level of statistical significance relates to the clinical significance should be predefined.

Criteria for the Termination of the Trial

Particularly if early termination, e.g. in a placebo controlled trial on a fatal/life threatening condition one treatment arm will have an obviously higher number of deaths. Procedure for accounting for missing, unused, and spurious data should be elaborated.

Procedures for Reporting any Deviation(s) from the Original Statistical Plan

Any deviation(s) from the original statistical plan should be described and justified in the protocol and/or in the final report, as appropriate. The selection of subjects to be included in the analyses (e.g. all randomized subjects, all eligible subjects, evaluable subjects) should be predefined.

TREATMENT SCHEDULES

It includes the treatment(s) to be administered, including the name(s) of all the product(s), the dose(s), the dosing schedule(s), the route/mode(s) of administration, and the treatment period(s), including the follow-up period(s) for subjects for each investigational product treatment group/ trial treatment group/ arm of the trial.

Product to be investigated, including source and its marketing status worldwide; who will supply it; dosage; route of administration; any special instructions e.g. reconstitution, storage conditions, shelf life and whether a scheduled drug. Similar information on placebos and reference comparator product(s), that are being used in the study have to be included.

It should also include details of blinding and decoding procedure and conditions for its use and management of serious adverse reactions. How patients will be treated after period of trial is complete, including continuing supply of investigational drug.

Concomitant Treatment/ Rescue Medications

Medication(s)/treatment(s) permitted (including rescue medication) and not permitted before and/or during the trial, needs to be specified. This often requires a lot of thought because of possible interactions or effects that could confound the results and conclusions. Rescue treatment may be standardized for the purposes of the trial.

Procedures of Monitoring Subject Compliance

The protocol should elaborate how blinding of subjects, researchers and assessors as appropriate will be achieved; and procedures such as watching subject swallow investigational product(s) and checking in their mouths afterwards (subject's return of packing of tablets for counting is never too convincing a method!); recording of patient compliance and follow-up will be conducted.

ASSESSMENT OF EFFICACY

Specification of the Efficacy Parameters

The author needs to state what measurements are being made, when, why and how. He needs to include all measurements and evaluations, giving references to validated measurement tools, e.g. Hamilton rating scale for depression.

Methods and Timing for Assessing, Recording, and Analyzing Efficacy Parameters

Provide an overall time and events schedule in a tabular form. It would include: screening assessments, pre-treatment or baseline and treatment assessments, assessments after treatment at each time point, specification of time points, follow-ups — what and when, where observations are to be recorded.

ASSESSMENT OF SAFETY

Specification of Safety Parameters

Highlight any expected adverse reactions on basis of known characteristics of drugs being used on the basis of the summary of product characteristics (SmPC), or pre-clinical and clinical data from previous trials. Adverse reactions can be detected by observing vital signs, staff observations, voluntary feedback from subjects and clinical laboratory data. Also elaborate SAEs that will require expedited reporting. Although there should be a focus on expected adverse reactions, procedures must facilitate the observation and recording of unexpected adverse reactions.

The Methods and Timing for Assessing, Recording, and Analyzing Safety Parameters

Objective measures should be made at specified time points to identify adverse reactions, e.g. blood pressure. Elaborate recording methods and location of all observations and measurements.

As adverse reactions may also be identified from clinical laboratory data these must be reviewed at regular and frequent intervals according to subject enrolment. Scoring systems to allocate the severity, and attribution of causality to the trial medication(s) should be defined.

Procedures of the management of serious adverse reactions, including definition, notification and timeframes for reporting to different parties must be defined. Many sponsors have standard pages for management of serious adverse reactions. It is important to clearly outline allocation of responsibilities for pharmacovigilance management and reporting particularly in the case of a mutlicenter trial, as only one centre must take responsibility for this. This will usually fall to the lead centre.

Procedures for Eliciting Reports of and for Recording and Reporting Adverse Event and Inter-current Illnesses

It is helpful to review this in advance, before the trial starts, because of the confusion that can arise from adverse reactions, the medical condition being treated and inter-current illnesses. The type and duration of the follow-up of subjects after adverse events must be specified.

NUMBER OF EVALUATIONS/VISITS/HOSPITALIZATION

The frequency of outpatient visits (or inpatient evaluations) during the treatment period is usually an issue that is evaluated in planning a clinical trial. Any factors will influence the decision of when patient visits (evaluations) are scheduled and whether the visits are to be equally or unequally spaced throughout the treatment period. In general, visits are often scheduled more frequently at the start of a trial and less often as the trial progresses. Each trial will have different factors to consider in determining the appropriate number of patient visits, but the additional time, cost, and energy that each visit entails must be considered for patient, staff, and investigator in addition to consideration of the value of the additional data that will be generated. It is often convenient to schedule patient visits n even multiples of days, weeks, or months (e.g., every 2 weeks for four visits, then every 4 weeks for the remaining visits). In studies involving patients suffering from life-threatening diseases or Phase I studies the duration of hospitalization and outpatient follow-up needs to be defined.

POST-TREATMENT PERIOD

Post-treatment refers to the time after the trial medicine has been discontinued. The major purposes of a post-treatment period are to check for any withdrawal effects and to ensure the patient's safety. The post-treatment period may also be useful to study residual effects of treatment. In evaluating the need for a post-treatment period in a clinical trial of a medicine (as well as its duration), one may consider previous experience with the medicine in similar patient population; whether the medicine dosage is being tapered slowly or abruptly stopped; the clinical status of the patients; whether patients are in a secure and/or controlled environment and the pharmacokinetic characteristics of the medicine.

Methods of Conducting a Post-treatment Evaluation

Clinic visits to conduct post-treatment evaluations may be scheduled as part of a clinical protocol. This is particularly relevant if withdrawal effects are expected or if the clinical trial is particularly designed to evaluate the return of original symptoms and signs of disease (e.g., how long does it take them to recur?). Ad hoc scheduled clinic appointments may be made. Another possibility is to assess one or more particular clinical end-points at annual clinic visits.

DIRECT ACCESS TO SOURCE DATA/DOCUMENTS

The sponsor should ensure that it is specified in the protocol or other written agreement that the investigator(s)/ institution(s) will permit trial-related monitoring, audits, regulatory review, and regulatory inspection(s), providing direct access to source data/documents.

QUALITY CONTROL AND QUALITY ASSURANCE

Provide assurance on good clinical practice, quality of data collection and refer to monitors and their role.

ETHICS

An early code for ethical behaviour is the famous Hippocratic oath. The Helsinki doctrine, which was approved by the World Medical association, is an important declaration, which has to be adhered while conducting clinical trials.

Ethics in research is used in a broad context that includes and overlaps with legal responsibilities in some instances and with routine obligations of a medicine trial's sponsor in other cases. Some of the major ethical issues in medicine trials concern informed consent and Ethics Committees/IRBs at the institution where the clinical trial is to be performed.

Four aspects of conducting a clinical trial that have ethical implications are briefly mentioned below.

Recruiting and Screening Patients for a Clinical Trial

There may be temptation for investigators or sponsors in some Phase II and III trials to stimulate patient enrollment by offering overly generous inducements. This view must be modified for Phase I clinical trials, plus selected other trials (e.g., pharmacokinetic trials) in which financial benefit is accepted as the primary motivating factor for many volunteers.

Providing Information to Referring Physicians

It is a responsibility of investigators to provide relevant clinical trial data and other information to colleagues who have referred patients for the trial.

Protocol Violation

Both investigators and sponsors must be sensitive to the issue of protocol violations. Although many minor deviations do not raise ethical issues, it is obvious that some deviations will raise significant dilemmas. These problems must be dealt with on a case-by-case basis in a prompt, sensitive, and effective manner.

Conducting Clinical Trials in Developing Countries

Some of the specific issues that should be considered in developing countries are:
- Are the patients, investigators, or hospitals being exploited in any way?
- Have all the practical and potential issues that would ensure patient safety been addressed?
- Will the medicine, if successful, be marketed eventually in that country or are patients being exposed to medicine that they can never obtain?
- Are the medicines being tested ones that the population would not wish to use (even if marketed) because of local traditions or style of medical practice (e.g., testing oral contraceptives in countries where they would not be used)?

INFORMED CONSENT

Informed consent may be defined as a patients being given adequate information about a clinical trial; understanding and voluntarily accepting the terms of a clinical trial and agreeing to cooperate in its conduct. The informed consent form presents information on which this concept is based and must be signed by the patient prior to enrollment in the study. The patient must be a competent individual who can evaluate the benefit-to-risk concept. In other words, the patient should be able to choose his or her best alternative.

DATA HANDLING AND RECORD KEEPING

This section should discus data retrieval, database management—data entry and validation, and security/storage, rules for handling non-compliant patients, determining evaluable data, etc. source data verification, audit, records retention – duration and location.

FINANCING AND INSURANCE

Financing and insurance should be discussed if not addressed in a separate agreement.

PUBLICATION POLICY

Publication policy should be discussed if not addressed in a separate agreement. Statements about documentation for the running of the trial and the reporting of the trial can be included here.

TABLES, FIGURES, AUTHORS AND DATE, REFERENCES AND SUPPLEMENTS

Separate sections should be devoted for tables, figures, authors and date, references and supplements.

PROTOCOL DEVIATIONS/ DROP-OUTS/ WITHDRAWALS/ STUDY TERMINATION

The methods to identify critical and non-critical deviations and ways to address it should be defined. In case of dropouts how these subjects would be dealt with should be specified in the protocol. The reasons for withdrawing patients from a study, needs to be elaborated. Specific criteria should be laid down for study termination whether done by sponsor or investigator.

APPENDICES

Based on the protocol relevant appendices as elaborated below should be attached:
- Summary of Product Characteristics (SmPC(s), data sheet(s)), for investigational products
- Measurement tools and their validation
- Pharmacy information such as dosage tables and information on reconstitution, storage information, shelf lives, dispensing procedures, etc.
- Methods for collecting patient samples, their storage, dispatch and handling conditions

- Clinical labs and tests (normal ranges if appropriate)
- Adverse reaction grading systems for particular safety parameters
- Scoring systems of efficacy parameters
- Analysis diagram – very important!
- Declaration of Helsinki
- Patient and parent/legal guardian consent form(s)
- Subject information sheet for informed consent
- Method of recruitment of patients/subjects to the trial, e.g. advertisement for Phase I trials

IMPROVING THE QUALITY OF A PROTOCOL

The most obvious technique for improving the quality of a protocol is for the author to review it as critically as possible. A fresh review after a lapse of time usually allows the author to view his or her own work more objectively. Peer review, institutional review and use of Trial Assessment Procedure Scale (TAPS) also help in improving the quality of a protocol.

CASE RECORD FORMS

The forms designed for collecting information during the clinical trial are also referred to as case report forms. One of the first decisions that must be addressed is whether or not to organize and group the forms on the basis of separate clinic visits or evaluations (e.g., Visit 1, Visit 2, Visit 3 etc.), with all forms for visit 1 separated from those for visit 2, etc. An alternative approach is to base the grouping on integration of similar or identical forms (e.g., forms for all physical examinations and vita signs are placed together, followed by the forms for all laboratory tests, followed in turn by the forms for all efficacy measures and so forth. In this approach, different copies of the same form (for any parameter) to be filled in on visits 1, 2 and 3 are all placed together. A third approach is to combine both of the approaches described above and to have some forms arranged in a visit-by-visit grouping and other forms integrated by type of examination, test or form.

PROTOCOL DESIGNING IN SPECIAL SITUATIONS

Protocol Designing for Herbal Remedies and Medicinal Plants

For the herbal remedies and medicinal plants that are to be clinically evaluated for use in the Allopathic System and which may later be used in allopathic hospitals, the procedures laid down by the office of the Drugs Controller General of India for allopathic drugs should be followed. This does not pertain to guidelines issued for clinical evaluation of Ayurveda, Siddha or Unani drugs by experts in those systems of medicine, which may be used later in their own hospitals and clinics. All the general principles of clinical trials described earlier pertain also to herbal remedies. However, when clinical trials of herbal drugs used in recognized Indian Systems of Medicine and Homeopathy are to be undertaken in Allopathic Hospitals, association of physicians from the concerned system as co-investigators/ collaborators/ members of the expert group is desirable for designing and evaluating the study.

Protocol Designing for Vaccines

Vaccines are usually developed to prevent disease in a healthy population. Most of the clinical trials conducted enroll healthy volunteers in all phases of vaccine testing. The enrollment of healthy volunteers warrants a very low tolerance for risk in vaccine clinical trials.

It is important to define the methods used to assess the severity of clinical and laboratory abnormalities in healthy adult and adolescent volunteers enrolled in clinical trials. It is recommended to use toxicity grading scale tables, as a guideline for selecting the assessment criteria. The grading system can also be useful in defining a particular study's stopping rules (e.g., a certain number of adverse events, as defined in the table, may call for stopping the study). Less extreme observations (e.g., mild) may not require discontinuing the study vaccine but can still contribute to evaluating safety by identifying parameters to focus upon in subsequent product development. Uniform criteria for categorizing toxicities in healthy volunteers can improve comparisons of safety data among groups within the same study and also between different studies.

Protocol Designing for Therapeutic Cancer Vaccines

Therapeutic cancer vaccines have characteristics that require a new paradigm for phase I and phase II clinical development. Effective development plans may take advantage of some of the following observations: Dose ranging safety trials are not appropriate for many cancer vaccines. Dose ranging trials to establish an optimal biologic dose are often not practical. An efficient design should be used to identify an immunogenic dose. Vaccine efficacy can be efficiently evaluated with tumor response as end-point utilizing a two-stage design with only 9 patients in the first stage. If no partial or complete responses are observed in the initial 9 patients, accrual to the trial is terminated. Optimization of vaccine delivery by comparing results of single arm phase II studies using immunological response as endpoint is problematic because of assay variation and potential non-comparability of patients in different studies. Randomized screening studies can be used to efficiently optimize vaccine immunogenicity. Efficiency in use of patients depends on having assay variation and inter-patient variability small relative to the difference in immunogenicity to be detected. Phase II studies using time to progression as endpoint are most interpretable if they employ randomized designs with a no-vaccine control group. Such designs may use an inflated type 1 error rate, and need not be prohibitively large if patients with rapidly progressive disease are studied. Interim monitoring plans may effectively limit the size of the trials by terminating accrual early when results are not consistent with the targeted improvement.

Protocol Designing for Medical Devices

A medical device is defined as an inert diagnostic or therapeutic article that does not achieve any of its principal intended purposes through chemical action, within or on the body unlike the medicated devices, which contain pharmacologically active substances, which are treated as drugs. Such devices include diagnostic test kits, crutches, electrodes, pacemakers, arterial grafts, intraocular lenses, orthopedic pins and other orthopedic accessories.

Depending upon risks involved the devices could be classified as follows:

1. *Noncritical devices:* An investigational device that does not present significant risks to the patients, e.g. thermometer, BP apparatus.
2. *Critical devices:* An investigational medical device that presents a potential serious risk to the health, safety or welfare of the subject—for example, pace markers, implants, internal catheters.

All the general principles of clinical trials described for drug trials should also be considered for trials of medical devices. The duration of the trial and extent of use may be decided in case to case basis by the appropriate authorities. However, the following important factors that are unique to medical devices should be taken into consideration while evaluating the related research projects:

- Clinical trial of medical devices is different from drug trials, as former cannot be done in healthy volunteers. Hence, phase I of drug trials is not necessary for trial on devices.
- Medical devices used within the body may have greater risk potential than those used on or outside the body, for example, orthopedic pins vs crutches.
- Medical devices not used regularly have less risk potential than those used regularly, for example, contact lens vs intraocular lenses.
- Safety procedures to introduce a medical device in the patient should also be followed as the procedure itself may cause harm to the patient.
- Informed consent procedures should be followed as in drug trials.

  The patient information sheet should contain information on procedures to be adopted if the patient decides to withdraw from the trial.

Protocol Designing for Hematopoietic Stem Cell Transplantation (HSCT)

Although no blueprint for designing a protocol of HSCT for autoimmune diseases can be laid out, the process should take into consideration the issues highlighted herein. The design of protocol of hematopoietic stem cell transplantation (HSCT) for autoimmune diseases requires investigators to address issues unique to this therapeutic approach and patient population. The proper composition of the protocol team is central to success. It is important to recognize that transplant physicians are no longer also the disease experts when transplanting patients with autoimmune diseases, and a close collaborative relationship between these groups early in the design stage must continue through the care of patients on trial to the assessment of toxicity and response. The early involvement of statisticians, expert in clinical trial design, and patient representatives are also vital to developing the optimal protocol. Each step in design and implementation requires particular consideration of the unique aspects of applying HSCT to autoimmune diseases. Some areas which need special focus are the role of disease and transplant databases in designing and analyzing clinical trials, design options for early-phase trials, maintaining clinical equipoise, eligibility criteria, blinding, outcome measures and statistical analysis.

Protocol Designing for Cell Transplantation into the Central Nervous System

Although initial excitement was raised in the medical and scientific communities by pilot trials using adrenal autografts (1980s) and fetal allograft (1990s), two controlled trials in Parkinson's disease (PD) patients, demonstrated negative results, with the conclusion that today, cell therapy cannot be recommended for PD. Nevertheless, trials are still in progress for diseases like Huntington's disease (HD), stroke, multiple sclerosis (MS), cord transection, epilepsy, and others. Human knowledge about the biology of stem cells and precursor cells is growing and we have more and more evidence that cell therapy could be useful in "repairing" brain lesions, not only by survival and integration of grafted neurons, but also by stimulation of resident precursors already present within the CNS.

As brain transplantation surges ahead as a new and promising treatment aimed at repairing disabled neural networks, patients in the very advanced stage of disease may desire to avail the opportunity of a "last chance" treatment. Whereas, from an ethical point of view, pilot trials were performed in severely disabled PD patients (stage IV and V according to the Hoehn and Yahr scale), the selection of the patients may define different groups. To ensure the validity of the results, the group of selected patients needs to have a minimal variability. The severity of the disease has to be defined according to the preclinical data and the assumed mechanism of action of the graft. Published series of PD patients indicates that the selection of patients younger than 60 years of age, and having a less severe disease (e.g., stage III), may allow better results. This can be drawn from pilot trials, and is of critical importance in controlled series. For graft procedures a choice has to be made among many different sources, from postmitotic fetal neurons to stem cells or adult cell lineages, genetically engineered. The administration of cells is not always carried out by stereotactic surgery. In the examples of stroke and MS, it may appear that intravenous injection of cells, if assumed to cross the blood-brain barrier, may permit to give a cell treatment quite soon after the lesion. This may also apply to spinal cord transection. The demonstration of possible fusion between injected cells and resident cells is a possible cause of misinterpretation of experimental results. For PD patients, the precise location of injected neurons within the striatum may be critical.

Pilot trials need to demonstrate the survival of the implanted neurons and the effectiveness of the postulated mechanism of action of graft itself. Several imaging techniques mainly PET imaging, are available at our disposal. Because of lack of appropriate tracing of grafted neurons in HD patients, regional glucose imaging has been used.

The clinical evaluation needs first to demonstrate a clinical effect, without the need for direct demonstration of the improvement in the quality of life. Timed tests were designed to achieve this goal for the example of PD. In HD patients, timed tests also showed rich promise to achieve this goal. It is of critical importance, in a given disease, to build a complex protocol to ensure a multiparametric evaluation of the results. The main objective of controlled trials is to demonstrate the efficacy of the treatment. Published trials demonstrated that controlled trials, with parallel-blinded cohorts, are now possible, but very difficult and expensive to build.

Protocol Designing for Radiotherapy

For designing a protocol for clinical trials of radiotherapy following EORTC guidelines exist:

The concept of a Master Protocol for phase III studies was raised at the Steering Committee of the EORTC Radiotherapy Group, in order to make the work of the study coordinators easier, when writing protocols and to give them more homogeneity. The Master Protocol defines and clarifies in a logical order the different steps, which must be taken when designing a randomized trial—from the rationale to the references. It pays particular attention to eligibility criteria, volumes of interest defined in agreement with ICRU report 50 (gross tumor volume, clinical target volume, planning target volume and organs at risk), simulation procedure, treatment technique, normal tissue sparing, dose computation, equipment, dose specification (also in agreement with ICRU report 50). Last but not least, the different procedures of quality assurance for protocols and patients are also defined (site visits, dummy run procedure, in vivo dosimetry, individual case review) to allow working plans to be made in advance.

Moreover, for every new trial, specific quality assurance procedures are an integral part of the preparation of the protocol and executed under the responsibility of the study coordinator. With the growing complexity of the radiotherapy techniques used in the framework of the more recent trials, quality assurance procedures have also become more complex including trial specific phantom based measurements. Future ways to evaluate all steps of the radiotherapy process using a common platform connecting all users with the internet are currently under development.

Protocol Designing for Genomic Profiling. Interplay between Clinical Epidemiology, Bioinformatics and Biostatistics

Determining the design of a study in a protocol is a first step to avoid impending pitfalls. The protocol should deal with the problem of understanding the complex reality behind genomic profiling. There are basic guiding principles, which can help handle the complex task of designing prognostic studies to find genomic signatures.

ICH-GCP GUIDELINES FOR CLINICAL STUDY PROTOCOL AND PROTOCOL AMENDMENTS

The contents of a study protocol should generally include the following topics. However, site specific information may be provided on separate protocol page(s), or addressed in a separate agreement, and some of the information listed below may be contained in other protocol referenced documents, such as investigator's brochure.

1. General Information

i. Protocol title, protocol identifying number, and date. Any amendment(s) should also bear the amendment number(s) and date(s).

ii. Name and address of the sponsor and monitor (if other than the sponsor).

iii. Name and title of the person(s) authorized to sign the protocol and the protocol amendment(s) for the sponsor.

iv. Name, title, address, and telephone number(s) of the sponsor's medical expert (or dentist when appropriate) for the trial.

v. Name and title of the investigator(s) who is (are) responsible for conducting the trial, and the address and telephone number(s) of the trial site(s).

vi. Name, title, address, and telephone number(s) of the qualified physician (or dentist, if applicable) who is responsible for all trial site related medical (or dental) decisions (if other than investigator).

vii. Name(s) and address (es) of the clinical laboratory (ies) and other medical and /or technical department(s) and/or institutions involved in the trial.

2. Background Information

i. Name and description of the investigational product(s).

ii. A summary of findings from non clinical studies that potentially have clinical significance and from clinical trials that are relevant to the trial.

iii. Summary of the known and potential risks and benefits, if any, to human subjects.

iv. Description of and justification for the route of administration, dosage, dosage regimen, and treatment period(s).

v. A statement that the trial will be conducted in compliance with the protocol, GCP, and the applicable regulatory requirement(s).

vi. Description of the population to be studied.

vii. References to literature and data that are relevant to the trial, and that provide background for the trial.

3. Trial Objectives and Purpose

A detailed description of the objectives and the purpose of the trial.

4. Trial Design

The scientific integrity of the trial and the credibility of the data from the trial depend substantially on the trial design. A description of the trial design should include:

i. A specific statement of the primary endpoints and the secondary endpoints, if any, to be measured during the trial.

ii. A description of the type/design of trial to be conducted (e.g., double-blind, placebo controlled, parallel design) and a schematic diagram of trial design, procedures, and stages.

iii. A description of the measures taken to minimize/avoid bias, including (for example):

(a) Randomization.

(b) Blinding.

iv. A description of the trial treatment(s) and the dosage and dosage regimen of the investigational product(s). Also include a description of the dosage form, packaging, and labeling of the investigational product(s).

v. The expected duration of subject participation, and a description of the sequence and duration of all trial periods, including follow up, if any.

vi. A description of the "stopping rules" or "discontinuation criteria" for individual subjects, parts of trial, and entire trial.

vii. Accountability procedures for the investigational product(s), including the placebo(s) and comparator(s), if any.

viii. Maintenance of trial treatment randomization codes and procedures for breaking codes.

ix. The identification of any data to be recorded directly on the CRF's (i.e., no prior written or electronic record of data), and to be considered to be source data.

5. Selection and Withdrawal of Subjects

i. Subject inclusion criteria.

ii. Subject exclusion criteria.

iii. Subject withdrawal criteria (i.e., terminating investigational product treatment/trial treatment) and procedures specifying:

a. When and how to withdraw subjects from the trial/ investigational product treatment.

b. The type and timing of the data to be collected for withdrawn subjects.

c. Whether and how subjects are to be replaced.

d. The follow up for subjects withdrawn from investigational product treatment/ trial treatment.

6. Treatment of Subjects

i. The treatment(s) to be administered, including the name(s) of all the product(s), the dose(s), the dosing schedule(s), the route/mode(s) of administration, and the treatment period(s), including the follow up period(s) for subjects for each investigational product treatment/trial treatment group/arm of the trial.

ii. Medication(s)/treatment(s) permitted (including rescue medication) and not permitted before and/or during the trial.

iii. Procedures for monitoring subject compliance.

7. Assessment of Efficacy

i. Specification of the efficacy parameters.

ii. Methods and timing for assessing, recording, and analyzing efficacy parameters.

8. Assessment of Safety

i. Specification of safety parameters.

ii. The methods and timing for assessing, recording, and analyzing safety parameters.

iii. Procedures for eliciting reports of and for recording and reporting adverse event and intercurrent illnesses.

iv. The type and duration of the follow up of subjects after adverse events.

9. Statistics

i. A description of the statistical methods to be employed, including timing of any planned interim analysis (ses).

ii. The number of subjects planned to be enrolled. In multicenter trials, the number of enrolled subjects projected for each trial site should be specified. Reason for choice of sample size, including reflections on (or calculations of) the power of the trial and clinical justification.

iii. The level of significance to be used.

iv. Criteria for the termination of the trial.

v. Procedure for accounting for missing, unused, and spurious data.

vi. Procedures for reporting any deviation(s) from the original statistical plan (any deviation(s) from the original statistical plan should be described and justified in the protocol and/or in the final report, as appropriate).

vii. The selection of subjects to be included in the analyses (e.g., all randomized subjects, all dosed subjects, all eligible subjects, evaluable subjects).

10. Direct Access to Source Data Documents

The sponsor should ensure that it is specified in the protocol or other written agreement that the investigator(s)/institution(s) will permit trial related monitoring, audits, M/IEC review, and regulatory inspection(s) by providing direct access to source data/documents.

11. Quality Control and Quality Assurance

Description of ethical considerations relating to the trial.

12. Ethics

Description of ethical considerations relating to the trial

13. Data Handling and Record keeping

14. Financing and Insurance

Financing and insurance if not addressed in a separate agreement.

15. Publication Policy

Publication policy, if not addressed in a separate agreement.

16. Supplements

(NOTE: Since the protocol and the clinical trial/study report are closely related, further relevant information can be found in the ICH Guideline for Structure and Content of Clinical Study Reports.)

SUGGESTED READING

1. Bolla M, Bartelink H, Garavaglia G, Gonzalez D, Horiot JC, Johansson KA, van Tienhoven G, Vantongelen K, van Glabbeke M, EORTC guidelines for writing protocols for clinical trials of radiotherapy. Radiother Oncol 1995;36(1):1-8.
2. Bredeson CN, Pavletic SZ, Considerations when designing a clinical trial of haematopoietic stem cell transplantation for autoimmune disease. Best Pract Res Clin Haematol 2004;17(2):327-43.
3. Friedman LM, Furberg CD and DeMets DL, Fundamentals of Clinical Trials, 3rd Edn., Springer: New York, 1998.
4. ICH Guideline for Good Clinical Practice available at- http://www.ich.org.
5. Indian Council of Medical Research, Ethical Guidelines for Biomedical Research on Human Subjects. 2000.
6. Mansmann U, Genomic profiling. Interplay between clinical epidemiology, bioinformatics and biostatistics. Methods Inf Med 2005;44(3):454-60
7. Pocock SJ, Clinical trials: A Practical Approach. 1983:John Wiley and Sons: New York.
8. O'Brien K and Wright J. How to write a protocol. Journal of Orthodontics 2002;29:58-61.
9. Simon R, Clinical trial designs for therapeutic cancer vaccines. Cancer Treat Res 2005;123:339-50.
10. Spilker B, Guide To Clinical Trials. Lippincott Williams and Wilkins: Philadelphia, 1991.

9

Sponsor's and Investigator's Responsibilities

Zinobia Madan, Anil Kukreja

SPONSOR

A sponsor in literal terms is defined as an individual or a company or an institution that takes the responsibility for the initiation, management and/or financing of a clinical study. In case an investigator independently initiates and takes full responsibility for a trial, he/she automatically assumes the role of a sponsor.

The clinical trials conducted are broadly divided in two classes — those conducted for regulatory purpose and those conducted as academic projects. For the trials conducted for regulatory purpose, the sponsor is generally the pharmaceutical company interested in evaluating a product for potential use in specific therapeutic indication/s. The sponsor as a pharmaceutical company conducts the clinical trial with a primary aim to ultimately seek manufacturing and/or marketing permission for the product evaluated for commercial purposes. For the clinical trials conducted as academic projects, the sponsor is the individual or institution interested in such a project for academic reasons, e.g. epidemiological studies, research projects conducted by students, professors, etc.

Sponsor's Responsibilities

Enlisted below are the sponsor's responsibilities in the management of a clinical trial:

Selection of Investigator and Clinical Trial Site

The sponsor is responsible for selecting the investigator(s)/clinical trial site(s) after ensuring the appropriateness and availability of the study site and facilities. The sponsor must assure itself of the investigator's qualifications and availability for the entire duration of the study. In the event of a need of a coordinating committee/coordinating investigator, sponsor is also responsible for organization of the same in case of multicentric studies.

Given below are enlisted factors involved in Investigator selection by a sponsor:

i. Reputation of the investigator in his/her field of expertise based on experience of conducting clinical trials as per GCP (Good Clinical Practice) guidelines, publications and several other factors.
ii. Availability of infrastructure at the clinical trial site for conduct of the study, e.g. equipment, adequately trained personnel, dedicated study co-coordinator
iii. Availability of subject population for timely enrollment of the subjects in the trial with no competing study requiring similar subject population
iv. Ease of accessibility of the trial site to the sponsor
v. Ability of the Ethics Committee (EC)/Institutional Review Board (IRB) to execute all its responsibilities expeditiously and fairly
vi. Anticipated time required to initiate and complete the trial
vii. Budgetary factors (i.e. cost of the trial to the sponsor)

Some of the relationships between Investigators, Sponsors and Contract Research Organizations (CROs) that may be established are depicted in Figures 9.1A to C.

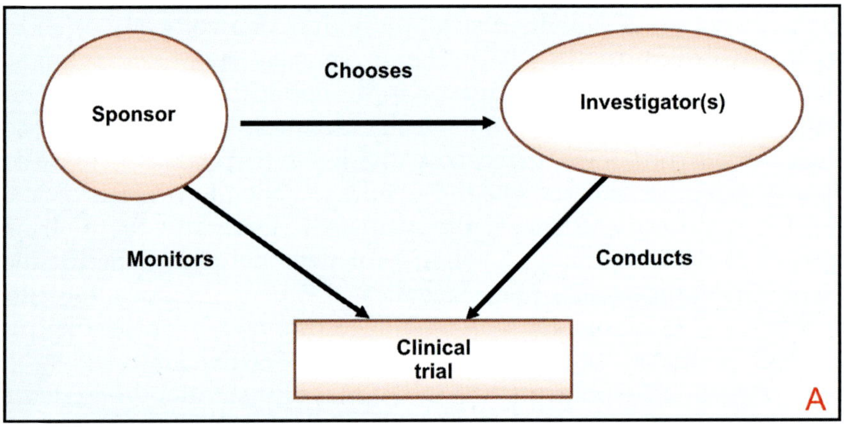

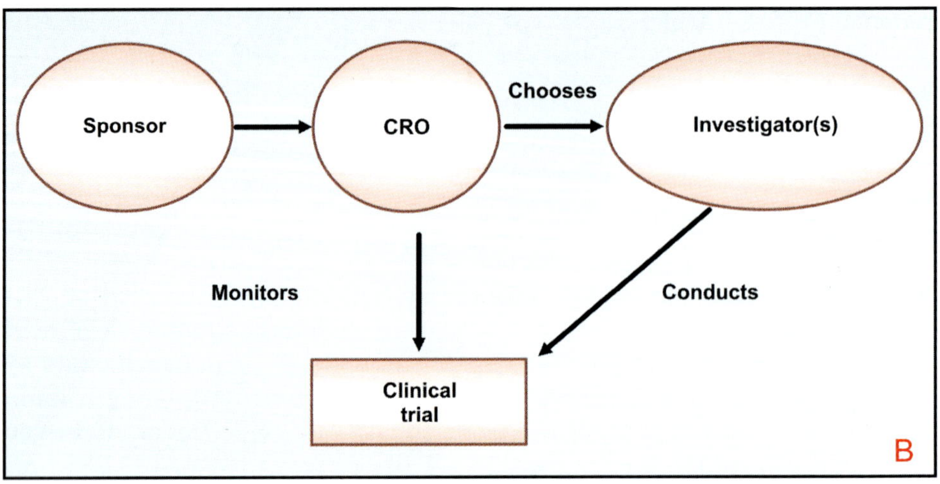

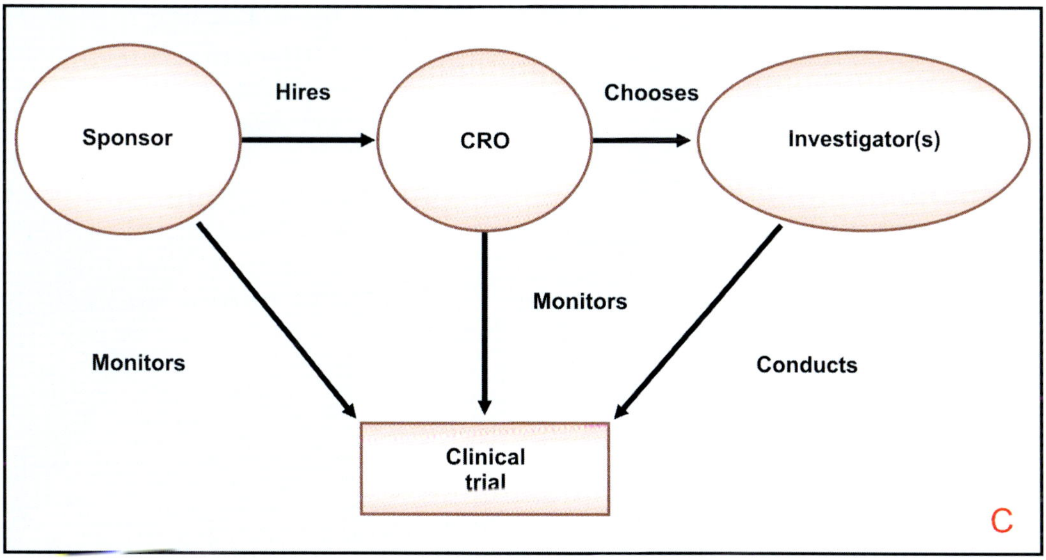

Figs. 9.1A to C: Relationships between investigators, sponsors and contract research organization (Adapted from: Guide to Clinical Trials, by Bert Spilker Lippincott Wiliams and Wilkins, 2000 ed, p. 408)

Preparation of Clinical Trial Documents

The sponsor holds a key responsibility of preparing all the clinical trial documents for submission to the investigator(s), which includes Investigator's Brochure, Protocol, Case Record Form, Informed Consent document and Subject Record Diary. These clinical trial documents are submitted to the Investigator(s) after getting a Confidentiality Agreement signed by them. Sufficient time should be provided to the investigator(s) for review of these clinical trial documents and in case the investigator(s) suggest any amendments to these documents, the same will be incorporated by the sponsor. Once the clinical trial documents are approved by all the investigators, the sponsor will procure undertakings from all the investigators for submission to the regulatory authorities.

As a prerequisite to planning of a study, the sponsor is responsible for providing the investigator(s) with an investigator's brochure. The brochure must contain the available chemical, pharmaceutical, toxicological, pharmacological and clinical data, which justifies the nature, scale and the duration of the study. In addition, the sponsor must bring any relevant new information arising during the period of study to the attention of the investigator(s) as well as the EC/IRB.

Agreement/Contract

The Sponsor holds the responsibility to enter into a formal and legal agreement/contract with the Investigator(s)/clinical trial site(s) on the following terms:

i. To conduct the study in compliance with GCP, the applicable regulatory requirements and as per the protocol agreed to by the sponsor and given approval/ favorable opinion by the ethics committee.
ii. To comply with the procedures for data recording, and reporting.
iii. To permit monitoring, auditing and inspection.
iv. To retain the study related essential documents until the sponsor informs the investigator(s)/clinical trial site(s) in writing that these documents are no longer needed.

The agreement should make a mention of the budgetary provision as mutually agreed upon between the sponsor and the investigator.

Standard Operating Procedures (SOP)

The sponsor is responsible for establishing detailed Standard Operating Procedures (SOP's) for the conduct of the clinical trial.

Allocation of Duties and Responsibilities

It is the sponsor's responsibility to define and allocate all study related duties and responsibilities to the identified person(s)/department(s)/organization(s).

Study Management, Data Handling and Record Keeping

i. The sponsor is responsible for the following activities related to the clinical trial. Alternatively, the Sponsor can involve another party and in this case the sponsor is responsible for securing agreement with the involved party/parties
ii. Access to all study related sites, source data/documents and reports for the purpose of inspection, monitoring and auditing by the authorised parties and inspection by national and foreign regulatory authorities
iii. Data processing
iv. Breaking of the code
v. Statistical analysis
vi. Preparation of the study report
vii. Preparation and submission of materials to the ethics committee, regulatory authorities and any other review bodies
viii. Reporting the ADRs, AEs to the ethics committee
ix. Quality assurance and quality control systems with written SOPs to ensure that the study is conducted and data are generated, documented (recorded), and reported — in compliance with the protocol, GCP and the applicable regulatory requirement(s).

Additionally, the sponsor is responsible to make arrangements for safe and secure custody of all clinical trial related documents and study material for an adequate period as per the applicable regulatory guidelines.

Compensation for Participation

The sponsor is responsible for making provision of compensation if any, to be paid to the subjects for the inconvenience, travel and time spent for their participation in clinical research. All payments, reimbursements and medical services to be provided to research subjects should be approved by the EC/IRB.

Confirmation of Review by the Ethics Committee

The sponsor is responsible for obtaining the documented approval/favorable opinion of the EC/IRB before the initiation of the study and the particulars about the members of the EC/IRB including their names and designations, from the investigator(s) and/or the clinical trial site(s). The sponsor is also responsible for procuring all the correspondence between the investigators and the EC/IRB.

Supply, Storage and Handling of Pharmaceutical Products

The sponsor is responsible for supplying the investigational products, including comparator(s) and placebo if applicable. The products should be manufactured in accordance with the principles of GMPs and they should be suitably packaged and labelled.

It is the responsibility of the sponsor to determine the acceptable storage conditions, reconstitution procedures and devices for product infusions if any, of the investigational product, including comparator(s) and placebo if applicable. The sponsor ensures that the site comply to these conditions by maintaining records.

The sponsor should not supply an investigator(s)/clinical trial site(s) with the product until the sponsor obtains all required documentation (e.g. approval/favorable opinion from EC/IRB and regulatory authorities).

The sponsor is responsible for procuring and maintaining documents related to adequate and safe receipt, handling, storage and dispensing of the product, retrieval of unused product from the subjects and return of unused product to the sponsor (or its alternative disposal procedure).

The sponsor is also responsible for maintaining sufficient samples from each batch and keeping the record of their analyses and characteristics for reference, so that if necessary an independent laboratory may be able to recheck the same.

Safety Information

The sponsor is responsible for evaluation of the safety of the product on an ongoing basis. In case of findings, which could potentially affect the safety of the subjects, the Sponsor should promptly notify all concerned and should take appropriate measures necessary to safeguard the study subjects.

Adverse Drug Reaction (ADR) Reporting

The sponsor holds the responsibility of providing ADR / AE reporting forms to the investigator(s) / institution(s) and to expedite the reporting to all concerned (including the ethics committee and the regulatory authorities) of all serious and/or unexpected ADRs.

Study Reports

It is the responsibility of the sponsor to ensure the preparation of a comprehensive final clinical study report as per the standards of the GCP guidelines for Format and Content of Clinical Study Reports (Refer ICH E3 for Structure and Content of Clinical Study Reports). The sponsor is also responsible for submitting any safety updates and/or periodic reports as prescribed by the regulatory authorities.

Monitoring

It is the sponsor's responsibility to ensure appropriate conduct and monitoring of the study. The monitoring should be carried out by adequately trained monitors or CRO appointed by sponsor, to supervise an ongoing study.

Audit

As a part of the QA system, it is the responsibility of the sponsor to perform an independent audit by appropriately trained and qualified audit personnel to ensure compliance with the protocol, SOPs, GCPs and applicable regulatory requirements. The same needs to be documented appropriately which can be made available for review by regulatory authorities. The sponsor is also responsible for initiating prompt action in case it is discovered that any party involved has not entirely complied with the GCP, SOPs, protocol and/or any applicable regulatory requirements.

Multicentric Studies

In case of multicentric studies, it is the responsibility of the sponsor to make special administrative arrangements, appointing a coordinating committee/coordinator and make arrangements to facilitate the communication between investigators at various sites, for the smooth conduct of the study. All investigators and other specialists should be given the training to follow the same protocol and systems. The sponsor should obtain written acceptance of the protocol and its annexes from each of the investigator and institution involved.

Premature Termination or Suspension of a Study

In case the sponsor chooses to or is required to terminate prematurely or suspend the study, then the sponsor should notify the Investigator(s), institution(s), the ethics committee and the regulatory authorities accordingly. The notification should document the reason(s) for the termination or suspension by the sponsor or by the investigator/institution.

Role of a Foreign Sponsor

If the sponsor is a foreign company, organization or person(s), it shall appoint a local representative or CRO to fulfill the appropriate local responsibilities as governed by the national regulations. The sponsor may transfer any or all of the sponsor's study related duties and functions in writing to a CRO but the ultimate responsibility for the quality and the integrity of the study data shall always reside with the sponsor.

Responsibilities of the Monitor Appointed by the Sponsor

The monitor is the principal communication link between the sponsor and the investigator and is appointed by the sponsor. The monitor should have adequate scientific qualifications and practical clinical trial experience. The main responsibility of the monitor is to oversee the progress of the study and to ensure that the study conduct and data handling comply with the protocol, GCPs and applicable ethical and regulatory requirements. The following are highlights of the responsibilities of the sponsor's appointed monitor:

- Verification of investigator(s) qualifications, expertise and the resources to carry out the study.
- Availability of investigator throughout the study period.
- Adequate and continued availability of institutional facilities like laboratories, equipment, staff, storage space, etc.
- Availability of sufficient investigational product(s) with proper storage facilities
- Ensure that the investigational product(s) are supplied only to eligible subjects at the specified dose(s) and time(s) and with proper instructions for handling.
- Ensure the documentation of the receipt, use, return and disposal of the product(s) at the site.
- Ensure that the investigator receives the current investigator's brochure and all supplies needed to conduct the study as per the protocol.
- Ensure compliance of protocol and maintenance of essential documents by the Investigator.
- Ensure appropriate training and further compliance to the protocol, SOPs and GCP guidelines by investigator and the study team.
- Ensuring that any of the trial tasks are not delegated to unauthorised individuals.
- Informing the sponsor in case of any unwarranted deviation from the protocol or GCP guidelines.
- Following predetermined written set of SOPs.
- Observing and reporting the subject recruitment rate to the sponsor.
- Visiting the site before, during and after the study to make assessments of the

protocol compliance and data handling in accordance with the predetermined SOPs.
- Assisting the investigator in reporting the data and results of the study to the sponsor, e.g. by providing CRF completion guidelines, etc.
- Ensuring that all CRFs are correctly filled out in accordance with original observations consistent with the source documents, are legible, complete, signed and dated.
- Clarifying any deviations, errors or omissions with the investigator, getting it corrected and explained on the CRF.
- Submitting a written report to the sponsor after each site visit and after all communications as prescribed by the SOPs.
- Ensuring the documentation of storage, handling, dispensing and return of investigational product as per the protocol and the SOPs.

INVESTIGATOR

Investigator: A person responsible for the conduct of the study at the trial site. Investigator is a person responsible for the rights, health and welfare of the study subjects.

Principal investigator: In case the study is conducted by a team of investigators at one site or at multiple sites, then the investigator who coordinates between the different investigators involved in the study is termed as the Principal investigator.

Co-investigator: A co-investigator is a person legally qualified to be an investigator to whom the investigator delegates a part of his/her responsibilities.

Investigator's Responsibilities

Enlisted below are the investigator's responsibilities in the management of a clinical trial:

Qualifying for being an Investigator

It is the responsibility of the investigator to participate in the study only if he/she is qualified as prescribed by the Medical Council of India (MCI). The investigator should provide a copy of the curriculum vitae and/or other relevant documents requested by the sponsor, the ethics committee, the CRO or the regulatory authorities.

Provision of Infrastructure and Resources for the Study

It is the investigators' responsibility to understand the time and other resource demands the study is likely to make and ensure they can be made available throughout the duration of the study. The investigator should also ensure that other studies do not divert essential subjects or facilities away from the study at hand.

Knowledge on Safety and Efficacy of Investigational Product (IP)

The investigator is responsible for being familiar with the safety, efficacy and appropriate use of the investigational product as described in the protocol, investigator's brochure and other information sources provided by the sponsor from time-to-time.

Compliance to Various Requirements

The investigator should be aware of and comply with GCPs, SOPs and the applicable regulatory requirements.

Medical Care of the Study Subjects

Investigator or a co-investigator for the study should be responsible for all study related medical decisions. investigator has to ensure that adequate medical care is provided to a subject for any adverse events including clinically significant laboratory values or any inter-current illness(es) during the study period. Investigator should also inform the subject's other attending physician(s) about the subject's participation in the study if the subject has another attending physician(s) and if the subject agrees to such other physician(s). Subsequent to the completion of the study or dropping out of the subject(s) the investigator is responsible for ensuring adequate medical care to the subjects. In case the subject is withdrawing prematurely from a study, the investigator should make a reasonable effort to ascertain the reason(s) while fully respecting the subject's rights.

Monitoring and Auditing of Records

It is the responsibility of the investigator to allow monitoring and auditing of the records, procedures and facilities, by the sponsor, the ethics committee, CRO or their authorized representative(s) or by the appropriate regulatory authority. The investigator should maintain a list of appropriately qualified person(s) to whom the investigator has delegated study-related duties and ensure that these people are adequately informed about the protocol, SOPs, the investigational product(s) and their study related duties and functions.

Communication with Ethics Committee

The investigator is responsible for ensuring that the essential study related documents (e.g. protocol, case record form, informed consent document, investigator's brochure, subject recruitment procedures such as advertisements, and any other written / verbal information to be provided to the subjects) have been reviewed and accepted in writing by the relevant ethics committee(s).

The investigator should promptly report to the ethics committee, the monitor and the sponsor:

a. Deviations from or changes of, the protocol to eliminate immediate hazards to the subjects
b. Changes that increase the risk to subject(s) and/or affecting significantly the conduct of the study
c. All serious and/or unexpected adverse drug reactions and adverse events
d. New information that may adversely affect safety of the subjects or the conduct of the study
e. For reported deaths the Investigator should supply any additional information, e.g. autopsy reports and terminal medical reports.

Compliance with the Protocol

The investigator/institution must agree and sign the protocol and / or another legally acceptable document with the sponsor, mentioning the agreement with the protocol, and confirm in writing that he/she has read and understood the protocol, GCPs and SOPs and will work as stipulated in them.

The investigator may implement a deviation from, or change of protocol to eliminate an immediate hazard(s) to study subjects without prior ethics committee approval/ favorable opinion. The implemented deviation or change, the reasons for it and if appropriate the proposed protocol amendment(s) should be submitted by the investigator to the ethics committee (for review and approval/favorable opinion), to the sponsor (for agreement) and if required to the regulatory authority(ies).

The investigator or person designated by him/her should document and explain any deviation from the approved protocol.

The investigator is responsible for following the study randomisation procedure, if any, and should ensure that the randomization code is broken only in accordance with the protocol. If the study is blinded, the Investigator should promptly document and explain to the sponsor any premature un-blinding, e.g. accidental un-blinding, un-blinding due to serious adverse event) of the investigational product(s).

Accountability of Investigational Product(s)

Investigator has the primary responsibility for investigational product(s) accountability at the study site(s) by appropriate documentation of the inventory at the site, the use by each subject, and the return to the sponsor or the alternative disposal of the unused product(s). These records should include dates, quantities, batch/serial numbers, specified storage conditions, expiry dates if applicable, and the unique code number assigned to the investigational product packs and study subjects. Investigator should maintain records that describe that the subjects were provided the dosage specified by the protocol.

The investigator is responsible for assigning some or all of his/her duties for investigational product's accountability at the study site(s) to his subordinate who is under the supervision of the investigator/institution.

Selection and Recruitment of Study Subjects

The investigator is responsible for ensuring the unbiased selection of an adequate number of suitable subjects according to the protocol and if required also seek the cooperation of other physicians; check the institution's records to assess the availability of a sufficient number of subjects. The investigator is responsible for maintaining a confidential list of names of all study subjects allocated to each study in addition to maintaining screening log and enrolment log.
The investigator is responsible for giving adequate information to subjects about the trial and the investigational product in accordance with the GCP.

Informed Consent Process

The investigator has the duty to:

i. Communicate to prospective subjects all the information necessary for informed consent. There should not be any restriction on subject's right to ask any questions related to the study as any restriction on this undermines the validity of informed consent.
ii. Exclude the possibility of unjustified deception, undue influence and intimidation.
iii. Seek consent only after the prospective subject is adequately informed.
iv. As a general rule obtain from each prospective subject a signed form as an evidence of informed consent (written informed consent) preferably witnessed by a person not related to the trial, and in case of incompetence to do so, a legal guardian or other duly authorized representative.
v. Renew the informed consent of each subject, if there are material changes in the conditions or procedures of the research or new information becomes available during the ongoing trial.
vi. Not use intimidation in any form, which invalidates informed consent. The investigator must assure prospective subjects that their decision to participate or not will not affect the patient-clinician relationship or any other benefits to which they are entitled.
vii. As part of the information provided to the subject, the investigator should supply subjects with, and encourage them to carry with them, information about their participation in the trial and information about contact persons who can assist in an emergency situation.

Records/Reports

The investigator holds the responsibility for ensuring accuracy, completeness, legibility, and timeliness of the data reported to the sponsor in the CRFs and in all required reports. Data reported on the CRF that are derived from source documents should be consistent with the source documents or the discrepancies should be explained.

Any change or correction to the paper CRF or electronic CRF should be dated, signed and explained (if necessary) and should not obscure the original entry (i.e. an audit trail should be maintained). The sponsor should provide guidelines to Investigators on making such corrections. The investigator should retain records of the changes and corrections.

Progress Reports

The investigator holds the responsibility of submitting the study status on periodic basis as requested by the sponsor/CRO. All reporting made by the Investigator should identify the subjects by unique code numbers assigned to the study subjects rather than by the subjects' name(s), personal identification number(s) and/or addresses.

Termination and Final Report

In case the investigator and sponsor agree to prematurely terminate or suspend the study for any reason, the investigator/institution should promptly inform the study subjects, the ethics committee as well as the regulatory authorities. The investigators should also ensure appropriate therapy and follow-up for the subjects.

However, if the investigator or the sponsor or the ethics committee decide to terminate or suspend the study without prior agreement of all parties concerned then the party initiating the suspension /termination should promptly inform all the concerned parties about such suspension/termination and suspension along with a detailed written explanation for such termination/suspension.

It is the responsibility of the investigator to maintain documents as specified in the essential documents' list and take measures to prevent accidental or premature destruction.

The study can be closed only when it is confirmed that all necessary documents are in the appropriate files.

It is the responsibility of the investigator to inform about the study completion to the institution, the sponsor and the ethics committee. The investigator should sign and forward the data (CRFs, results and interpretations, analyses and reports, of the study from his/her center to the sponsor and the ethics committee. Investigator should submit his signed and dated final report to the institution, the ethics committee and the sponsor verifying the responsibility for the validity of data. In case of a multicenter study – the signature of the coordinating investigator may suffice if agreed in the protocol.

In case the Investigator is the sponsor then he/she assumes the responsibilities of both the functionaries.

CONCLUSIONS

Both the sponsor and investigator play key roles in conduct of a clinical trial. This means that the roles of both the sponsor and the investigator are so crucial that in the event of their not executing their defined responsibilities, the clinical trial would be compromised significantly. During the conduct of any clinical trial, it is vital that the sponsor and the investigator have adequate interactions and communications to ensure smooth conduct of the trial. Effective planning at both the sponsor's and investigator's end is crucial for a successful clinical trial. Failing to plan at both the ends is planning to fail. Thus to summarize, adequate planning, appropriate infrastructure and successful execution of the responsibilities both by the sponsor and the investigator would go a long way in contributing to the success of a clinical trial.

SUGGESTED READING

1. Bert Spilker, In Guide to Clinical Trials, Lippincott Wiliams and Wilkins, 2000.
2. Good Clinical Practices, Guidelines for Clinical Trials on Pharmaceutical Products in India, Central Drugs Standard Control Organization, Directorate General of Health Services, 2001.
3. ICH Topic E6. Note for Guidance on Good Clinical Practice, CPMP/ICH/135/95.

10 Patient Recruitment and Retention in Clinical Trials

Suhasini Sharma, Rashna Cama

INTRODUCTION

The process of new drug development is extremely time consuming and expensive. It is estimated that for a new molecule that is discovered it would take approximately 10-15 years to reach the market at an approximate cost of $ 500 – 800 million. Of these 10-15 years, it is estimated that recruitment of subjects takes up 30 percent of clinical timelines.[1] Therefore, recruiting of appropriate subjects is an issue that must be considered before the study and throughout the duration of the study and investigators must be realistic when determining feasibility of recruiting patients into a particular study.

For a long time patient recruitment was neglected as studies were conducted at large hospitals where it was presumed that a large patient database already existed. However, soon realization set in that these studies were taking an enormous length of time and pharmaceuticals began looking for novel and faster ways of patient recruitment. Thus began the advent of professionalizing recruitment activities.

Internationally, recruitment and retention of clinical trial patients are a big challenge. More than 80 percent of global trials fail to enroll on time, with 52 percent delayed by 1-6 months. Failure to recruit patients on time leads to loss of over 85-95 percent of days in a clinical trial.[2]

Patient recruitment today is considered the "key bottle-neck" of clinical trials. It is the leading cause of missed clinical trial deadlines and it costs more and consumes more time than any other aspect of clinical trials. Due to this reason patient recruitment is being focused upon by pharmaceuticals as reducing the time for recruitment would eventually reduce total costs of drug development and make treatments available to the consumer at an earlier date and at more affordable prices.

BACKGROUND

Over the years the number of patients required to undergo clinical trials on a new drug is steadily increasing. As the number of New Drug Applications (NDAs) increase the number of subjects per NDA also increases. Presently approximately 5,300 subjects are needed per NDA.[3] With 80,000 clinical trials underway in the US alone, the search for appropriate subjects continues and sponsors are scrutinizing recruitment plans before entrusting a clinical trial to a particular site (Fig. 10.1).

As there is lot of competition for clinical trial patients in the western world (US and Europe), pharmaceutical companies and Clinical Research Organizations (CROs) are increasingly turning to Eastern Europe, Latin America and Asia for speeding up patient recruitment and clinical development of their new drugs. India is attracting global attention in this field due to availability of a large and essentially treatment-naïve patient pool, besides having other advantages such as low costs and satisfactory medical infrastructure and scientific talent. However, most trials in India take place at a few well-known urban hospitals. As the number of clinical trials in India increase, we too may face similar challenges in patient recruitment and retention.

A basic fact about clinical research is this: even though a study may be very well designed and well funded, it cannot bring a drug to the market without the availability of suitable subjects.[4]

Difficulties faced in the recruitment process may be due to a variety of reasons. Recruitment strategies are rarely considered early enough and should be considered during protocol design. Frequently the inclusion/exclusion criteria are so narrowly defined that it makes one wonder whether such patients actually exist! Many a times, the budgets allocated for effective recruitment are inadequate or enrolment deadlines are not realistic. Sometimes, the investigator may lack a basic knowledge about recruiting patients and may not have staff dedicated for the recruitment process. An investigator may assume that he will rely on his own database for recruitment and in actuality this may be inadequate to recruit the required number of patients. These difficulties in recruitment may be further aggravated by negative publicity from the media, which tends to highlight the failures and underplay the advantages of research.[4]

The consequence of delayed recruitment and not meeting enrollment timelines is tremendous for the drug company and the costs involved are staggering. Says Siporin,

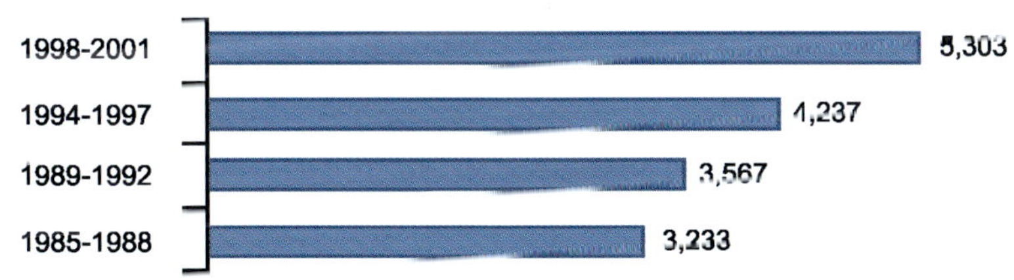
1998-2001
5,303
1994-1997
4,237
1989-1992
3,567
1985-1988
3,233

Source: Tufts center for the study of drug development, 2002.
Food Drug Law Journal, 1997.

Fig. 10.1: Number of patients per NDA

"The average cost of a phase III clinical trial ranges between $4 million and $20 million for one trial, and you have to run a minimum of two phase III trials. A delay for a drug that is to be a moderate success can cost a company $1 million a day in lost sales. A delay for a billion-dollar-a-year blockbuster product can cost upwards of $3 million a day in lost sales."[5]

Therefore, timely recruitment of patients in clinical trials and their satisfactory retention assume critical importance in containing the cost of new drug development, and ultimately, the price consumers would pay for that medicine when it reaches the market.

BASIC PRINCIPLES OF PATIENT RECRUITMENT

Why do Patients Join Clinical Trials?

Understanding why a patient chooses to participate in a clinical trial is helpful not only in recruiting the subject but also in retaining the particular subject in the trial. Patients choose to join clinical trials for a variety of reasons including wanting to help advance knowledge of the disease in the interest of society. However, besides a few altruistic individuals the main reasons for participating include – a lack of available therapy, improved medical care, lack of health insurance, advice from the family physician, financial reasons, etc.

What are the Barriers to Participation?

A Harris Interactive Survey reported that of patients who are aware of an appropriate clinical trial, 71 percent of eligible patients choose not to participate.[6]

Reasons for not participating could be:

i. Risk of side-effects
ii. Concern about getting placebo
iii. Center too far away
iv. Unable to find a trial
v. Not eligible
vi. Inconvenient hours
vii. Not enough information.

Patient concerns are generally of the following nature:

i. What if I change my mind and decide to drop out?
ii. Will I get a placebo or the real thing?
iii. What is in it for me?
iv. Will I be taken advantage of?
v. What is in it for my doctor?

What Motivates the Patient to Participate in a Clinical Trial?

i. Access to promising therapies
ii. Access to greater medical expertise
iii. Close individualized medical attention/care
iv. Emotional support
v. Something to do (break boredom)
vi. Altruism (usually limited to phase I).

ETHICAL ISSUES IN PATIENT RECRUITMENT

Confidentiality and Privacy of Personal Health Information

Any information by which a patient can be identified is called identifying information. As a part of the recruitment process an investigator has access to a patient's health information. In the USA, this health information is protected by a federal law called HIPAA, i.e. the Health Insurance Portability and Accountability Act. This was passed in the US in April 2003 to avoid misuse of health information. There are 2 parts to HIPAA: The HIPAA privacy rule and the HIPAA security rule. The HIPAA privacy rule applies to all paper and the security rule applies to all electronic Personal Health Information (PHI). In order to use a patient's PHI an authorization from the patient is mandatory. Hence, today, all informed consent forms carry a statement indicating that the patient's health information will be shared with the monitor and other staff involved in the research work.

Advertising for Clinical Trial Patients

Advertising for patients is permitted and is one of the ways of recruiting protocol-suitable patients in clinical trials. Various media such as newspapers, radio, television, mail-shots, posters or flyers can be used for the purpose. There are guidelines laid down by ICH GCP, Indian GCP and clinical trial regulations of respective countries on the use of advertising for subject recruitment in clinical trials. All the advertising material (print ads, scripts for radio or television ads with the visuals, posters, flyers, letters, etc.) proposed to be used for subject recruitment in a clinical trial must be submitted to the IRB/IEC for review and approval before it can be used.

When an application is made to an IRB/IEC for approval of a study, the IRB/IEC will not only go through the protocol and design of the study but will also scrutinize all recruitment material including GP mailshots (letters from GP to patients informing them about the study), letters to patients and all advertising material for their content and accuracy. The IEC's aim is to see that patients are not misled with false promises of a "new drug", nor are they coerced with monetary gains.

Therefore, recruitment materials are reviewed by the IEC to ensure that:

i. They are neither misleading nor coercive to potential subjects.

ii. They make no claims that might lead a subject to believe that an investigational treatment is proven safe and effective and/or equivalent or superior to other treatments.
iii. The advertisement does not use terms such as "new treatment," "new medication" or "new drug" without explaining that the test article is investigational. Phrases such as "receive new treatments" or "receive new therapy" mislead study subjects to believe they will be receiving newly improved products of proven benefit.
iv. They do not promise "free medical treatment," when the intent is only to state that subjects will not be charged for taking part in the study.

Undue Influence

Offering excessive, unwarranted, inappropriate or improper compensation as an attraction to enroll or remain compliant in a clinical trial is called using undue influence, e.g. Rs. 4,000 for a 4-day, treatment of common cold. To prevent undue influence compensation must be reasonable and must not influence a patient's decision to enroll in a trial.

In contrast, coercion is a threat of adverse consequences should the patient decline to participate. An example of coercion would be prisoners under threat of being denied parole if they refuse to cooperate for a clinical trial.

Vulnerable Population

Patients who cannot be expected to choose what is right for themselves, i.e. those who have limitations on their capacity or freedom is termed a vulnerable population. These include children, patients who are mentally disabled, i.e. with dementia or other psychiatric disorders and prisoners. Sometimes the elderly, and students and employees of the investigator are also classified as vulnerable groups. For these vulnerable groups the informed consent form may be signed by a legally acceptable representative (LAR), however, the patient's "assent" is very important. Every effort must be made to explain the study to the subject up to the level of his understanding. If a child capable of assenting indicates an unwillingness to participate in the study, he should in no way be intimidated or enrolled in the research.

METHODS OF PATIENT RECRUITMENT

Scientific planning of recruitment strategy and budget during protocol design is the key to cusure that a particular study will have the appropriate subjects within the specified timeframe.

Investigator Database

Investigators or investigative sites are chosen because of their expertise in a particular therapeutic area. Therefore, the first point of recruitment starts with the investigator's own database and a fair number of appropriate subjects would be available from this. However, investigators always tend to overestimate the number of patients they would be able to enroll. This is often because they are looking at the number of subjects with the general overall diagnosis, e.g. hypertension, without weighing the exclusion criteria, due to which many subjects would fail screening.

Clinician Referrals

A database of clinicians (GPs, Consultants) who are supportive of research should be identified at an early stage in the recruitment process. Collaborations must be initially established and then maintained. For pre-study promotion, special presentations, meetings and forums can be arranged.[7] The clinicians must be made aware of the eligibility criteria and recruitment materials must be provided. Recruitment material may be in the form of posters, flyers, and mail shots, which the clinician can send to prospective subjects. All these materials must be initially approved by the IEC and recruitment letters must have an 'Opt-in" or an "Opt-out" option.

Opt-out Procedure

The recruitment letter should include a telephone number to call or a postcard to return if the subject is not interested in participating in the study. If no telephone call is received or postcard returned, the subject might then be contacted by the investigator to determine whether or not the subject is interested in learning more about and/or participating in the study.

Opt-in Procedure

The recruitment letter should include a telephone number to call or a postcard to return if the subject is interested in learning more about and/or participating in the study. The investigator may not contact subjects who have not called or returned a postcard indicating interest in learning more about the study.

Having established collaboration with clinicians, it is important to maintain this collaboration. This may be achieved by a research staffer telephoning or visiting the referral site, keeping the clinician informed about the progress of the trial and his individual patient's clinical details and showing appreciation for the help received. If a clinician feels good about the way he and his patient have been treated throughout a study, it will ensure his repeat participation in future recruitment efforts.

Advertising

Mass media campaigns for clinical trials include newspaper advertisements, radio or TV advertisements. Media campaigns may also include press releases, mass mailings, billboards, bus stop signs, public service announcements etc. All advertising material must have prior approval from the IRB/IEC before it can be used.

In order for an advertisement to be approved by an ethics committee it needs to fulfill certain criteria. It is important that the advertisement is neither misleading nor coercive to potential subjects; that they make no claims that might lead a subject to believe that an investigational treatment is proven safe and effective and/or equivalent or superior to other treatments. The advertisement should not use terms such as "new treatment," "new medication" or "new drug" without explaining that the test article is investigational. Phrases such as "receive new treatments" or "receive new therapy" mislead study subjects to believe they will be receiving newly improved products of proven benefit. The advertisements should not promise "free medical treatment," when the intent is only to state that subjects will not be charged for taking part in the study.

Certain key elements that should be present in any advertisement for research include:

i. Name of research facility;
ii. Purpose of the research and eligibility criteria (briefly stated);
iii. Time commitment and remuneration, if any
iv. Contact person for more information
v. The word "research" somewhere in the advertisement
vi. If monetary compensation is offered, it must not be presented as an inducement to participate.

Advertising needs to be targeted at a particular section of society depending on the study in question. For example, if a study involves only adult men, it would be appropriate to put a newspaper ad in the sports section of the paper or if it targeted only women it would be more appropriate in the lifestyle section of the paper. Similarly if a radio advert targeting people between ages of 20-40 were to be run at 11:00 am, it would be quite useless as this section of the population would probably be at work and hence unable to catch the ad. Hence, proper placement and timing of ads (media buying) is important in finding the appropriate subjects.

The success of advertising in patient recruitment depends on therapeutic indication. It is more in certain indications where patients have limited existing treatment options (cancers, some rare diseases); or when patients are not satisfied with their current treatments, and would not mind trying alternative solutions (e.g. common cold, allergies, headaches, acidity); or in conditions which patients are hesitant to share with their doctors for fear of embarrassment (e.g. sexual dysfunction, urinary incontinence).

Community Based

Recruitment may be stepped up by organizing health camps. These camps would target populations having the disease under study. For example, if there is a study on osteoporosis, an investigator would organize an osteoporosis screening camp. At this camp, potential patients would be made aware of a study on osteoporosis, and if interested they could be invited for a further screening check. Similarly speaking at a meeting for a disease-specific support group could increase the target audience's awareness about a clinical trial in their particular disease-related area and this may enhance recruitment for an investigator.

Web-based

Today there are several companies listing clinical trials on the web. centrewatch.com and clinical trials.gov are just a few of the sites. In addition companies are proclaiming trials on their own web sites. On-line partnerships with search-engines like Yahoo and Google enable sponsors to provide a lead to prospective subjects. Customized web sites are now being used to post the pre-qualifying questionnaire and to prescreen subjects online through a secure network setup.

Call Centers

Sponsors are increasingly looking towards call centers to centralize the recruitment process. They form the first point of contact for a patient in the recruitment process and health information data is obtained during the telephone screen. This data can be rapidly processed and filtered to spread the recruitment over several sites. Call centers can also help identify which modalities of advertising are working so that rapid solutions can be developed to aid the recruitment process. Some call centers will even help by giving the first appointment to a patient at a convenient center.

However, call centers have their limitations. Call center operators need intensive training to ensure accurate recording of data. Also, for a multinational study language specialists may be needed. Occasionally for studies in areas such as HIV and AIDS the center may be inundated with calls and be unable to handle the large volumes. Keeping a person on hold would put some people off. Data confidentiality could also be an issue with call centers though now Institutional Board review is required for all call guides. Which recruitment method/s or what proportion of a mix of different methods will be used for a particular trial requires prior planning and will depend upon the therapeutic indication, target population and understanding and experience of the investigative team and sponsors in patient recruitment.

RECRUITMENT METRICS

With so many possible methods of patient recruitment comes the understanding that recruitment success has to be me asured, and that accountability is destined to become standard practice. Accountability involves a complete tracking of each point of contact, starting with the prescreening call through scheduling of the first screening visit, then recruitment, enrollment, retention, and linking these actions to the referral source. Through continuous measurement of these actions, meaningful metrics will take shape (Fig. 10.2).

i. Patients identified	-	1000
ii. End of prescreening	-	400
iii. End screening (incl/excl)	-	250
iv. Randomized	-	150
v. Qualified/evaluable	-	100

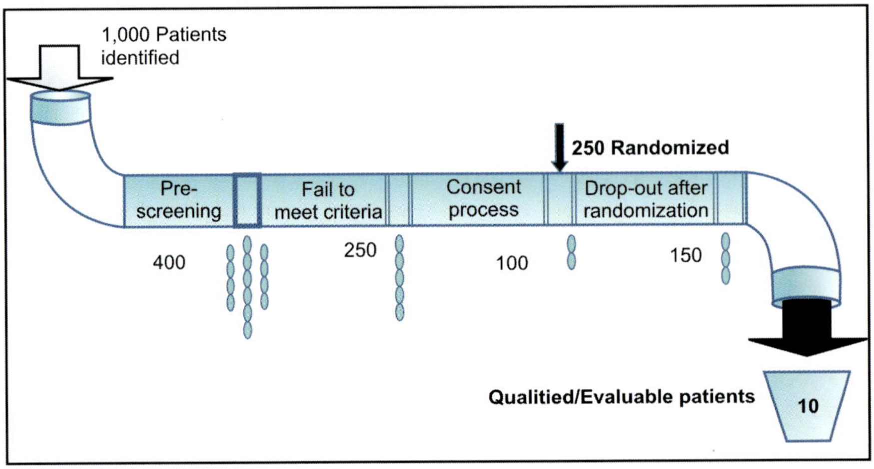

Source: Harper B, Moench L: Patient Focused Performance Driven Clinical Trial Management, December 1997, Vol.6, Number 12

Fig. 10.2 The recruitment metrics

THE RECRUITMENT FUNNEL

Prior to starting a recruitment campaign, an investigator needs to project how many patients he would need to see in order to get 'n' number of patients for screening and what percentage of that he would ultimately be able to enroll for a particular study. This leads to the development of a "recruitment funnel" on the basis of which ultimate study performance would be analyzed. From various prior studies it has been found that on an average only 1 in 20 patients who respond to a recruitment promotion ever complete a study and only 1 out of 5 who respond ever show up for an initial screening.[8] The recruitment funnel is also the basis for setting up budgets for a trial (Fig. 10.3).

STEPS IN THE RECRUITMENT PROCESS

Identify

Protocol suitable patients need to be identified by mining the investigator's database, helping GPs mine their database, through telescreens and prescreens.

Approach

Once protocol suitable patients are identified, they need to be told about the study and their voluntary participation sought. This is done by the investigator who would explain the study to them including the risks and benefits. The patient information sheet is given to them to discuss with members of their family or their personal physician and if they are agreeable to participate they come back for signing the informed consent form and for screening.

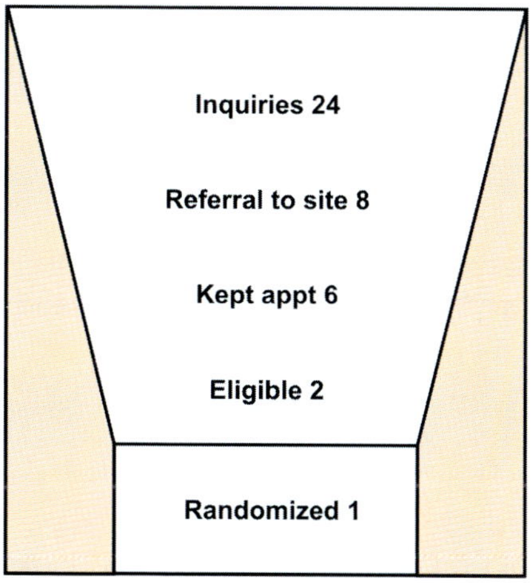

Source: Brescla BA, Budgeting and Contracting in Patient Recruitment, A Guide to Patient Recruitment and Retention by Diana L. Anderson, 143-156

Fig. 10.3: The recruitment funnel

Informed Consent and Screen

Having signed the informed consent patients then undergo screening, which includes a thorough medical history for inclusion/exclusion criteria, a medical examination, lab work, ECG, etc.

Assess

Once the lab reports come in a final assessment is made regarding the suitability of the subject for a particular protocol. If the patient passes the screening tests, he is finally enrolled into the study and randomized.

Enroll—Recruited

Having undergone the above rigorous 5 steps, a patient is enrolled/recruited into a study.

PROFESSIONAL APPROACH TO RECRUITMENT

Planning

Planning for recruitment should start with the initial stages of protocol design so as to make it easy for investigators to recruit patients. Protocols should not be designed so as to make an investigator wonder whether such patients actually exist. Throughout the duration of the study recruitment strategies need to be monitored and assessed and modifications made as per the evaluations. For example, in some studies advertising may bring in far more patients than referrals. In such cases a larger portion of the budget should be allocated for advertisements, which should be given more frequently.

Budgeting

Typically 10-15 percent of a study budget is allocated to recruitment. For some studies this may go to as high as 25 percent.[3] Sponsors currently spend approximately $520 million each year on patient recruitment programs[9] and are increasingly allocating greater portions of this budget to patient recruitment initiatives over and above recruitment through investigators. Budgeting for patient recruitment must start in the early planning stages so that expenses can be anticipated, allocated and contained. Though previously budgeting was decentralized, i.e. individual sites received independent promotional budgets, today the trend is towards centralized recruiting and budgeting where the sponsor is very much aware and in control of recruitment expenditure.

Monitoring and Tracking

All recruitment activities should be monitored for their effectiveness. For different studies, different recruitment methods would work and tracking recruitment that occurs through the various channels would help define the best strategy for that particular study.

Unfortunately at the beginning of a study it is difficult to guess which strategy would be best. If that can be predicted through efforts at previous studies in a particular therapeutic area, planning for recruitment would become a much easier and predictable task.

Metrics

The collection of metrics begins with the first phone call and entails measuring and analyzing the success of various recruitment methods. To evaluate the effectiveness of a recruitment program, not only tracking and monitoring but also recruitment metrics need to be identified. This helps to identify strategies, which are not working so that modifications and remedial measures may be undertaken to salvage enrollment timelines.

Training

Training for recruitment and retention occurs at 2 stages. The first is where the sponsor trains the investigator sites in patient recruitment methodology and for centralized recruitment initiatives. Call center employees involved in the initial telescreens need intensive training in the therapeutic area of the field of study. The second level of training occurs at investigator site, which ensures that the investigative site staff understands the protocol and procedures, and agrees with the recruitment initiatives. They also need to be trained in the informed consent process and the ethical issues involved. Staff is also encouraged to read literature about the condition being studied. The goal of training is to allow the staff to be more proactive throughout recruitment and retention. Training of staff is shown to boost morale and improve confidence leading in the end to better performance.

RETENTION OF STUDY SUBJECTS

The only thing harder than recruiting patients is retaining them in a study. Just as recruitment of study volunteers needs careful planning and well developed strategies, retention of patients for the study duration also needs and deserves attention as a very high dropout rate would make a study statistically invalid. Overall drop-out rates for a study are approximately 25 percent.[10] This rate increases to approximately 30 percent for phase III studies due to their long time commitments.

In order to formulate a good retention plan, several key factors need to be considered including

i. *Patient profile*– Demographics and personal attributes – is the patient educated, is his personality compatible with remaining compliant?
ii. *Key influence*– Patient's primary reason for participating - is the patient participating for the free medication and investigations, is his participation altruistic – to serve mankind or is it that there is no effective therapy for the condition under study?
iii. *Barriers to participation*– What are the patients concerns regarding participation - is he worried about getting time off from work, is he worried he may be getting a placebo?
iv. *Motivators for participation*– What would make the patient happy - small items of appreciation, pre-arranged transport to and from the facility?

There are numerous reasons why volunteers drop out of a clinical trial. Some of the most common reasons include lack of efficacy of the study drug, adverse reactions, too long a study duration, need for invasive procedures, or unfriendly site staff! Occasionally patients may drop out due to time constraints, lack of transportation or if the protocol is too complex and difficult for him to follow.

Retention of study volunteers is linked to how valued they feel and how well they are treated at each point of contact, i.e. showing respect and delivering good customer service. Subjects want and deserve personal attention from everyone they come in contact with at the site. They want their questions answered. Subjects who adhere to a study are generally ones who are well informed about the study, those who have regimen aids, and are well compensated for their travel and time. They also have a sense of commitment and a sense of belonging. Several retention tools such as newsletters, appointment reminders with phone calls or mail, follow-up phone calls, education material, and appreciation items at intervals help in retaining subjects through a long study.

RECENT ADVANCES

Professional Recruitment Providers

Professional recruitment providers today often work with sponsors, CROs and SMOs to improve recruitment efforts at a site. These companies can structure media campaigns, design and place adverts and follow-up the strategy as the study unfolds.

Increased Use of Market Research

Sponsors are increasingly turning toward market research strategies to increase patient recruitment. Market research can segment populations based on demography (age, gender, ethnicity and education levels), geography (urban, rural, state), psychology (attitude, lifestyle, hobbies) and behavior. With market research sponsors can gain access to the media behavior of their cluster of patients and therefore focused media campaigns can be developed for the target audience. Therefore, market research can ensure that the advertisements are placed with the right message in the right media so that members of the target group are exposed to the message repeatedly.

Informatics

Informatics is a database driven approach to finding good potential subjects. An informatics service could provide de-identified data obtained from pharmacies, physicians, hospitals, insurance companies, etc. This service would be able to say whether a particular condition is more prevalent in a particular area or if the inclusion/exclusion criteria are too narrow. Once the population is defined an informatics service provider would target it with a direct mail campaign.

Centralized Recruiting

Centralized prescreening means that there is one centralized location for all information regarding potential participants. The goal is to ensure that only the most suitable candidates are scheduled at the various research sites. This procedure facilitates accurate tracking and analysis of recruitment activities.

Development of Metrics – "The Leaky-pipe Analysis"

To evaluate the effectiveness of a recruitment program, recruitment metrics need to be identified. The "Leaky-pipe Analysis" is a visual aid.[11] Once identified, the leaky areas of the pipeline need to be repaired. This not only helps in tracking the recruitment process but also helps to repair when damages are done.

CONCLUSIONS

As the number of clinical trials increase, the number of patients needed for clinical trials continues to increase. Traditional recruitment methods have failed to deliver recruitment goals within the specified timeframes, making sponsors look for newer innovations for recruitment. Thus, recruitment of subjects today has become a partnering process between the sponsor and an investigator site. Exploring the difficulties of recruitment and retention helps in growing, learning and improving on the next project.

REFERENCES

1. Cutting Edge Information, Accelerating Clinical Trials: Budgets, Patient Recruitment and Productivity, May 2004.
2. Hirschhorn WM, Understanding the Protocol as a Foundation for developing a viable Patient Recruitment Campaign, Aug 2, 2004, www.temple.edu/ovpr/oct/doc/understanding_the_protocol.doc.
3. Tufts Centre for Study Drug Development. Food Drug Law Journal 2002.
4. New Approaches to Patient Recruitment, ARCP White Paper, 2002.
5. Kittredge CA. Shrinking Target, Ip-Health, April 2005, http://www.the- scientist.com/2005/4/11/46/1.
6. Barriers to Clinical Trial Enrollment-National Cancer Institute, www.cancer.gov/clinical trials/developments.
7. Patel MX et al, Challenges in recruitment of Research Participants, Advances in Psychiatric Treatment 2003, vol 9,229-38.
8. Patient Recruitment Strategies, NIH Training Workshop, December 2003, www.nichd. nih.gov/about/ncmrr/workshops/Recruit.pdf.
9. Centerwatch Survey, 1999, 2000.
10. Centerwatch Survey, 2002.
11. Anderson DL, The Patient Recruitment Market: A History and Overview of Today's Issues, A Guide to Patient Recruitment and Retention, 3-11.

11 Project Management in Clinical Trials

Arun Bhatt

INTRODUCTION

The discovery and development of a new drug costs $800-1000 million and takes longer than 10 years. Clinical development, the most important step prior to a drug entering the market, takes over five years. Each day's delay in completing the drug development and launching the product in the market means a revenue loss of $1.5 million. With the increasing cost and time pressures, the clinical trials are an important area where project management techniques are applied. The pharmaceutical companies use project management techniques and tools to plan for a timely and successful entry of a new product in the market. This chapter reviews the current concepts of project management.

EVOLUTION OF PROJECT MANAGEMENT

The concept of project management traces its origins to development of planning techniques such as Gantt chart, Program Evaluation and Review Technique (PERT) and Critical Path Method (CPM). The Gantt chart is named after Henry L Gantt, who was awarded a US presidential citation for his application of this type of chart to ship building during World War I. The PERT was developed by the United States Department of Defense. The department, faced with the sputnik crisis, needed to speed up the military project process. In 1958, they invented the PERT, as part of the Polaris missile submarine program. This was a massive project involving over 3000 contractors. As most of activities had never been done before, there was an uncertainty about the time estimates. The PERT was developed to handle these uncertainties. Around the same time, the DuPont Corporation created a new project management tool called Critical Path Method (CPM) for scheduling maintenance shutdowns at their chemical processing plants. Over the years, the features that distinguished CPM and PERT have diminished. These concepts, because of their inherent utility in the product development, were quickly adopted by the industry.

PROJECT

A project is defined as a series of related activities or tasks usually directed toward some major output and requiring a significant period of time to perform. A project is a temporary venture undertaken to create a unique product e.g. drug or service e.g. clinical trial. The term temporary implies that the project has a distinct start and a distinct end. Typical projects might include the construction of a factory, or the development of a software program, or development of a new drug. The duration of a project is the time from the beginning to completion, which may take several days, months or years.

Project Management

Project management includes the planning, supervising, and managing resources (manpower, money, materials, and machines) to meet the technical, cost, time and quality requirements of the project. The project management is the process to quantify the resources — amount of time and budget — a project will cost. The goal of the project management in a clinical trial is to control the key variables: time, quality and cost. The planning, implementation and monitoring of a major project requires setting up a competent project team.

Clinical Trial Project Team

The clinical trial project team (Fig. 11.1) consists of

- Project manager
- Medical adviser
- Clinical research associate/s
- Data manager

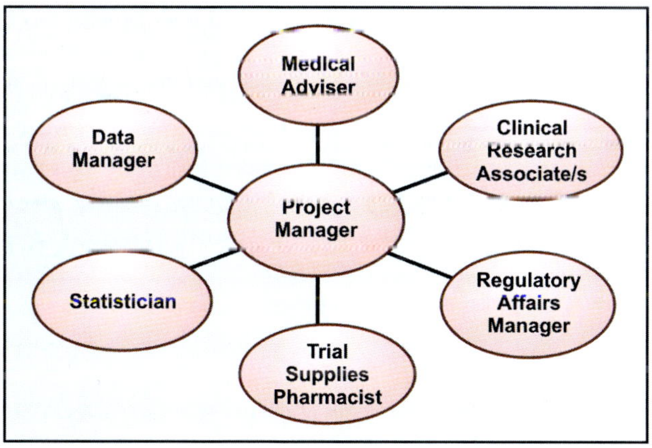

Fig. 11.1: Project team structure

- Statistician
- Regulatory affairs manager
- Trial supplies pharmacist.

Each member has a specific role in the team.

Project Manager

The project manager is the person who has the overall responsibility for the successful planning and execution of any project. Most project managers oversee two or three projects. The project managers usually have a life science background and have over five years' experience in a pharmaceutical company or a contract research organization (CRO).

The project manager's important responsibilities are;

- Leading the project team
- Developing the project budget
- Coordinating and tracking project activities
- Creating and controlling project timelines
- Directing team meetings
- Managing project resources
- Preparing agendas and minutes for meetings
- Handling project communications.

The project manager, to shoulder these wide responsibilities, requires training in several areas:

- Drug development
- Leadership
- People management
- Cost and budget management
- Time management
- Problem solving
- Communication
- Effective presentations
- Negotiation.

S/he requires a thorough understanding of the planning process and an appreciation of the critical elements in the integrated trial management function both from local and global viewpoint. S/he should be able to consider the strategic, tactical and operational issues and options, and the practical management of projects by critical path analysis.

Project Team Members

Each member of the project team has a specific and well defined role. For instance, the medical advisor is responsible for the preparation of protocol and supporting medical aspects of the trial, whist the regulatory affairs manager looks after regulatory approval of the clinical trial. The team members are responsible to tracking progress of their task in their own functions and reporting.them to the project manager. Each team member should have broad knowledge of drug development, in depth understanding of his/her own special function and its impact on other functions. Besides, they also must be proficient in communication, interpersonal, and time management skills.

MANAGING THE PROJECT

The project manager, along with his/her team, sets up the project and runs it. The different stages in the process are:

- Project initiation
- Project planning
- Project execution
- Project monitoring
- Project completion.

Project Initiation

The major activities are:

- Development of project proposal
- Deciding the objectives of the project

A project begins as a project proposal, which includes a written description of the objectives of the project, a brief statement of the work to be done and a proposed schedule specifying the start and completion steps and the written reports to be provided. The project proposal provides a description of budget, measures of performance, and project milestones (specific events to be reached at points in time) and work break down structure (WBS). The WBS defines the hierarchy of the project tasks, subtasks and work packages. The WBS is important in organizing a project because it breaks down the project into manageable pieces. The number of levels - tasks, subtasks, work package — will vary depending on the complexity of the project. A task is a subdivision of the project, which is usually no longer than several months and performed by one function, e.g. trial supply pharmacy. The task may be further split into subtasks.

A work package is a group of activities, which can be assigned to a single functional unit in a company. For example, the task of regulatory approval will include the key activities such as preparation of investigational new drug (IND) application. The activities are chunks that consume time but may not always require effort from a team member, e.g. making copies of documents for ethics committee submission.

Project Planning

The purpose of project planning is to develop a project management plan that a project manager can use to track the progress of the tasks.

The steps in developing a plan are:

i. Determine the exact end points for the success of the project to be completed or to terminate the project. In clinical trials, the success of the project depends on the completion of required number of patients in the expected time frame. The project may get extended if the completed patient numbers are not achieved. In case a planned interim analysis shows the drug to be unsafe, the project may be terminated.

ii. Describe all the key tasks to be done by each team member and assess how much time it will take to complete each activity. This requires a discussion with all the project team members. Each major task will be split into subtasks of shorter duration. For example, the task of obtaining regulatory permission is subdivided into several subtasks as follows:

- Collection of regulatory documents, e.g. chemistry, manufacturing, control data; preclinical; clinical data
- Preparation of protocol, case record form and consent documents
- Obtaining consent and undertaking from the investigators
- Compilation of IND application
- Submission of IND application.

The time required for each of the subtask can affect the final outcome–clinical trial permission.

iii. Describe how the tasks depend on each other and the required sequence of activities. Identify the immediate predecessors linked to each activity. The immediate predecessors are the activities that need to be completed immediately before an activity. For example, the IND application cannot be made unless all the required documents are available. Once the dependencies are identified, the project manager can sequence the tasks into the likely completion order, and create a project network.

iv. Determine the critical path. Assess the minimum time the project will require. This is the longest path through the project network from the start to finish. This path is the critical path. Any delay in any critical path activity will automatically delay the overall deadline of the project. If a single estimate of the time required to complete an activity is not reliable, the best procedure is to use three time estimates. The estimated activity time is calculated using a weighted average of a minimum, maximum, and most likely time estimate.

v. Identify the resource requirements - manpower, money, and materials-to complete each of the tasks. One key resource is the cost. The project management creates a time-cost model - the link between time to complete an activity and the financial resources required. The basic assumption is that there is a relationship between activity completion time and the cost of a project. The time-cost model tries to develop a minimum-cost schedule for an entire project and to control expenditures during the project. On one hand, it costs money to expedite an activity; on the other it costs money to sustain or lengthen the project. The costs include the time and efforts of manpower employed on the project and resource related, e.g. buying of equipments.

vi. Develop a project schedule in the form of project control charts and milestones. Milestones are major time points and stages in a project's life. For projects involving clinical trials, these usually include:
   1. Project start date
   2. Document completion dates
   3. Approval dates
   4. Site initiation
   5. First patient first visit
   6. Recruitment of 50 percent of subjects
   7. Last patient first visit
   8. Last patient last visit
   9. Database lock
   10. Report

vii. Anticipate the problems and plan for risk management.

viii. Discuss the plan with the team members and obtain their commitment.

Project Control Charts

Gantt Chart

This is a bar chart (Fig. 11.2) showing both the amount of time involved and the sequence in which activities can be performed. This type of chart is easily understood and widely used. The Gantt chart is able to relate to activities to time in a usable fashion for small projects. However, it is not suitable for large and complex project that include more than 25 activities. As the number of activities increase, it becomes difficult to visualize the interrelationship of activities. Besides, the Gantt chart does not provide any direct procedure for determining the critical path.

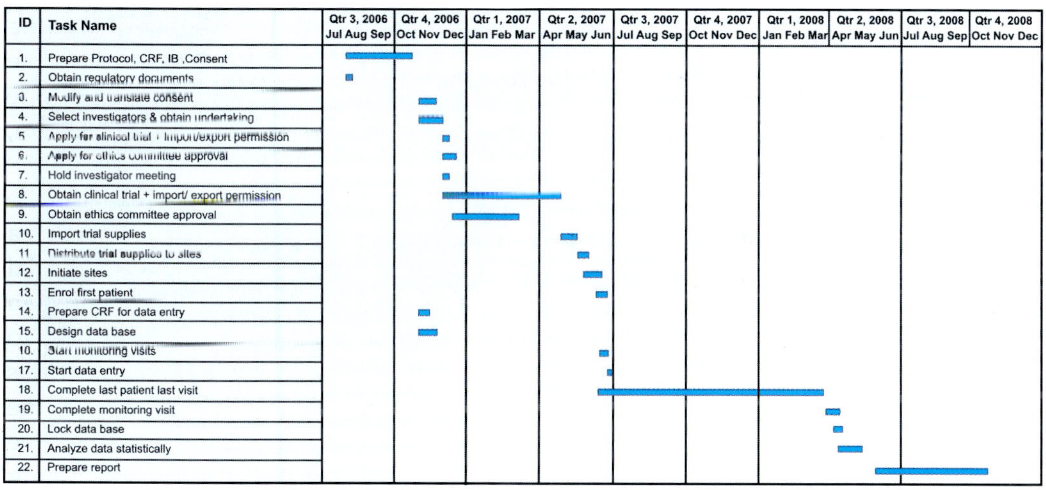

Fig. 11.2: Gantt chart of a clinical trial

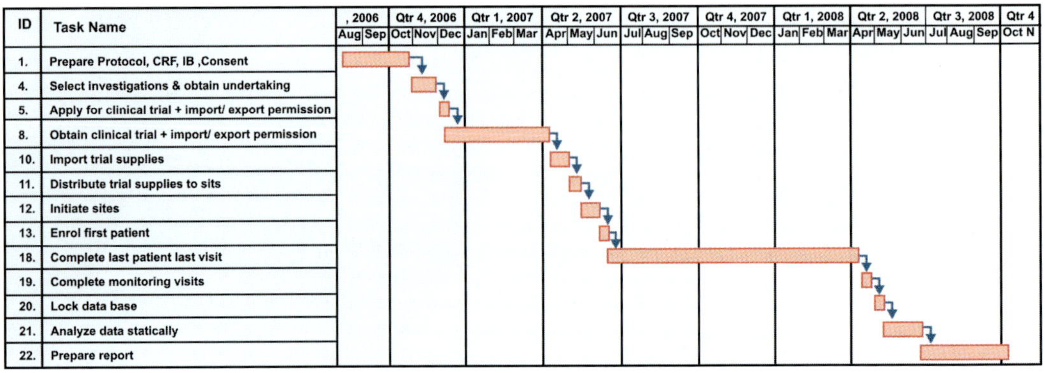

Fig. 11.3: Critical path for a clinical trial

CPM

The CPM (Fig. 11.3), referred as network method, is more complex compared Gantt chart, as it illustrates and documents how multiple processes are interdependent and can be followed in each project. The CPM is based on the assumptions that project activity times can be estimated accurately. The objective of CPM is to determine scheduling information about each activity in the project. The critical path of activities is the sequence of activities that form the longest chain in terms of time to complete. This method calculates when an activity must start and end, together with whether the activity is part of the critical path. The CPM is usually accompanied by a listing of all of the separate activities shown. It is desirable to list activities for each individual function responsible for those activities, e.g. regulatory, trial supplies etc. These lists may then be used by the respective functions as planning tools.

The Gantt chart and CPM are constructed using soft wares such as MS Project or Primavera SureTrack. MS Project aids in scheduling, allocating and tracking as well as in monitoring the costs and producing presentation quality graphs and reports.

Critical Path Activities for a Clinical Trial Project

The activities on the critical path (Fig. 11.3) are:

- Prepare protocol, CRF, IB, consent
- Select investigators and obtain undertaking
- Apply for clinical trial + import / export permission
- Obtain clinical trial + import / export permission
- Import trial supplies
- Distribute trial supplies to sites
- Initiate sites
- Enroll first patient
- Complete last patient last visit
- Complete monitoring visits
- Lock data base

- Analyze data statistically
- Prepare report

These tasks further depend on the sub tasks e.g. regulatory permission depends on availability of regulatory documents. Besides, some task can only be done after an earlier task is completed, e.g. site initiation can be done only after the regulatory and ethics approval are available. In contrast, there are other tasks, which are important, but can be completed in parallel to the above critical tasks, e.g. holding investigator meeting.

Project Execution

The focus of this stage is on:

- Running the project as per the plan
- Reporting the achievement of milestones
- Reviewing and modifying the project plan, if needed.

During this stage, the project is tracked by a tracking Gantt chart. This tracking chart superimposes the current schedule onto the planned schedule so that the deviations can be visualized and managed.

Project Controlling

This is the key responsibility of project manager. S/he has to monitor the project in terms of time and resources, and plan risk management. A risk is a possible event, which can negatively affect the schedule or cost or quality. The risk management would involve making decisions. The decisions could be:

a. Changing the project timelines.
b. Adding more resources e.g. funds.
c. Terminating the project if in spite of changing time-cost variables, the project goals are impossible to achieve.

For example, the project manager should be able to judge early in the project whether the selected sites will be able to achieve the target recruitment rate of patients. If this appears unlikely, s/he may need to consider adding more sites.

Project Closeout

This stage is the conclusion of the project. The project manager will report on the successful completion of the project. The report would capture:

- Achievements vis-à-vis objectives,
- Time taken vs. the scheduled time
- Costs incurred vs. the budget
- Problems faced and solved.

SUCCESS OF PROJECT

The project management is the heart and soul of any project. Effective project management requires scheduling and tracking the critical path, and a committed team working under a competent project manager. The success of a project depends on excellent communication within team, a simple and timely reporting by team members, and clear delimitation of responsibilities of each team member and above all leadership from a talented project manager.

SUGGESTED READING

1. Chase RB, Aquilano NJ, Roberts Jacobs F, Operations Management for Competitive Advantage, 9th (ed) Tata McGraw-Hill New Delhi 2002; pp 56-87.

12

Pharmacovigilance in Clinical Research

Moin Don

INTRODUCTION

Pharmacovigilance—International Scenario

Pharmacovigilance has always been considered a critical activity by almost all the key stake holders, associated with drugs, and its high place in organizational priorities has never been questioned. From time to time, episodes like thalidomide tragedy (1962) and cardiovascular risks posed by COX 2 inhibitors (2005), only add emphasis to this ever evolving medico-regulatory discipline.

Traditionally speaking, the science of pharmacovigilance has been a discipline more focused on the post marketing or post authorization period. As a part of 'Risk Management Tool' it has not only an important role to play in patients' safety, but it has also assumed astronomical significance, to safeguard pharma industry against possible loss of revenue through damaging litigations and declining share value. However, as biological sciences have evolved, pharmacovigilance has also become an integral part of new drug development process. The new regulations require that the would be marketing authorization holders submit in the application dossier, a comprehensive review of the safety profile of the new drug, and how the potential risks will be further investigated and/or minimized during life cycle of medicines.

Most of the regulations that describe safety reporting from clinical trials (CTs) focus on the expedited reporting of the individual case safety reports (ICSRs). ICH guidelines E2A which is generally considered the standard for the information to be sent, stipulates that sponsors should submit suspected adverse drug reactions that are both serious and unexpected to the regulators within 7 (if fatal or life threatening) or 15 calendar days in an appropriate format.[1]

Expedited single case reports from clinical trials (CTs) are accepted by majority of the Regulatory Authorities (RAs) on the CIOMS I or similar form. With the adoption of ICH Guidelines E2B[2] and then E2B(M), [3] which define standard data elements for electronic ICSRs, some RAs have begun to require the electronic submission of expedited reports in the post marketing scenario.

More recently, the European Union (EU) and Japan have begun requiring electronic submission of the expedited reports from CTs as well.

While the time frames and reporting criteria, that are Suspected, Unexpected, Serious, Adverse, Reactions (SUSARs) for expedited reporting are mostly consistent across the ICH regions, there are authorities that require expedited reporting of suspected SADRs, regardless of 'expectedness'.

The CIOMS VI Working Group endorses the ICH Guidelines E2A for expedited reporting and recommends that, *"Under exceptional circumstances and on an ad hoc basis, should sponsor be expected to report on an expedited basis SADRs that are considered expected"*.[4] The diversified reporting requirements are summarized in Box 12.1.[5]

Box 12.1: Requirements for diversified expedited reporting

Country	
US	SUL (serious unexpected local)+SUF (serious unexpected foreign)
UK	SUL + SUF
Japan	SUL+SEL (serious expected local)+SUF; also SEF if fatal or life threatening
France	SUL+SUF+SAEs having potential effect on trial designs (if studied in France)

As evident from the table, it is only 'SUSARs', are eligible for expedited reporting to the regulators in the above named countries, with the lone exception of Japan. Such regulation then pre-empt submission of weird unrelated cases, such as hip fracture, nerve injury involving machine accident, enteric fever, to the regulators.

On the international front the Council for International Organizations of Medical Sciences (CIOMS), which, has proposed common policies for international postmarket drug, adverse event reporting over the last 20 years, recently moved to consider surveillance and safety reporting related to clinical trials. Recently the CIOMS VI working group on managing safety information from clinical trials of medicinal products issued a final report offering recommendations for implementing common safety information reporting systems around the world. The report addresses expedited and periodic safety reporting and draws from the provisions in ICH documents, World Health Organization guidelines, and relevant EU directives and guidelines.

The report advises the research community to replace the current practice of sending large numbers of individual case reports to IRBs and IECs. *Sponsors instead should submit "periodic and ad hoc communications" to investigators and ECs, with expedited communications focusing on "significant new safety information" that has "implications for the conduct of the clinical trial."* This approach follows the European policy of expedited reporting of serious and unexpected suspected adverse reactions (SUSARs), but still leaves it to investigators to decide what events warrant more aggressive reporting [6].

Spontaneous reporting and Periodic Safety Update Reports (PSURs) form the backbone of the traditional, post marketing surveillance activities throughout the pharma world. US FDA's MedWatch forms and MHRA's 'Yellow Cards' have almost become synonyms with spontaneous reporting. While US FDA recommends voluntary spontaneous reporting of all serious suspected ADRs through form 3500A, for health care professionals, it makes such reporting mandatory for the marketing Authorization Holders (MAHs) and draws very stringent timelines and reporting requirements.

The international expedited reporting requirements, in post authorization era are summarized in Box 12.2.[5]

Box 12.2: Requirements for international expedited reporting

Country	
US	SUL (serious unexpected local)+SUF (serious unexpected foreign)
Canada	SUL + SEL + SUF
UK	SUL + SEL (within MS) / SUF + SEF (from other EU) / SUF (Non EU)
Japan	SUL + SEL + SUF + non serious unexpected local (NUL)
France	SUL + SEL (within MS) / SUF (Non EU)

All other adverse events/reactions, which are not reported to regulators, in an expedited manner are included in periodic clinical trial reports (in case of pre-marketed development phase) and for marketed products in form of PSURs.

A PSUR is "a formal, structured update of the worldwide safety experience for a registered medicinal product (per ICH E2C standards), prepared for submission to regulatory authorities at defined times post authorization". The contents of a PSUR (as per EU requirements) are as follows;

1. Introduction.
2. Worldwide market authorization status.
3. Update of regulatory authority or Market Authorization Holder (MAH) ↔ actions taken for safety reasons.
4. Changes to reference safety information.
5. Patient exposure data (marketed use, clinical trials, post marketing studies).
6. Presentation of individual case histories.
7. Studies.
8. Other information.
9. Overall safety evaluation (R/B Analysis).
10. Conclusions.
11. Appendices.

The periodicity and contents as required in US and EU can be summarized as follows:

EU requirements

- Even if not marketed
- Six-monthly – first 2 years
- Annual – subsequent 2 years
- At the first renewal, and then
- 5-yearly at renewal thereafter
- Based on IBD

Contd...

Contd...

- One PSUR for each active substance
- To be submitted within 60 days of last data lock

US requirements

- Pre-approval PSUR–4 months after application
- Post-approval for each approved NDA/ ANDA/BLA
- Quarterly– for first 3 years
- Then annual interval / on request
- Within 30 days of the close of quarter
- Annual reports within 60 days
- Divided into 4 sections
- Section – 1: 15 day alert reports
- Actions taken (labelling changes/new studies)
- Line listing of reporting form (other than above)
- FDA forms 3500A.

The US FDA and EMEA, now have gone, a step beyond these well known current pharmacovigilance practices, by asking Marketing Authorization Applicants (MAAs) to submit Pharmacovigilance Plan (as per ICH- E2E guidelines) as a part of a larger Risk Management Program (RMP) during the approval process itself.[Article 8 (3)(ia) of Directive 2001/83/EC]. To assist MAAS and MAHs in complying with the requirements the EMEA has published the 'Guidelines on risk management system'.

[EMEA/CHMP/96268/2005] which incorporates the concepts of ICH-E2E guidelines. Hence, risk management, (a proactive approach to the safety profile of a medicines, which is continuously updated throughout the lifecycle of the product), is an important advance in the sphere of pharmacovigilance and would have great implications and impact on all the important stakeholders in time to come.

Clinical Trials and Pharmacovigilance: Indian Scenario

Clinical research is currently in the news for its immense business potential in India. The current 30 million US dollar business is likely to increase ten fold by the year 2010. The only possible hurdle, which could seriously hamper such a development, is the apprehension in the minds of outsourcing companies about the quality of data and acceptance of such data by the global regulatory authorities, in general and the US FDA, in particular. And this apprehension stems from the fact that only a fraction of about 500,000 doctors are trained in ICH-GCP, which could mean inadequate documentation and inaccurate safety profiling of the New Chemical Entity (NCE).

According to the US FDA Federal Regulation of 1938, establishing the safety of a new molecule is a pre-requisite for obtaining a marketing approval. This was further corroborated by the infamous thalidomide tragedy (phocomelia among pregnant women) in 1962, which amply demonstrated that the "Safety" consideration Must take precedence over the "Efficacy" consideration of NCE. Ever since, all the regulators and health care authorities, worldwide have established very stringent codes for conducting clinical trials. These guidelines have undergone constant evolution, starting from the Helsinki declaration adopted by the World Medical Assembly (WMA) in 1964 to the current ICH-GCP guidelines. The only aim of these directives is to safeguard the rights and well-being of the trial subjects.

"Efficacy" of a new molecule can be demonstrated through 'positive findings' (results) that indicate its therapeutic usefulness. On the other hand "Safety" of the new molecule can only be established by its 'lack of relative risk' to the patients. This can be done only if the trial subjects on study medications are closely and diligently monitored for 'possible' adverse experiences / reactions (refer the section on definitions) during the study. The timely and continuous analysis of the safety and efficacy data in terms of 'Risk/Benefit Ratio' of the NCE is very critical to the conduct of the study involving the new molecule.

It is important that irrespective of the, seriousness, expectedness or causality assessment (see definitions section) , all adverse events experienced (and not only ADRs, where causality is implied) are monitored , documented adequately and accurately and then reported in a pre-decided timely manner. Medical evaluation of the safety data, alone would ensure safety and well-being of the trial subjects.

Though it is critical to monitor and collect maximum possible information about the patient (demographic details, medical history), medication (concomitant as well as study medication), and the event itself (temporal relationship, concurrent illnesses, if any), its all the more necessary that the Serious Adverse Events (SAEs) are reported by the investigators to the sponsor in the prescribed format within pre-defined timelines, in an expedited manner. This is essential in order to comply with the strict regulatory requirements all over the world. (see schedule Y and international regulations of expedited reporting requirements). Often it is necessary to do a follow up of the ongoing Adverse Event (AE), till its resolution and the causality assessment from the investigator is most desirable.

Pharmacovigilance: Basic Concepts and Definitions

Pharmacovigilance

"This is the science of collecting, monitoring, researching and evaluating data on the effects of medicinal drugs, biological products, herbals and traditional medicines with a view to identifying new information about adverse reactions and preventing harm to patients."[7]

Aims of Pharmacovigilance[8]

The aims of the pharmacovigilance can broadly be described as follows;

- Improve patient care and safety in relation to the use of medicines and all medical and paramedical interventions

- Improve public health and safety in relation to use of medicines
- Contribute to the assessment of benefit, harm, effectiveness, and risk of medicines, encouraging their safe, rational, and more effective use
- Promote understanding, education and clinical training in pharmacovigilance and its effective communication to public.

Adverse Event/Adverse Experience (AE)

Any untoward and undesirable medical experience in a patient or clinical investigation subject administered a medicinal product and that does not necessarily have a causal relationship with this treatment.

The WHO defines an AE as [9]—

"Any untoward medical occurrence that may present during treatment with a pharmaceutical product but which does not necessarily have a causal relationship with this treatment."

Adverse Drug Reaction (ADR)

'A response to a drug which is noxious and unintended, and which occurs at doses normally used for the prophylaxis, diagnosis or therapy of disease, or for the modification of physiological function.'[9]

To this basic definition, the European Union adds the following:

'A reaction, contrary to an event, is characterized by the fact that a causal relationship between the drug and the occurrence is suspected, i.e. judged possible by the reporting or reviewing healthcare professional.' 'An adverse drug event that is judged to be caused by the drug'.[10]

Serious Adverse Event (SAE)[11]

A Serious Adverse Event is any untoward medical occurrence that at any dose:

- Results in death
- Is life-threatening
- Requires inpatient hospitalization or prolongation of existing hospitalization
- Results in persistent or significant disability or incapacity
- Is a congenital anomaly or birth defect.

Medical and scientific judgment should be exercised in deciding whether expedited reporting is appropriate in situations where none of the outcomes listed in the serious adverse event definition occurred. Important medical event that may not be immediately life threatening or results in death or hospitalization but may jeopardize the patient or may require intervention to prevent one of the other outcomes listed in the definition above should also usually be considered serious.

A list of "critical terms" compiled by WHO may be used as a guiding document to assess seriousness of such an Adverse Event that may be considered medically important.

1. *Seriousness and Severity*

At this juncture, it is worthwhile to understand the difference between these two important terms, which cause lot of confusion and often results in erroneous reporting.

Seriousness serves as a guide for defining regulatory reporting obligations, whereas Severity describes the intensity of the event (mild, moderate, severe), and may be of relatively minor medical significance.

2. *Side Effect*[12]

A non-specific term used to describe an unwanted effect of a drug. Note that the term is sometimes used to imply an ADR predictable on pharmacological grounds, i.e. a type A reaction.

A side effect is defined by the World Health Organization as 'Any unintended effect of a pharmaceutical product occurring at doses normally used in man which is related to the pharmacological properties of the drug'. [13]

The term usually, but not necessarily, implies an undesirable effect. For instance, in the treatment of peptic ulcer with atropine, dryness of the mouth is a side effect and decreased gastric secretion is the desired drug effect. If the same drug was being used to inhibit salivation, dryness of the mouth would be the therapeutic effect and decreased gastric secretion would be a side effect.

3. *Spontaneous Report*[14]

"An unsolicited communication to a company, regulatory authority or other organization that describes an adverse drug reaction in a patient, given one or more medicinal products, and which does not derive from a study or any organized data collection scheme".

4. *SUSAR (Suspected, Unexpected, Serious, Adverse, Reaction)*

This term (acronym) was introduced by EU Clinical Trial Directive in connection with expedited reporting: All suspected adverse reactions related to an Investigational Medicinal Product and comparator, that are both 'Unexpected' (see definition below) and 'Serious' are subject to expedited reporting." These are also known as 15 Days reports, to be disseminated to other participating investigators with 'Dear Investigator Letter (DIL)'. For detail guidance: http://pharmacos.eudra.org/F2/pharmacos/docs)

5. *Unexpected AE/ADR*[15]

"An AE/ ADR, is one for which the nature, or severity, is not consistent with information in the relevant source documents, domestic labeling or market authorization, or expected from characteristics of the drug."

Under 21 CFR 314.80 the FDA defines, an unexpected ADE as:

"Any ADE that is not listed in the current FDA approved labeling for the drug or licensed biological product. It also includes an AE that may be symptomatically and pathophysiologically related to an event listed in the labeling, but differs from the event because of greater severity or specificity.

Causality Assessment

The Food and Drug Administration (FDA) define a causality assessment as;

"Determination of whether there is reasonable possibility that the product is etiologically related to the adverse experience. Causality assessment includes, for example, the assessment of temporal relationships, dechallenge/rechallenge information, association (or lack of association) with underlying disease, and the presence (or absence) of a more likely cause and physiological/pathological plausibility".

Causality assessment of AEs is the structured and standardized assessment of individual patients/case reports for the likelihood of involvement of suspected drug in causing particular event in a given patient. Basically, it is an exercise to assess whether there is a reasonable possibility that the adverse event is associated with the marketed product or study medication?

This question is asking if there was a reasonable possibility that the drug under question, caused or may have contributed to causing the adverse event. There are two different questions concerning causality.

1. Is it possible that the drug can cause the AE?
2. Has the drug actually caused the event in given patient?

For fair medical evaluation of every case, it is important that the reporting physician's assessment of causal relationship is obtained. In order to medically evaluate the cases for causality, the following criteria can be made use of;

1. Pharmacological plausibility.
2. Temporal relationship between administration of suspect drug and onset of ADR.
3. Response to rechallenge.
4. Response to dechallenge or presence of established risk factor/s.
5. Alternative explanation to ADR .

In assessing causality, the above mentioned criteria can be further elaborated as follows[16];

- Timing or temporal relationship (time interval between taking the drug and the appearance of the AE/ADR, i.e. plausibility and consistency of time to onset between cases)
- Dose-response relationship (positive dose response, known effect in drug overdose cases)
- Pharmacology (there is a known mechanism, the drug is known to affect the same body system as the AE/ADR, pharmacokinetic evidence, recognized class effect of the drug, similar findings in animal studies, biological/pharmacological plausibility)
- Withdrawal (positive dechallenge)
- Reproducibility of event upon re-exposure (positive rechallenge)
- Pattern/previous cases (evidence from clinical trials and/or post-marketing surveillance studies, similar AEs/ADRs already recognized for the drug, clear-cut easily evaluated cases (e.g. index cases), high frequency of reports, recognized consequence of drug overdose)

- Opinion of reporter (reports being of high status (credibility))
- Absence of alternative causes (lack of confounding factors, lack of obvious alternative explanations, concomitant medication being unlikely to have played a role).

The expression 'reasonable causal relationship' means that there is evidence of reasonable arguments that might suggest a causal relationship.

From a regulatory point of view, all cases judged by either the reporting doctor or the marketing authorization holder (MAH)/licensed manufacturer as having a reasonable suspected causal relationship to the medicinal product qualify as suspected adverse reactions. The classification given by the doctor cannot be overruled by the MAH. If the MAH/licensed manufacturer disagrees with the causality classification of the reporter, they should provide a comment in the report submitted to the regulatory authority. The opinions of both the reporter and the MAH/licensed manufacturer should always appear on the reporting / declaration form. In clinical trials, causality assessment is the judgment of either the investigator or the sponsor's safety department. The final decision of the investigator conducting a clinical trial of the causality assessment between the AE and the investigational product is final and may not, normally, be changed. Again, the classification given by the doctor should not be overruled by the sponsor. If the MAH/licensed manufacturer disagrees with the causality classification of the investigator, a comment from the MAH/licensed manufacturer should be provided.[17]

Dechallenge[16]: The clinical decision to withdraw / discontinue a drug treatment after a possible ADR has occurred. The response to dechallenge is a major factor used in the evaluation of causality assessment. A dechallenge is positive or suggestive if the reaction abates, partially or completely when the drug is withdrawn and is considered to be 'negative' or 'against' if the reaction does not abate when the treatment is stopped. A dechallenge is positive if the event/reaction appears after each dose and abates after a time. Dechallenge may not be evaluable (e.g. reaction resulted in death) or may be irreversible. It is also not applicable where;

- Drug is one dose treatment (vaccine)
- Reaction occurred after the drug was discontinued
- Lack of efficacy, congenital anomaly.

Rechallenge[17]: The deliberate or inadvertent administration of a further dose(s) of the same medicinal product to a person who has previously experienced an adverse event / adverse drug reaction that might be drug-related. The Food and Drug Administration (FDA) defines rechallenge as the 'reintroduction of a suspect product suspected of having caused an adverse experience following a positive dechallenge. Failure of the product, when reintroduced, to produce signs and symptoms similar to those observed when the suspect drug was previously introduced implies a negative rechallenge, while recurrence of similar signs and symptoms upon reintroduction of the suspect product implies a positive one.

The response to rechallenge is a major factor used in the causality assessment of drug causality.

A rechallenge is not applicable if:

- The suspect drug was a one-dose treatment
- The drug was not discontinued and reintroduced
- The event/reaction occurred after the product was discontinued.

For ethical reasons, deliberate rechallenge is rarely performed, but it may be carried out when the results are in the interest of the patient suffering the reaction, particularly when there are no suitable alternative drugs.[21]

There are two (2) stages of causality assessment;

1. Causality assessment-1st stage: Assessment of individual case reports.
2. 2nd stage: Interpretation of aggregated data.

Different methodologies and algorithms are employed to assess and describe the causality of the AEs, of which the most commonly used are;

1. WHO assessment scale: After consulting with all participating countries, the Uppsala Monitoring Centre of WHO has established 6 defined causality categories, namely[18];
   - Certain
   - Probable
   - Possible
   - Unlikely
   - Conditional
   - Unassessable/ unclassifiable
2. Naranjo's scale: a method for estimating the probability of ADRs.[19]
3. The European ABO System.[20]

"The CIOMS VI Working Group recommends that the investigators be asked to use a simple 'Binary Decision' for drug causality ('Related' or 'Not Related') for SAEs."

RESPONSIBILITIES OF THE STAKE HOLDERS

Sponsors of the clinical trials, the investigators, the Ethics Committees (Including IRBs) and the Local Regulators, all of them have great responsibilities, towards the safety of the trial subjects. Unless these are understood properly and due care taken for diligent monitoring is taken safety of trial subjects can not be ensured. That's why it essential that the sponsors and the investigators particularly and the other stake holders like Ethics Committees and the Regulators diligently heed for their responsibilities, the gist of which is summarized here under:

Responsibilities of the Sponsor

Some of the main responsibilities of the sponsor (not all inclusive) are as follows;

1. To have proper Standard Operating Procedures (SOPs), which would discuss and ensure.

- Protocol designs w.r.t safety aspects
- Process involved and
- Timelines in safety reporting.

2. It is also the responsibility of the sponsor to train
   - Study team and
   - Investigators in the process of safety reporting.
3. To have resources and Infrastructure to monitor, document and communicate safety information.
4. Compilation and evaluation of safety reports on an ongoing basis to assess benefit/ risk.
5. Dissemination of information (e.g. AEs/safety updates/PSURs) to all concerned parties such as regulators, investigators and ethics committees.

Responsibilities of Investigator

At the same time one more important party that is the investigators and his team has a set of responsibilities, which can be summarized as under;

1. To understand the protocol requirements, particularly in relation to safety reporting (e.g. there could be some exceptions where SAEs could be study outcomes, and need not be reported in an expedited manner).
2. To train his team members on safety monitoring, reporting and oversee the safety monitoring.
3. To provide necessary resources and infrastructure to monitor, document and communicate safety information (fax machine, telephone lines, e-mailing and internet facilities)
4. To whom it may concern: Monitor, capture and documents all adverse events
5. To report the safety information, accurately and legibly in prescribed formats, and within the timelines as per the protocol.
6. To disseminate safety information to concerned parties, such as ECs and IRBs. Besides, it is expected of the investigator and his team.

- To provide medical care to the subject, in case of an AE
- To follow up the AEs till resolution, or till such times deemed necessary
- To whom it may concern: Respond to queries
- And archive the records for 15 years.

Responsibilities of Ethics Committees and Regulators

To put it simply, the greatest responsibility of the Ethics Committees and Health Authorities (Regulators) is to, "To keep a check on ongoing clinical trials to ensure the safety and well-being of the trial subjects".

This can be done by;

1. Evaluating trial documents for scientific rationale and design of the study.
2. Evaluating measures outlined in the trial documents regarding patients' safety.
3. Timely reviewing reported adverse events, in particular, the serious adverse events and adverse events of special interests.
4. Evaluating benefit/risk of the study on an ongoing basis.
5. Initiating appropriate and timely action.

Data and Safety Monitoring Board (DSMB)

A monitoring board may be required for certain studies to determine safe and effective conduct and to recommend conclusion of the trial when significant benefits or risks have developed or when the trial is unlikely to be concluded successfully. The DSMB is an expert committee, independent from the investigators and the sponsor of the trial, which periodically examines the safety data accumulated during progress of the trial and ensures that the benefit/risk ratio remains acceptable for participating patients. A DSMB will be required for;

- Multicenter trials
- All phase III clinical (interventional) trials
- Studies that involve vulnerable populations, blinded, and are considered high risk.

For studies requiring a DSMB, a description/charter for the DSMB must be provided in the Data Safety Monitoring Plan (DSMP).

The meeting frequency of the DSMB, its composition and its responsibilities will be tailored to the design and risks of each trial. The board should include a group of individuals with sufficient expertise to make safety decisions for the trial at hand. Clinicians, statistician, ethicists, epidemiologists, scientists from other fields, and members from outside the institution not directly affiliated with the study may be needed.

NATIONAL AND INTERNATIONAL REGULATORY REPORTING NORMS

Indian Regulatory Requirements as per Amended Schedule Y

With the latest amendment (dated 20th Jan 2005) to the Schedule Y of Drugs and Cosmetic Act 1945, the reporting of adverse events from clinical trials has become clearer and unambiguous. According to the amended Schedule Y, the responsibilities of the sponsors vis-à-vis safety reporting are given in clause 2; which is as follows:

"Any unexpected serious adverse event (SAE) (as defined in GCP guidelines) occurring during a clinical trial should be communicated promptly (within 14 calendar days) by the Sponsor to the Licensing Authority and to the other Investigator(s) participating in the study (see Appendix XI)".

Whereas the responsibilities of the investigator(s) vis-à-vis safety reporting are given in clause 3, which are as follows:

"Investigator(s) shall report all serious and unexpected adverse events to the sponsor within 24 hours and to the ethics committee that accorded approval to the study protocol within 7 working days of their occurrence".

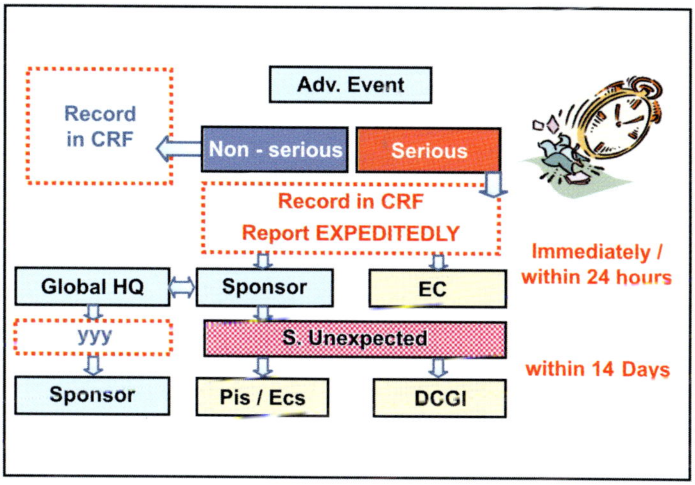

Fig. 12.1: Adverse event information flow (India)

Though the requirements of the regulations demand that, the investigators report only unexpected SAEs to the sponsors in an expedited manner, but in line with the ICH – GCP guidelines, the industry practice has been to report, in an expedited manner all SAEs irrespective of the association with the study medication and labeling status of the adverse event (Fig. 12.1). Most pharmaceutical companies use their own formats to document and collect SAEs from the investigators, but by and large CIOMS I forms are used to report qualifying SADRs of foreign origin (Refer Annexure).

Appendix XI [Format for ICSR submission to DCGI]

Data elements for reporting serious adverse events occurring in a clinical trial are as follows:

1. Patient Details (Identifiers) - Mandatory
   - Initials and other relevant identifier (hospital/OPD record number etc.)-
   - Gender
   - Age and/or date of birth
   - Weight/height.
2. Suspected Drug(s) - Mandatory
   - Generic name of the drug
   - Indication(s) for which suspect drug was prescribed or tested
   - Dosage form and strength
   - Daily dose and regimen (specify units - e.g., mg, ml, mg/kg)
   - Route of administration

- Starting date and time of day
- Stopping date and time, or duration of treatment
- Other treatment(s).

Provide the same information for concomitant drugs (including non prescription/ OTC drugs) and non-drug therapies, as for the suspected drug(s).

3. Details of Suspected Adverse Drug Reaction(s)
    - Full description of reaction(s) including body site and severity, as well as the criterion (or criteria) for regarding the report as serious. In addition to a description of the reported signs and symptoms, whenever possible,
    - Describe a specific diagnosis for the reaction - Mandatory
    - Start date (and time) of onset of reaction
    - Stop date (and time) or duration of reaction
    - Dechallenge and rechallenge information
    - Setting (e.g., hospital, out-patient clinic, home, nursing home)
4. Outcome

    Information on recovery and any sequelae; results of specific tests and/or treatment that may have been conducted. For a fatal outcome, cause of death and a comment on its possible relationship to the suspected reaction; any postmortem findings.

    Other information: anything relevant to facilitate assessment of the case, such as medical history including allergy, drug or alcohol abuse; family history; findings from special investigations, etc.
5. Details about the Investigator – Mandatory
    - Name and address/telephone number
    - Profession (specialty)
    - Date of reporting the event to Licensing Authority
    - Date of reporting the event to Ethics Committee overseeing the site
    - Signature of the Investigator.

International Reporting Requirements

Most of the regulations that describe safety reporting from clinical trials focus on the expedited reporting of the individual case safety reports (ICSRs). ICH Guidelines E2A, which is generally considered the standard for the information to be sent, stipulates that sponsors should submit suspected adverse drug reactions that are both serious and unexpected to the regulators within 7 (if fatal or life threatening) or 15 calendar days in an appropriate format.

Expedited single case reports from clinical trials are accepted by majority of the Regulatory Authorities (RAs) on the CIOMS I or similar forms. With the adoption of ICH Guidelines E2B and then E2B (M), which define standard data elements for electronic submission, some RAs have begun to require the electronic submission of expedited reports in the post-marketing scenario. More recently, the European Union (EU) and Japan have begun requiring electronic submission of the expedited reports from CTs as well. While the time frame and reporting criteria for expedited reporting are mostly consistent across the regions, there are authorities, which require expedited reporting of suspected SADRs, regardless of 'expectedness'.

The CIOMS VI Working Group endorses the ICH Guidelines E2A for expedited reporting and recommends that, "Under exceptional circumstances and on an ad hoc basis, should sponsor be expected to report on an expedited basis SADRs that are considered expected". [21]

CIOMS Working Group VI Recommendations[21]

On the international front, the Council for International Organizations of Medical Sciences (CIOMS), which has proposed common policies for international post market drug adverse event reporting over the last 20 years, recently moved to consider surveillance and safety reporting related to clinical trials. Last month, the CIOMS VI working group on managing safety information from clinical trials of medicinal products issued a final report offering recommendations for implementing common safety information reporting system around the world. The report addresses expedited and periodic safety reporting and draws from the provisions in ICH document, World Health Organization guidelines, and relevant EU directives and guidelines.

The report advises the research community to replace the current practice of sending large numbers of individual case reports to IRBs and IECs. Sponsors instead should submit "periodic and ad hoc communications" to investigators and ECs, with expedited communications focusing on "significant new safety information" that has "implications for the conduct of the clinical trial." This approach follows the European policy of expedited reporting of serious and unexpected suspected adverse reactions (SUSARs) still leaves it to investigators to decide what events warrant more aggressive reporting.

It is interesting to note the latest recommendations of CIOMS VI Working Group are contrary to the common belief and understand which favours overreporting.

It states that *"The group does not believe that increasing the number of expedited reports, by lowering the threshold for considering an adverse event a suspected adverse reaction, would contribute to the protection of trial subjects or the overall assessment of safety"*. To the contrary individual case reports are generally not an effective means of communicating important new safety information. The CIOMS VI Working Group recommends that regulators adopt the phrase "a reasonable possibility of a causal relationship" and consider dropping the phrase" a causal relationship cannot be ruled out" from the definition of suspected adverse reaction.

Pragmatic Approaches: Recommendations and Proposals[21]

A number of proposals for improving AER quality and for limiting report volume were presented at the FDA meeting by sponsors, IRBs, research organizations, investigator groups, and others, demonstrating the complexity of the issues. Some of which can be summarized as follows:

i. Establishing a central IRB for multisite studies that would receive and analyze all AERs. Local IRBs would be responsible for assessing only those AERs filed by its investigators, which then would be sent on to the central IRB.
ii. Sponsors to provide periodic (probably quarterly) summaries of all other AERs to IRBs and investigators, in addition to the annual reports required by FDA. However, some IRB officials feel that sponsors are not sufficiently objective to handle this task and that third party should review safety reports.
iii. Promoting the concept and the role of independent Data Safety Monitoring Boards (DSMBs) to periodically analyze the safety and identify new issues, if any. DSMBs recommendations though not mandatory, but may prove decisive in the conduct of the Clinical Trials.

PROCESSES AND PROCEDURES

Practical Tips for Safety Monitoring and Reporting during Clinical Trials

In order to monitor, document, disseminate and evaluate safety information (issues) in clinical trials, a simple checklist of 'Dos' is as follows:

1. Prepare SOP, encompassing the entire process of safety during the trial.
2. Design the SAE reporting form.
3. Have the necessary infrastructure in place, which should include the following equipments, but not limited to;
   - Multi-connection telephone, cell phone
   - Computer (database, word processor)
   - Printer (computer linked)
   - Fax
   - E-mail
   - Photocopier.
4. Include safety reporting details in the protocol and monitoring plan.
5. Train all the stakeholders, like internal team –members, investigators and his team members.
6. Ensure that the sites have infrastructure necessary for safety monitoring and reporting.
7. Check for adverse events while monitoring.
8. Ensure that all AEs are recorded on the CRFs.
9. Ensure that all SAEs are reported in an expedited manner to the sponsor.
10. Create database and documentation system for the incoming safety information.

11. Investigator to forward all such SAEs to the respective IRB/ EC.
12. Sponsor to report all SAEs to global team (applicable to multinational studies).
13. Report to local regulator, in the prescribed format and timelines all those cases which qualify for such reporting.(Like in case of India; all Unexpected SAEs to DCGI's office in format appendix XII of Schedule Y, in 14 calendar days).
14. File acknowledgement received from the regulatory authority.
15. Disseminate all such cases submitted to local health authorities to other investigators and ECs.
16. Obtain and file acknowledgements from the ECs.
17. Forward all '15 day IND – Safety Alerts' (SUSARs and DILs) received from global team to all the investigators participating in the study.
18. Obtain acknowledgement from the Investigators/ ECs.

CIOMS I Form

The sponsor needs to submit the Individual Safety Case Report (ISCR) to regulatory agencies in CIOMS I form, (for a foreign case) which also provides the regulators, the sponsor's perspective about the issues involved (see Annexure).

Category	*No*	*Data elements*
M	1	Identifiable patient
	2	Identifiable reporter
	3	Suspected medicinal product
	4	Adverse event(s) Verbatim Coded using MedDRA
A	5	Daily dose of suspected medicine and regimen
	6	Route of administration
	7	Indication
	8	Starting date
	9	Full description of reaction
	10	Seriousness criteria
	11	Onset of reaction
	12	Time interval between drug administration and reaction onset
	13	Treatment duration
	14	Time lag after cessation of treatment
	15	Outcome / recovery
	16	Dechallenge information
	17	Rechallenge information
	18	Cause of death and possible causality
	19	Causal assessment
B	20	Stopping date / time
	21	Concomitant treatment· • Daily dose • Stopping date
	22	Other specific tests
	23	Setting (hospital, OPD, home, etc)
	24	Autopsy / PM findings(if available)
	25	Hospital discharge summary
	26	Medical history
	27	Other etiological factors

However, additional, need based information can also be sought through, specially designed forms. The CIOMS I format, more or less complies with the Indian regulatory requirements as mentioned in Appendix XI of the amended Schedule Y, except for the signature of the investigator.

Good Case Management (Follow-up) Practice[22]

CIOMS Working Group V developed a recommended set of data elements that should be sought during follow up of post marketing, mostly spontaneous cases. For that purpose the elements were prioritized according to three categories of cases; 1- non-serious expected cases; 2 - serious expected and non-serious unexpected cases; and 3 - serious unexpected and special interest cases.

It will be appropriate to recall that for a valid ADR report the first four (4) data elements are 'Mandatory' (M category); whereas for category 2 (serious expected and non-serious unexpected cases) besides category M, data elements from category A are desirable. For the third (3) category of events (serious unexpected and special interest cases), it is most desirable to collect all data elements that are included under category M + A + B.

For safety monitoring during clinical trials, however, in practice it is desirable that most or all the data elements recommended be collected; besides some more information such as, study code/protocol number, action taken as a result of AE, suspected drug sub classification (active, comparator, placebo) may be necessary.

REGULATORY INSPECTION[23-25]

Inspections by regulatory authorities (e.g. FDA, MHRA) is a common practice, and sponsors and investigators should always be in a 'Audit-Ready' mode. An audit conducted by a regulatory authority is termed as an 'Inspection'.
Definition of an Audit:

"A systematic and independent examination of trial-related activities and documents to determine whether the evaluated trial-related activities were conducted, and the data were recorded, analyzed and accurately reported, according to the protocol, sponsor's SOP, GCP and the applicable regulatory requirement(s)." *(ICH-GCP 1.6)*

The inspections can be Clinical Trial related or Pharmacovigilance related, as a part of routine regulatory process (e.g. GCP compliance, GMP compliance, new drug approval process) or a targeted ' for-cause' (e.g. specific ADRs investigations, or Recall related) audit. Hence, there can be specialist inspectors with a given task or inspectors during a routine surveillance activity. Table 12.1 summarize the salient features of Regulatory Inspections.

Table 12.1: Salient feature of regulatory inspections

Topics	*Salient features*
• When to expect?	• Routinely • For cause (Batch Recall) • Specific issue (Specific safety/ADR issues)
• Notice or Arrival	• Prior notice • Surprise visit • Presents credentials • Form FDA 482
• Methodology	• Check facility • Interview • Check documents • Debrief regularly
• Molecules of interest?	• NCE • Approved in last 3 years • Of special interest • Of suspect BA/BE
• Documents of interest?	• Organogram • Job descriptions • CVs • Training records • SOPs • Contractual agreements • SOPs • Forms/appendices/flowcharts • Training manuals and records
• What else they may look at?	• Handling adverse events reporting • System compliance • Data verification • Data quality • Archival • Database validation • Data security • Report tracking • Query processing and follow-up procedures • Documentation of affiliates or subsidiaries
• AEs of interest?	• Unexpected SAE/fatal or hospitalization • Incomplete unexpected SAE or unexpected AEs without outcome • Periodic reports • 15 Days reports
• AEs handling process?	• Reporting compliance • Timelines • Completeness • Accuracyo Availability of information – Was all information included in form

Contd...

Contd...

Topics	*Salient features*
	– Initial receipt date supplied to FDA is correct – Was new FU info obtained for better evaluation – Annual reports contents meet requirements
• Outcome?	• Debriefing • Voluntary compliance • Form FDA - 483 – Failure to submit – Failure to promptly investigate – Inaccurate information – Incomplete disclosure – Lack of written procedures – Failure w.r.t reporting requirements. • Initiate regulatory action
• Guidance	www.fda.gov/ora/compliance_ref/www.fda.gov/cder/aers/chapter53.htmlEU paper on compliance PV regulatory obligations – Jan, 2002; CPMP/PhVWP/1618/01.

It is important to know that inspectors only expect that a company has performed what is reasonable. They cannot expect 100 percent in everything – only the key areas of reporting timelines and administrative adequacy. They would however see that when mistakes occur there are processes in place to enable timely action.

LIMITATIONS OF CLINICAL TRIALS IN SAFETY PROFILE OF AN NCE

Despite best of the efforts, one must always remember that the safety profile of the new chemical entity is always incomplete and provisional. The well-known limitations of the clinical trials can be summarized as follows;

1. A very limited number (about 3000 – 5000) subjects are being exposed to the NCE. The number of subjects enrolled is based on statistical significance keeping in mind the efficacy parameter and not the safety criteria.
2. Only a select band of subjects, is being enrolled as per the inclusion and exclusion criteria of the protocol, which does not include sub populations like infants, children, old, nursing mothers, women in child bearing age group, and immunologically suppressed.
3. The exposure to the NCE is for a very short period of time, and hence does not really give any idea about its long-term usage in a chronic condition.
4. Rare adverse reactions and ADRs with latency periods are never discovered during a clinical trial

And hence, 'Post Marketing Surveillance' is not only essential but now is being considered as mandatory by most of the health authorities.

Annexure: CIOMS FORM

SUSPECT DRUG
ADVERSE REACTION REPORT

I. REACTION INFORMATION

1. PATIENT INITIALS (first, last)	1a. COUNTRY	2. DATE OF BIRTH			2a. AGE	3. SEX	4-6 REACTION ONSET			8-12 CHECK ALL APPROPRIATE TO ADVERSE REACTION
		Day	Month	Year	Years		Day	Month	Year	

7+13 DESCRIBE REACTION(S) (including relevant tests/lab. data)

☐ PATIENT DIED

☐ INVOLVED OR PROLONGED INPATIENT HOSPITALIZATION

☐ INVOLVED PERSISTENCE OF SIGNIFICANT DISABILITY OR INCAPACITY

☐ LIFE THREATENING

II. SUSPECT DRUG(S) INFORMATION

14. SUSPECT DRUG(S) (include generic name)

20. DID REACTION ABATE AFTER STOPPING DRUG? ☐ YES ☐ NO ☐ NA

15. DAILY DOSE(S)

16. ROUTE(S) OF ADMINISTRATION

17. INDICATION(S) FOR USE

21. DID REACTION REAPPEAR AFTER - REINTRODUCTION? ☐ YES ☐ NO ☐ NA

18. THERAPY DATES (from/to)

19. THERAPY DURATION

III. CONCOMITANT DRUG(S) AND HISTORY

22. CONCOMITANT DRUG(S) AND DATES OF ADMINISTRATION (exclude those used to treat reaction)

23. OTHER RELEVANT HISTORY (e.g. diagnostics, allergies, pregnancy with last month of period, etc.)

IV. MANUFACTURER INFORMATION

24a. NAME AND ADDRESS OF MANUFACTURER

24b. MFR CONTROL NO.

24c. DATE RECEIVED BY MANUFACTURER

24d. REPORT SOURCE ☐ STUDY ☐ LITERATURE ☐ HEALTH ☐ PROFESSIONAL

DATE OF THIS REPORT

25. REPORT TYPE ☐ INITIAL ☐ FOLLOW UP

REFERENCES

1. ICHE2A: Guidelines for Industry: Clinical Safety Data Management: Definitions and Standard for Expedited Reporting, Step 5 as of Oct 1994
2. ICH E2B: Guidance on Data Elements for Transmission of ICSRs, Step 5 as of July 1997.
3. ICH E2B: Clinical Safety data Management: Data Elements for Transmission of ICSRs, Step 5 as of Nov 2000.
4. Management of Safety Information from Clinical Trials CIOMS Working Group VI report.
5. Current challenges in pharmacovigilance and pragmatic approaches.
6. Management of Safety Information from Clinical Trials – CIOMS Working Group VI.
7. Viewpoint: Part I, – UMC publication 2004.
8. The Erice Report.
9. WHO Technical Report No 4998 (1972).
10. Strom Brian L, Pharmacoepidemiology, 3rd edition, Wiley, 2000.
11. E2A Guidance Document, CPMP/ICH/377/95, June 95.
12. Alghabban A , Dictionary of Pharmaceutical Medicine, 1st (edn). Edinburhcovigilance.
13. WHO Collaborating Centre for International Drug Monitoring: Guidelines for setting up and Running a Pharmacovigilance Centre. Uppsala: WHO, 2000.
14. E2C Guidance Document, CPMP/ICH/377/95.
15. E2A Guidance Document, CPMP/ICH/377/95 June 95.
16. Alghabban A, Dictionary of Pharmaceutical Medicine, 1st (edn). Edinburh.
17. Alghabban A, Dictionary of Pharmacovigilance; 1st edn. USA.
18. Edwards IR, et al. Harmonisation in pharmacovigilance. Drug Safety 1994;10:93-102.
19. Naranjo et al; Clinical Pharm Ther.1981;30: 239-45.
20. Meyboom RHB, et al. Drug Safety 1997;16:355-65.
21. Management of Safety Information from Clincal Trials: Report of CIOMS Working Group VI – Geneva 2005.
22. Current challenges in pharmacovigilance: Pragmatic Approach – CIOMS V Working Group Report; Geneva.
23. www.fda.gov/ora/compliance ref/
24. www.fda.gov/cder/aers/chapter53.html
25. CPMP/PhVWP/1618/01.

Role of Contract Research Organization in Clinical Research Management

13

Chetan Tamhankar, Anand Bidarkar

INTRODUCTION

The pace of drug discovery in recent years has resulted in an enormous pressure on the drug development process. The inability of the conventional development pathways to deliver on the demands has for the first time ever transformed the industry from 'discovery constrained' to 'development constrained.

Outsourcing or contracting of clinical research to third parties is being increasingly viewed as an effective option to partially overcome the development related constraint. In fact this option has been around for a long time now, in various forms, since the late seventies to be precise. That was a time when outsourcing was not a very common term, contracting was; that's how the name stuck–Contract Research Organization (CRO).

Contract research is a very broad term comprising of any type of research outsourced, including discovery related or other market related research apart from clinical research. To provide for this specificity in identification, the term clinical research organization came in to vogue. However, the abbreviation CRO remains the same – so the confusion continues. For the purpose of this chapter we use CRO as an abbreviation for contract clinical research organization.

CROs conduct clinical research on behalf of the pharmaceutical, biotechnology, and medical device industries (sponsors). Clinical trials are a CRO's core competency just as a pharmaceutical company's core competency is usually developing drug pipelines and marketing. CRO professionals bring their scientific, regulatory and information management expertise to bear for the completion of timely, accurate, cost-effective trials. By outsourcing, the drug and device companies gain the benefits of CRO experience, even while controlling costs and reducing the research and development timeline.

In the Code of Federal Regulations (CFR), the US Food and Drug Administration regulations state that a CRO is "a person [i.e., a legal person, which may be a corporation that assumes, as an independent contractor with the sponsor, one or more of the obligations of a sponsor, e.g., design of a protocol, selection or monitoring of investigations, evaluation of reports, and preparation of materials to be submitted to the Food and Drug Administration." [21 CFR 312.3(b)]

It is estimated that, roughly 25 percent of all clinical trials are outsourced. Of phase I-III trials not conducted in-house by the sponsor, CROs are involved in about 64 percent, while approximately 36 percent are conducted in academic medical centers. This was not always the case; the contract clinical research industry has an interesting history.

HISTORY OF CONTRACT CLINICAL RESEARCH INDUSTRY

As the R and D costs increased steadily in the late 1970s, a few service organizations emerged to provide specific tasks for pharmaceutical companies, such as identifying investigator sites, monitoring data processing, statistical analysis, and regulatory support. By mid-1980, a few of these companies, had grown to several hundred employees to provide an almost full-range of services to the pharmaceutical industry.

In the late 1980s and early 1990s, pharmaceutical companies faced enormous pressure from health care reform in the USA. This forced a large number of them to limit in house clinical research staff to the minimum possible level and to use the services of the CROs to supplement their resource needs. The outsourcing of clinical research to CROs was established as a branch of the service industry when G H Besselaar was acquired by Corning Glass Works in 1989.

The Tufts Center for the Study of Drug Development (Tufts CSDD) estimates that global biopharmaceutical companies spent $5.5 billion on contract clinical research services in 2004, an annual increase of 15 percent since 2001. During this same period, overall biopharmaceutical company spending on all global development activities grew 11 percent each year. Moreover, the largest and oldest CRO companies report that their clinical research headcount has grown by nearly 6 percent annually since 2001.

To get a better idea of the contributions CROs have made: in 2004, leading CROs managed 23,000 Phase I-IV trials worldwide, monitored more than 150,000 clinical investigators, and enrolled more than 640,000 new subjects, according to the Tufts study.

According to the Association of Clinical Research Organizations (ACRO), major CROs contributed 29,849 clinical research personnel in 2004, a 5.5 percent annual increase since 2001. These employment trends suggest that CROs are a primary mechanism utilized by sponsor companies to augment rising global capacity needs and contain development costs.

The growth of the CRO sector has been largely performance driven. According to sponsors, projects with high CRO usage stay closer to schedule: in general, high CRO usage projects are submitted more than 30 days closer to their projected submission date than are low CRO usage projects.

The above figures were obtained from an analysis of 83 NDAs and BLAs submitted to the FDA between 2000 and 2005 and provide impressive figures complementing the Contract Research Organization (CRO) industry. "Clinical outsourcing offers a development speed advantage at comparable quality," according to Ken Getz, senior research fellow at Tufts CSDD (Fig. 13.1). What it comes down to is that if a company is involved in drug development, it needs a CRO. Now that we know a bit of history about CROs let us delve deeper in to the structure of a typical CRO.

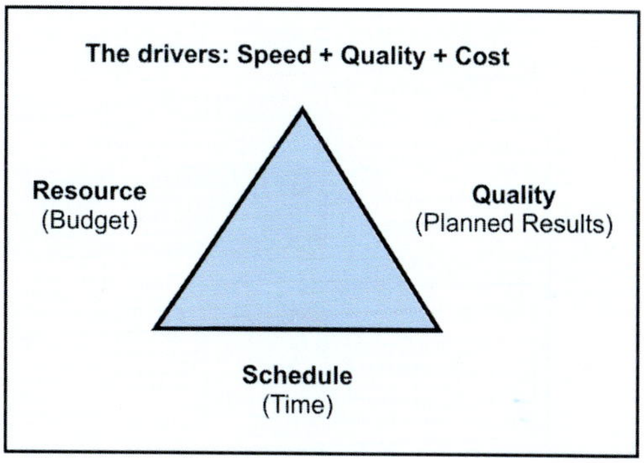

Fig. 13.1: The three most critical factors in drug development

THE CRO FUNCTIONAL SET-UP

A typical CRO's functional set-up consists of four major departments. These include clinical operations, clinical project management, biomedical operations and medical affairs. Quality control is usually an independent department, or an independent part of each department.

SERVICES OFFERED BY CROs

When Contract Research Organizations (CROs) were first formed, pharmaceutical companies outsourced to them only certain aspects of the conduct of their clinical trials. At first CROs were highly specialized entities, providing, for example, either biostatistical advice, clinical research associates who monitored investigational sites for regulatory compliance, or regulatory support. Gradually, full service CROs emerged, offering a full range of services for clinical trials, including the selection of investigators and investigational sites, assistance with patient recruitment, safety surveillance and reporting, site audits, and data management and biostatistics (Fig. 13.2).

ANALYSIS OF THE FACTORS LEADING TO OUTSOURCING

Over the last few years, the pharmaceutical industry has seen large companies use 'downsizing' strategies more and concentrate resources on core skills. As industry margins come under increasing pressure, companies could begin outsourcing aspects of their development, manufacturing or marketing processes so as to concentrate on their core specialties (Fig. 13.3).

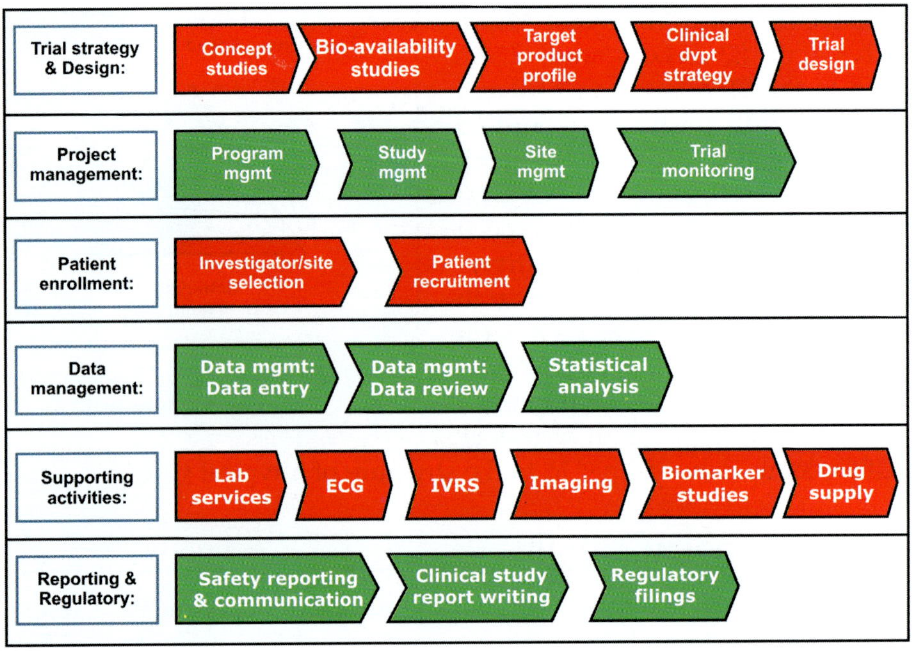

Fig. 13.2: Typical services offered by the CROs range from trial strategy and design to project management and regulatory reporting

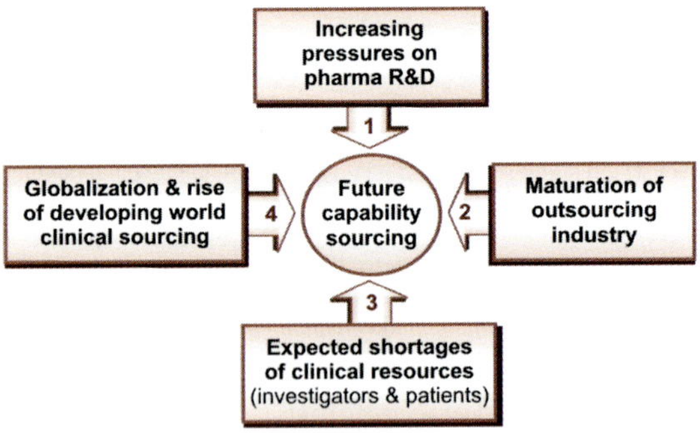

Fig. 13.3: Why are companies increasingly outsourcing?

Despite operating environment changes that require more capacity, major pharmaceutical and biotechnology companies are not increasing their own clinical research headcount. According to the Pharmaceutical Research and Manufacturers Association (PhRMA), member companies in 2004 employed 28,783 people who were engaged in global Phase I–III programs. This figure is lesser from the 28,992 clinical research personnel employed in 2001.

Outsourcing an operation is a means of converting the fixed costs of maintaining the necessary personnel, infrastructure and expertise into the variable costs of paying a sub-contractor to perform that process when it is required. Outsourcing also gives companies the flexibility to acquire skills and technologies in a cost and time efficient way, thus avoiding having to get heavy financial backing to develop them in house. This strategy has been particularly influential in the pharmaceutical industry as the success of a large pharmaceutical company depends on competence in fields as diverse as combinatorial chemistry, computer integrated manufacturing and marketing medicines direct to consumers.

The drug discovery and development process is extremely time-consuming and expensive. The Tufts Center for the Study of Drug Development estimates that the cost to develop a new prescription drug increased from $231 million in 1987 to $897 million in 2003, and it typically takes between 10 and 15 years to develop a new prescription drug and obtain approval to market it in the United States.

The clinical stage is the most time-consuming and expensive part of the drug development process, making up over 38 percent of the total research and development expenditure (Fig. 13.4).

It is estimated to cost between $1 million to $ 1.3 million each day a drug's approval is delayed, based on lost revenue potential for a top-selling drug. Because it is not always financially practical to maintain redundant development staffs, drug companies commonly rely on outsourcing to CROs to shorten product development time and cut fixed overhead costs, leading to timelier drug introduction and greater sales revenues over time.

There are three major reasons why such companies might take the decision to outsource some of their services: lack of capacity, skill deficiency and cost control. However, external cost pressures have also acted as a major driver for the pharmaceutical outsourcing market. At bottom, the outsourcing market has developed in response to the downward and upward cost pressures exerted on pharmaceutical manufacturers' profit margins.

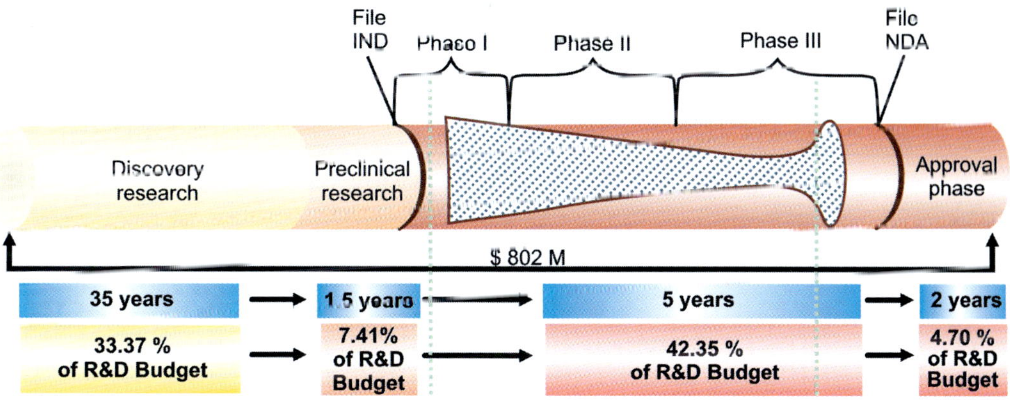

Fig. 13.4: Time and expenses involved in drug development

Given that such pressures are likely to increase in the future, Clinical Research Organizations (CROs) will become more and more important strategic partners for pharmaceutical companies.

TYPICAL OUTSOURCING ISSUES THAT SPONSORS CONSIDER

- When to outsource
- Vendor selection
- Retaining in-house expertise
- Cost-effectiveness
- Patient recruitment
- Regulatory and ethical issues.

While cost is also a determinant for selecting a service provider, it typically ranks at or near the bottom of survey responses for outsourcing selection criteria. Key selection criteria usually include such elements as expertise in a specific therapeutic area, ability to deliver study participants, speed and a strong reputation (Fig. 13.5).

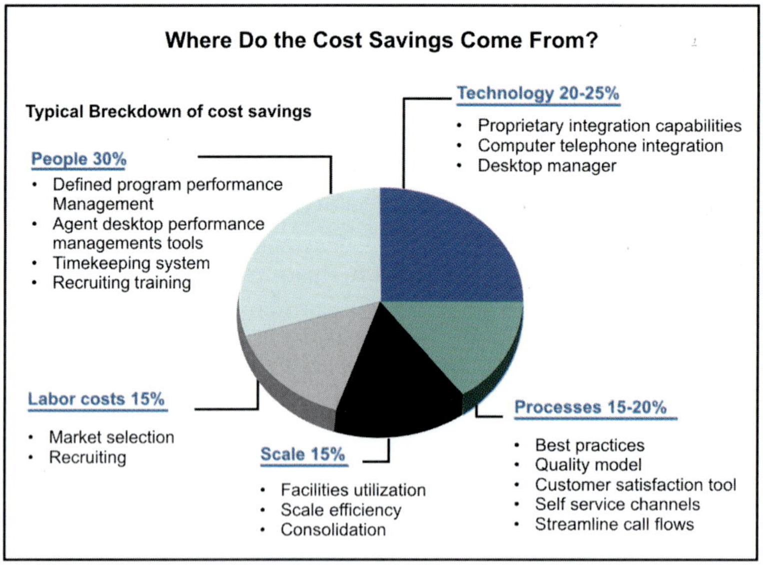

Fig. 13.5: Role of CROs in reducing costs

Answering "yes" to all of these questions would mean the work stays in house, while a "no" answer to any of the questions would advise outsourcing.

- Do we have in-house resources?
- Are the resources available?
- Would these resources be optimally employed on this project?
- Is it cost-effective to do the project in-house?
- Can we do it fast enough?

WAYS IN WHICH CROs ADD VALUE

CROs add value to the sponsor's clinical research projects in multiple ways. These include (Fig. 13.6):

- Reduces the time (8 to 15 years) required to develop and bring a new drug to market
- Sponsor can convert the fixed costs of maintaining the personnel, expertise and facilities like data management) necessary for clinical trial management into variable costs.
- Substitute for non-availability of services in-house
- Provide knowledge of regulatory affairs in a particular country of interest
- Manage increased complexity of clinical trials
- Obtain increased amount of data required from clinical trials
- Facilitate multinational and multi-center nature of current clinical trials
- Fulfill large requirement of patient populations
- Can manage trials for regionalized diseases.

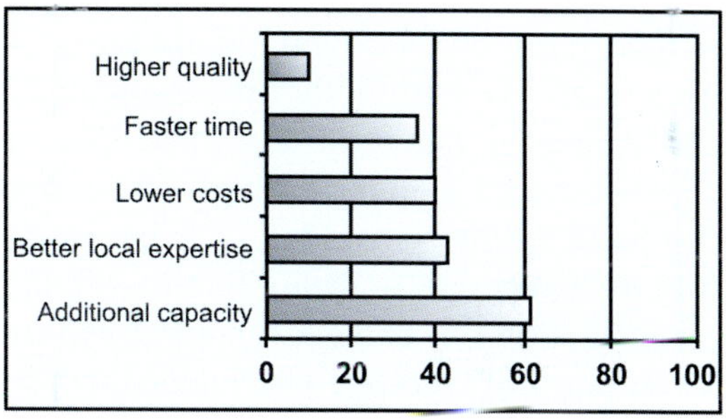

Fig. 13.6: Percentages, the higher the better

OUTSOURCING MODELS AND SPONSOR — CRO ENGAGEMENTS

Outsourcing Tactics

A sponsor may either outsource certain processes in a study or the entire study. The decision is usually a factor of the expertise of the CRO as well as the size and the internal resources of the sponsor (Fig. 13.7).

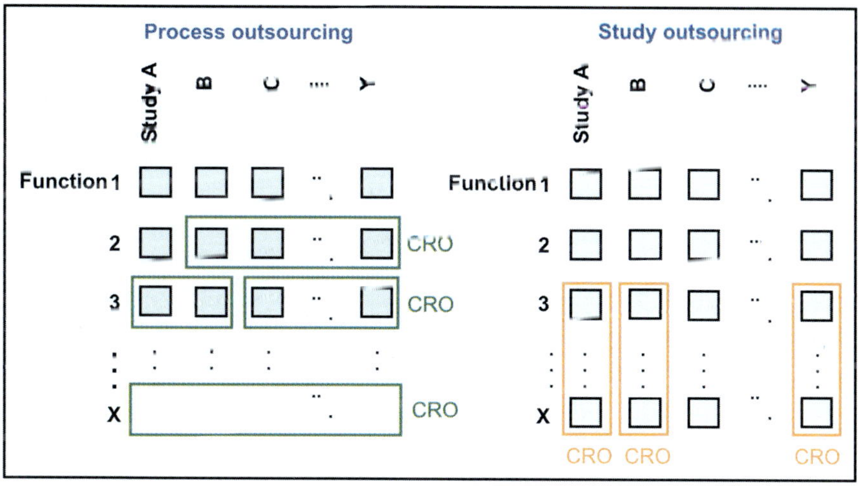

Fig. 13.7: Outsourcing tactics

Sponsor–CRO Engagement Models

1. Full Time Equivalent (FTE) outsourcing
2. Functional Service Provider (FSP)
3. Individual Project outsourcing

In the Full Time Equivalent (FTE) model, the sponsors outsource the job of developing the facility, offices and human resources (FTEs) to the CRO. The sponsor usually provides hardware, software and arrange for their installation and training. This model is essentially an extension to the contract staffing model as the service provider provides both the office and manpower.

This model demands a high initial investment and provides an opportunity for the local service provider to learn on the sponsor's systems. This model usually has a provision for the CRO to act as a Functional Service Provider (FSP) on project/protocol basis after a certain number of years.

In the FSP model, CRO also provides training, functional supervision and assumes a greater degree of responsibility and risk. This model has several advantages like:

- Faster initiation of work
- Lower negotiated service costs
- Reduced risk
- Reduction of required sponsor project management
- Long-term planning–increases transparency and capacity
- Overheads associated with contracting needs are reduced.

Sponsor –CRO engagement models will continue to evolve toward a best-of-breed, selective sourcing approach. Depending on the need of the sponsor, they will increasingly engage services from providers that offer a high level of expertise in a narrow knowledge domain. Sponsors will procure services from a combination of CROs that makes the most sense for their business.

ROLE OF CROs IN THE CLINICAL RESEARCH INDUSTRY

Sponsor Expectations from CROs

1. *Security:* Confidence in the secure transaction and storage of customer information.
2. *Reliability:* Ability to provide consistent support and service around customer needs in all types of business scenarios.
3. *Redundancy:* Ability to seamlessly shift interaction from one center to another with no impact on the service level or type.
4. *Scalability:* Capable of ramping or declining support and service per customer (peak and valley) demands.
5. *Training:* Leveraging cross-trained agents to facilitate multi-functional roles within the enterprise.
6. *Industry expertise:* Having industry specific knowledge around customer facing business processes.

ROLE OF CRO: SPECIFIC AREAS OF CONTRIBUTION

Patient recruitment

Internationally, recruitment and retention of clinical trial patients are a big challenge. More than 80 percent of global trials fail to enroll on time, with 52 percent delayed by 1-6 months. Failure to recruit patients on time leads to loss of over 85-95 percent of days in a clinical trial (Fig. 13.8).

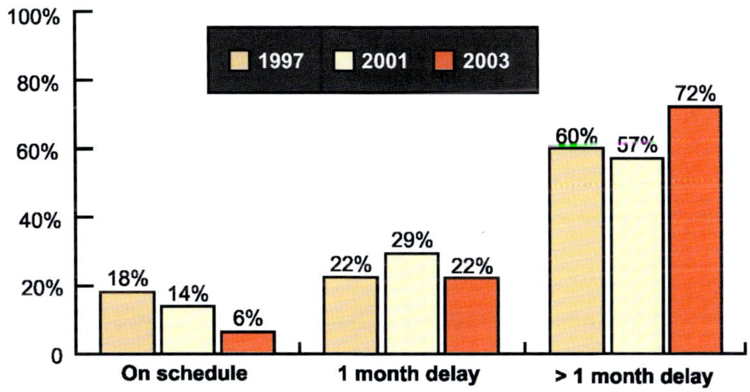

The number of U.S. Clinical trials with delays of more than one month has risen 15 percent during the past two years.
Patient recruitment has been cited as the major stumbling block, with statistics showing more than 80 percent of research trials are delayed because of a lack of research volunteers.

Sorurce; Center watch surveys of investigation sites

Fig. 13.8: US Clinical trial enrollment delays worsen

When implemented effectively, clinical trial recruitment (CTR) initiatives can be highly successful. Time lines can be dramatically reduced and recruitment targets can be met ahead of schedule; every day saved in the progression to marketing authorization can equate to millions of pounds made in patent-protected sales revenue.

However, great care is needed in the development of a CTR program. Considerable ethical scrutiny is applied to all patient recruitment materials and initiatives. For example, in 2002 the European Commission issued guidelines for consultation which require patient advertising and details of recruitment initiatives to be submitted to appropriate ethics committees.

Unfortunately, there is no simple code of practice established and no unified regulatory body and no recourse to appeal. If an ethics committee does not like what a CRO has planned, the CRO cannot use it. In Europe, this aspect has yet to be effectively addressed.

Enhancing CTR is obviously an area in which great caution is required. Some investigating doctors, for example, question the need for extra activities as, they claim, there are sufficient numbers of suitable patients among those already attending their clinics. However, practical experience has shown that this is an over-estimation of the number of patients physicians will be able to recruit and it is estimated that only about 10 percent of a physician's patients will actually wish to enroll in a clinical trial.

A review of recent press coverage also highlights a deep skepticism of industry involvement in clinical research. If not approached ethically, a firm's CTR campaign can leave them wide open to aggressive media criticism and adverse advocacy relationships.

Over the past several years these problems have been addressed in the US, where clinical research receives more and more active support of government bodies, advocacy groups, charities and patient groups. This provides a collaborative environment and ensures that there is always an independent counterpoint when the integrity of industry-sponsored studies is attacked.

Traditionally, direct access to patients has been the preserve of the clinical investigator. While industry found and selected investigators, CROs did relatively little to help investigators find patients. Forward-thinking clinical research associates were quick to prepare standard letters for investigators to mail to patients, and laminated checklists of inclusion/exclusion criteria for investigators to carry around with them.

The model was simple and straightforward and was successful for many years, but as competition for investigators and their patients has intensified, a more sophisticated model is being evolved. Unfortunately, evolution leaves much to chance, so perhaps it is now time to more actively direct the patient recruitment process.

There are many tactics CROs can use to increase their chances of successful recruitment efforts.

- Create competition among investigational sites and principal investigators.
- Reward the investigators for successful recruitment;
- Design communication aids explaining the research for investigators and patients;
- Target patients with recruitment materials that recognize what they may be facing in terms of the disease or condition, other options and the trial they're being recruited for.
- Be proactive by identifying and addressing potential enrollment issues upfront;
- Perform a pilot program to evaluate recruitment strategies; and
- Develop a backup plan.

The driver for optimal patient recruitment is clearly the potential for a knock-on delay to market of valuable new medicines, something that impacts on patients and health care providers as well as suppliers. This situation could get worse. Reports suggest that the number of NCEs likely to be developed each year is set to show anything from a two- to an eight-fold increase over the next three to five years.

While these numbers are inconsistent, it is likely that combinatorial chemistry, high throughput screening and pharmacogenomics will create a huge number of potential targets for the global drug development pipeline. In response, the pharma industry (and its suppliers) must accelerate the means by which it establishes the safety and efficacy of new products, using efficient models to complete clinical activities. Improved patient recruitment is fundamental to this goal.

Ensuring Patient Safety

For all CROs, the most critical task is to ensure the safety of those participating in clinical trials. Researchers must monitor and regularly assess whether programs are being conducted properly. Patient protections should be in place regardless of whether a trial is funded by government, industry, or academia.

While pharmaceutical companies, regulators, researchers and others involved in product-development have an intrinsic commitment to safety, they are under intense pressure to ensure the well-being of patients in all phases of research, distribution and use. In particular, the US. Food and Drug Administration is under unprecedented scrutiny by members of the US Congress, and most observers expect the agency to increase its focus on safety issues. All of this makes the process of moving a drug from laboratory to market more complex than ever, and has given CROs the opportunity to demonstrate not only their expertise in, but their commitment to, patient safety.

Safety is particularly important during the initial phase of a clinical trial, Phase I, which involves a drug's first use in subjects. Where in later phases, patients often volunteer to test a potential new treatment, Phase I subjects are usually healthy people who take part simply to ensure a medicine is as safe in the real world as has been indicated in the laboratory.

As allowed by regulations and scientific ethics, CROs compensate subjects for the time, effort and inconvenience that may be part of participation in a Phase I trial. At the same time, they must be careful not to offer undue incentives to potential volunteers, or to link payment in any way to the level of risk in the trial. Further, CROs should ensure that the investigators make every effort to ensure that volunteers understand the requirements of participation and can give fully informed consent.

Greater emphasis on post-trial activities and post-market studies also will deepen the involvement of CROs in the product life cycle. A drug's side effects often do not appear until the medium or long term, or until the product's been used by a larger universe of patients than is seen during a trial.

ROLE IN EDUCATION OF THE CLINICAL RESEARCH WORKFORCE

Traditionally most pharmaceutical companies provide training programs to teach the basics of drug development to new monitors and in-house study coordinators. These courses tend to last two to five days and only cover the most important procedures and regulatory aspects intrinsic to the research process.

Intensive training is expensive and, therefore most companies provide very little. Therefore, monitors initially gain experience by traveling with experienced monitors, as finances permit. However, there is usually great pressure on supervisors to limit the number of such training trips. In-house coordinators often receive less job instruction than monitors, because it is assumed that they will have ample opportunity to ask peers for assistance as questions arise.

Investigators usually have little formal introduction to clinical research methodologies, and thus rely heavily on guidance from the coordinators they hire and the monitors they encounter. Unfortunately, coordinators, monitors, and physicians often have similar levels of research education and training. So it is not uncommon for those engaged in research to guide each other through the complex process and the maze of regulatory requirements.

As a result, there is a great need for educational opportunities outside the traditional academic sphere. Several CROs have developed internal processes to impart ongoing and intensive training to their clinical research staff. Investing in such training might not be feasible for many pharmaceutical companies, CROs can help by providing training to 'Industry monitors' and share their experiences.

Maintaining Ethics in Clinical Trials

The ethical conduct of research, like the scientific conduct of research, requires careful consideration, planning and attention to detail.

CROs should be dedicated to ethical and lawful behavior in performing clinical research. They should follow a code of ethics that emphasizes patient safety, integrity, confidentiality, and public education. A CRO should be committed to improving public understanding of the clinical research process, and strengthening the public's confidence in the process and those who undertake it.

Contract research organizations scout out the "best" test sites and the countries with the easiest approval process and access to the largest markets. CROs make up a huge and growing industry in their own right. Many countries hope to attract pharmaceutical and biotech investments by relaxing the guidelines governing clinical trials. Countries are competing with one another — and even within countries, jurisdictions are falling over each other to entice investors.

At a minimum, most research carried out must go through review by an interdisciplinary IRB or meet stringent criteria for exemption from review. IRBs evaluate several aspects of a proposed study, including its risks, benefits, consent process, confidentiality issues, recruitment practices and the importance of the knowledge to be gained.

If an institution has an IRB, that IRB should review the protocol. Local review is important because a committee whose members are drawn from the institution and the community is best prepared to assess a study's risks and benefit in light of the unique needs and concerns of that institution's patient population. For all of these reasons, CROs should make sure that the protocol is reviewed by their hospital's IRB. All proposed clinical research, regardless of the source of support, should be approved by the local IRB to assure that the research plans are reasonable and that the research participants are adequately protected.

If clinicians are not affiliated with an institution that has an IRB, they must rely on the IRB affiliated with the CRO to provide ethical oversight. Although this CRO-based review process should be objective, it lacks understanding of the local patient population required for adequate review. An outside IRB may not scrutinize studies as carefully as a local IRB, which needs to maintain community relations and patient trust. Therefore, clinicians who participate in research should be aware that they will have to take on the role of the local IRB to some degree, particularly by ensuring that the consent information is appropriate for their patients. Clinicians without access to an IRB may wish to contract with a nearby academic medical center IRB that may be willing to review protocols for a fee which could then be billed to the CRO.

Another factor to be considered by the CROs is the investigators' loyalties. An investigator's loyalties should lie with the participants. The selection of clinical trial investigators needs to be carried out with due diligence. The ultimate control of the trial is in the hands of the investigator so CROs need to be absolutely confident about their choice.

It is essential to be sure that chosen investigators completely understand and respect good clinical practice (GCP), the consent process and the need for documentation of the consent process, as well as the ethics involved in clinical trials. CROs can have a process of independent auditors to interview the research participants in confidence.

Patient Education and Management

Patient education is an important aspect of the CROs role. Besides the obvious moral issues, if patients aren't completely aware of the clinical trial process they may not follow the protocol correctly and this could render any data useless. Surprisingly, hardly anyone seems to be educating the people about their role in the research.

Apart from knowing their rights, patients ought to have a say in deciding what research is worth doing. It is often said that "The greatest potential for improving research may lie in greater public involvement." Over the past few years, the pharmaceutical industry's image has significantly impacted the public trust. And building a foundation of public trust necessitates both action and value on the part of industry stakeholders, CROs have a major part to play in ensuring this.

The Association of Clinical Research Organizations (ACRO) has adopted the following principles to ensure ethical and lawful behavior in performing clinical research:

1. Members are dedicated to the protection and maintenance of the rights and safety of human participants in all aspects of clinical research;
2. Members conduct their services with objectivity, accuracy and integrity;
3. Members adhere to applicable local, national, and/or international laws and regulations in performing clinical research;
4. Members monitor changes in laws and regulations affecting the rights and safety of human participants in clinical research and the integrity of data to ensure that their policies and procedures conform to those changes;

5. Members support laws and regulations that enhance the rights and safety of human research participants and safeguard the integrity of data;
6. Members strive to identify and address potential conflicts of interest that may affect the rights and safety of human participants in clinical research and the integrity of data;
7. Members respect the confidential nature of the health information obtained from individual study participants, as well as the proprietary information of their clients; and
8. Members promote good clinical practices through appropriate educational initiatives.

Ensuring Quality Control

CROs need to have a high degree of focus on quality control throughout the clinical trial process to ensure the safety of patients and the integrity of results.

Maintaining accuracy and quality throughout a clinical study is a continual, dynamic process. Although study requirements are carefully set forth initially in detailed documents such as an approved clinical protocol, a data management plan, and an accompanying project plan, expectations and requirements can change during a study. This ongoing process requires revising mechanisms and communicating these revisions clearly to all investigators and support staff. A well oiled and standardized communication process at the CROs can ensure that such changes do not compromise on the acceptability of the trial results.

For a CRO managing the quality of clinical data includes the following:

- Ensure management of compliance with the protocol, SOPs, and GCP.
- Enable systemic problems to be resolved before the end of the study.
- Help reduce data queries.
- Identify ways to reduce cycle times for various processes.
- Ensure data integrity throughout the study's course and that the data collected are the data required by the protocol.
- Ensure the accuracy and consistency of data from entry into the CRF to final datasets reported in the final CSR
- Play a critical role in dealing with instances of nonconformity while carrying out clinical trials.

Evolution of Technology

CROs should use information technology to streamline the clinical trial process by speeding the transmission of results between physicians, researchers and sponsors, and to improve the quality of information available to patients and others.

Liaison with the Government and Regulatory Authorities

Government regulation is an important component of a CRO's work. A CRO should work diligently to develop dialogues with government regulators that are professional and credible. They should have appropriate access to regulators and often provide input on the development and revision of legislation and regulations.

CROs, like sponsors, are subject to heavy regulation by governments across the world. They must follow applicable state laws, must respect international guidelines, and are obliged to follow their own operating procedures. Moreover, they are judged by the industry on the basis of the scope and quality of services provided, including the degree of adherence to the research protocol, regulatory requirements, and timelines; the quality of the professional working relationships with investigators and institutions, both academic and community-based; and the validity of the data.

Further, CROs are subject to comprehensive audits by sponsoring companies, US or local FDAs, and other regulatory authorities. For all these reasons, CROs are being tasked with strict vigilance of all stages of the clinical trial process to ensure that the laws, regulations, and industry standards designed for the protection of human subjects and data integrity are maintained.

EMERGING ROLES FOR CROs

Recent industry discussion has focused on moving contract research organizations (CROs) from the traditional role of supplemental capacity supplier to strategic and collaborative partner with pharmaceutical companies. Increasing needs to maximize the value of existing products as well as a rise in poor clinical-trial results attributable to formulation have led to redefined CRO-sponsor relationships and a greater reliance on CRO expertise in product reformulation and lifecycle management.

Traditional pharmaceutical, specialty pharmaceutical, and biopharmaceutical companies must now shift their attention to product life cycle management tactics from as early as preclinical development throughout market life. Forward-thinking CROs provide strong evidence for the new dynamic by offering innovative solutions to product reformulation challenges for a variety of pharmaceutical dosage forms and by working to identify and execute strategies that are closely tied to client needs at every phase of the product life cycle.

Small and medium specialty pharmaceutical companies as well as some biopharmaceutical companies rely on CRO expertise as a survival strategy in all aspects of product life cycle management. CROs that have successfully aligned their capabilities to match increasingly complex client demands are positioned to provide sponsors with a competitive edge.

Beginning as early as preclinical development, these CROs offer strategies for accelerating drug development such as expedited formulation and direct-fill of active pharmaceutical ingredient (API) into capsules for early clinical proof-of-concept studies.

During pre-launch and the patent exclusivity period, CROs can work with sponsors to build prelaunch awareness and develop a product launch strategy that enables sponsors to maximize initial sales and product profitability through line extensions, product reformulation, and identification of new active ingredient forms.

CRO STRATEGIES FOR EXTENDING THE EXCLUSIVITY PERIOD

Key strategies for extending the patent exclusivity period include product reformulation, alternative dosing regimens, novel delivery mechanisms, combining complementary in-house actives into a new product, combination products involving alliances between companies, creation of branded generics, and pediatric or orphan indications. A recent report indicates that product reformulation is the most cost-effective way to extend the lifeline of most brand-name therapies.

With careful attention to patent expiration dates and intelligence about competitive products, sponsor pharmaceutical companies and CROs can work together to develop a strategic plan for extending the market life of an existing branded product through product reformulation. Key strategies focus on the reformulation of the drug product in novel ways and may include modifying the release profile, developing alternative dosing forms of the API for niche markets, or applying novel or proprietary delivery mechanisms to improve accuracy, efficacy, or patient compliance

Combination products are another trend in the pharmaceutical industry because of rapid sales uptake, significant patent protection, and sufficient barriers for generic competitors. The complex nature of development objectives for combining complementary active ingredients into a totally new product is served particularly well by experienced CROs.

Finally, CROs can gather competitive intelligence and work with sponsors to develop a strategic plan for extending the patent exclusivity period through product reformulation, new dosing regimens, or novel delivery mechanisms.

LOOKING AHEAD: CHANGES AT THE CROs

To address emerging challenges and pave the way for continued growth, CROs are taking a number of steps. These include continued geographical expansion, deepening of service offerings and enhancement of technological expertise.

Regulators around the world are increasingly asking for more detailed safety assessments on drug candidates. In addition, regulators ask for details about the molecular effects of new scientific approaches. This requires more carefully designed studies evaluated by teams with greater expertise in specific therapeutic and scientific areas.

Pharmaceutical firms are consolidating in an effort to enhance their own efficiency. When this happens, RandD projects are often re-evaluated and outsourced research may be temporarily suspended, resulting in cancellation of CRO contracts. This can wreak havoc with CRO staffing, as contract research companies are usually unable to re-deploy staffers to other projects quickly. In the past, such fluctuations have led to industry-wide cycles of staffing-up and staffing-down as CROs adjust their personnel levels to correspond to changing workload.

Another strategy is deepening service offerings through acquisition of specialized providers and experts in various therapeutic areas. This has resulted in some CROs being able to offer a far more complete range of pre-clinical or clinical services than competitors, thus positioning them for strong future growth.

Lastly, CROs continue to upgrade their technical capabilities through the acquisition of time saving technologies such as voice-response data collection systems and web-based clinical trial platforms. Such enhancements position CROs as cutting-edge service providers who can deliver technological advantages not readily available clients on their own.

It is predicted that the following will occur in the near term:

- CROs will reexamine their go-to-market strategies and group services into classes based on changing sponsor needs.
- Consulting and business process outsourcing relating to clinical development will increasingly be facilitated by vendors which are experienced in evaluating the processes of clinical development organizations in order to drive operational improvements.
- The roles and capabilities of clinical staffing and project management firms will blur with those of CROs.
- Clinical operations executives will shift their focus toward managing multiple vendors.
- The provisioning of data management services will increasingly move to countries like India to take advantage of its low-cost, skilled labor force. In addition, outsourcers will continue to ramp up and more aggressively market their clinical development domain expertise.

THE ROLE OF CROs IN INDIA

Much has been said about the attractiveness of India as a clinical trial destination. A recent Australian study puts India on the top of the list in meeting the timelines for clinical trials. Currently almost all of the fortune 500 pharmaceutical companies process one or more parts of their trial components in India. The current status is an outcome of concerted effort by several stakeholders over the past decade or so.

The cost advantage and the patient pool are often stated to be the key reasons for driving clinical trial business to India; however these would be meaningless without the expertise that has been developed in carrying out the clinical trials, a positive regulatory climate and the infrastructure to facilitate the trials. CROs in India have played a crucial part in developing all aspects of clinical research.

CONCLUSIONS

Since the 1980s, pharma companies have been able to complement their own resources by calling upon Contract Research Organizations (CROs) to avoid delays caused by lack of resources or inexperience in a particular therapeutic area. More recently, technology and centralized dispatch systems have been used to ensure the timely, reliable distribution of clinical trial supplies to sites actively recruiting patients, while electronic data capture offers the potential to speed up data management and create a real-time study database.

The integral role now played by contract service providers and their apparent contribution to development performance suggests that we reevaluate the conventional notion that CROs are simply vendors providing capacity on a specific project. Given the current climate for managing and conducting global clinical research, the importance and potential impact of establishing more effective alliances with CROs is paramount. CROs must be viewed less as a necessary evil to be micromanaged and beaten down for better cost savings, and more as an essential partner, capable of assisting sponsor companies in maximizing the performance of well-coordinated internal and external resources.

Already a small but growing number of sponsor companies recognize the opportunity to rethink their CRO partnerships and to apply their implications. Companies have implemented, or plan to implement, new approaches designed to streamline contracts and initiate projects; to better match and optimize internal and external functional capabilities; and to avoid setting unrealistic and limiting budgets under which their CROs must still deliver speed and high quality.

The growing use of CROs during the past decade to support the development enterprise has enabled pharmaceutical and biotechnology companies to build a larger drug pipeline and to complete projects faster without compromising data quality. The current outsourcing renaissance offers insights into the direction that CRO partnerships must take if sponsors are to address the keys to their survival: improving development performance while achieving higher levels of development efficiency. Ultimately, through more effective CRO collaborations, growing pipelines of new medical treatments hold greater promise for patients worldwide.

SUGGESTED READING

1. A.T. Kearney.Fishing for Opportunities. Successful Clinical Trials Management. PharmaExec.Jun 1, 2006
2. Ashis Kumar Mukherjee. Emerging trends for contract research and manufacturing partnering companies in India. Pharmabiz.com website accessed at http://www.pharmabiz.com/default.asp
3. Clinical Research Organizations Expand Speed and Capacity of Pharmaceuticals' Product Development Pipeline, Tufts Study.PharmaLive.com, January 23, 2006. website accessed at http://www.pharmalive.com
4. Clinical Research Services Multilingual Life Science Solutions from Translations_com.htm. website accessed at http://www.translations.com/index.html
5. Cullen T. Vogelson. Learning the ins and outs of clinical research doesn't have to be experimental. Modern Drug Discovery. March 2001, Vol. 4 No. 3, pp 28–30, 32, 34. website accessed at http://pubs.acs.org/journals/mdd/index.html
6. Cullen T. Vogelson. The art and science of monitoring. A quick and dirty "how-to" for the uninitiated.Modern Drug Discovery. March 2001. Website accessed at http://pubs.acs.org/subscribe/journals/mdd/v04/i03/toc/toc_i03.html

7. Dr V V L N Sastry. Potential and trends of CRO industry: An analysis. Wednesday, August 04, 2004. Pharmabiz.com.website accessed at http://www.pharmabiz.com/default.asp
8. Ethics case study: When are industry-sponsored trials a good match for community doctors? ACP-ASIM Observer.March 2001. website accessed at http://doctorsforadults.com/index.html
9. Garrett D. Smith.Evaluating Challenges to Clinical Trial Execution. Next Generation Pharmaceutical.http://www.ngpharma.com
10. Glass, Harold E. Patterns in Prescribing Behavior: The Potential Hidden Costs of Using CROs.Drug Information Journal 2004. website accessed at http://findarticles.com/p/articles/mi_qa3899
11. Jane Baguley. The Challenge of Patient Recruitment. website accessed at http://www.samedanltd.com
12. Joe Feldkamp.Customer Care Operations Anxieties:Cost, Quality, Control and the Role of the Outsourcer. Convergys Corporation
13. Julia Lloyd-Parks.Drug Information Association (DIA), 38th Annual Meeting reports. website accessed at http://www.samedanltd.com
14. Kenneth A. Getz. Insights from Today's CRO Renaissance. Applied Clinical Trials June 1, 2006. website accessed at http://www.actmagazine.com/appliedclinicaltrials/
15. Kristin Brooks. CRO Industry Update: Growth Expansion and New Opportunities. Contract Pharma. http://www.contractpharma.com/index.php
16. Mahadev Murthy. Clinical Trials in India: Current Trends and Future Opportunities. August 2006: Globalization Regulatory Update. Regulatory Affairs Focus Magazine. website accessed at http://www.raps.org/
17. Martin Valania. Quality Control and Assurance in Clinical Research. A system of checks and examinations that helps ensure the quality of clinical trials. Applied Clinical Trials. Mar 1, 2006. website accessed at http://www.actmagazine.com/appliedclinicaltrials.
18. Martin Valania. Quality Control and Quality Assurance in Clinical Research. Pharmanet.
19. Nick Trythall. Offshoring Within Pharma.World Pharmaceutical Frontiers • Providing a global perspective on the pharmaceutical industry • website accessed at www.worldpharmaceuticals.net
20. Sandhya Srinivasan. Clinical Trials - Part III: 'India is being projected as a global hub for clinical trials'. InfoChange News and Features, December 2005. Website accessed at http://www.infochangeindia.org/index.jsp
21. Scott Lundstrom. Clinical Industry Developments. Have Wyeth and Pfizer Changed the Market? Contract Pharma. Website accessed at http://www.contractpharma.com/index.php
22. Ted Agres. 2004 Pharma Challenges Line Up. Drug Discovery and Development. website accessed at http://www.dddmag.com/default.aspx
23. The Association of Clinical Research Organizations (ACRO). website accessed at http://www.acrohealth.org/
24. Thomas Lander and Tom Johns.Improving Efficiency in Drug Development Impact of Project Management and Strategic Outsourcing.1st International Athens Conference on Project Management Best Practices Athens, July 1st, 2006. Business Management Consultants.
25. Toby Jane Hindin, Public Education and Clinical Trials:Minutes from an industry working group on educating the public about clinical trials. Applied Clinical Trials. Jan 1, 2006. website accessed at http://www.actmagazine.com/appliedclinicaltrials
26. Tony Craig. Factories, call centres — and now clinical trials outsourced to India. National Review of Medicine. July 30, 2004, Vol 1 No 44.
27. Wai Lang Chu. CRO's drug RandD contribution never been more significant.25/09/2006. Drug Researcher.com.website accessed at http://www.drugresearcher.com/news/ng.asp?id=70787.
28. World Contract Research Organizations (CROs) Market: Poised for strong growth despite challenges. Frost and Sullivan. 22 August 2003. http://www.frost.com/prod/servlet/research.pag

14 Outsourcing Clinical Research

Mohanish Anand

WHAT IS OUTSOURCING?

Outsourcing is the act of transferring some of an organization's recurring internal activities and decision rights to outside providers, as set forth in a contract.

WHAT CAN BE OUTSOURCED IN "CLINICAL RESEARCH"?

In a nutshell every aspect of clinical research! Organizations outsource complete clinical development program. Depending on need of the organization it is possible to outsource a study or its parts viz. protocol design and development, case report form design, regulatory activities, safety reporting, study report writing, investigator qualifications and recruitment, investigator grant administration, meeting management, site selection, clinical monitoring, data processing and data management, laboratory sample processing or statistical analysis of study results. This is by no means an exhaustive list. There are a number of other areas in conduct of clinical research, which involves interaction with service providers and have an element of outsourcing. These may include data management, central laboratories, translation services, CRF printing, site supplies, couriers, drug distribution and IT resources including EDC vendors, hardware requirements, and software requirements.

WHY OUTSOURCE?

There are many surveys floating around that give you the "Top five" or "Top Ten" reasons to outsource any activity in your organization. Not surprisingly the results vary. Just as the probability of another persons shoe fitting you is remote so is the probability of another organization's reasons to outsource fitting yours equally remote. What is important is to understand the reasons for considering outsourcing and the benefits your organization seeks.

Here are some examples of the reasons to outsource:

- *Needed expertise:* No learning curve. Do not recreate the wheel
- *Needed manpower:* Do not have enough staff
- *Time requirements:* Running out of time to get job done
- *Needed economics:* Overall cost savings
- *Removing stumbling blocks:* Keeping the work flowing.

The central themes around outsourcing decision focus on core competence. The key considerations in determining core competence are:

- Complexity of task
- Resources required
- Strategic importance
- Cost to build vs. outsource
- Ability to standardize components of the activity.

For an organization determining its outsourcing strategy it is good to ask these questions:

- Based on time, quality, and cost: does it make sense to build or buy the service? What types of skills do we have and what do we need to acquire or develop to build or sustain a core competency?
- Are these skill sets easily acquired?
- Is there an ample supply on the market?
- Does our organization have the lead time/patience to develop the core competency?
- How does building the core competency impact the current organizational structure and strategy?
- How do we maximize company revenue by developing as many compounds as possible?
- How do we minimize company expenses by building only those competencies, which add strategic value?

Whether you should outsource or not would depend on the answers to above questions. A few other key parameters while taking outsourcing decision are:

i. Resources vs their strategic importance: The Figure 14.1 takes an example of a clinical development program and classifies activities based on resources required to perform an activity and the strategic importance of activities. Those activities that require higher level or resource and have a low strategic importance are ones that can be outsourced.

ii. Standardization vs Strategic Importance: Highly standardized activities that have a lower strategic importance are the ones more likely to be outsourced (Fig. 14.2).

iii. Cost to outsource vs cost to build: Activities that have a higher cost to build and a lower cost to outsource are again the ones that should logically be outsourced.

In all three parameters above design of a clinical study is one that has a high level of strategic importance, requires lower level of resources, is difficult to standardize and not so expensive to develop as a competence. This is not an activity that most companies would outsource.

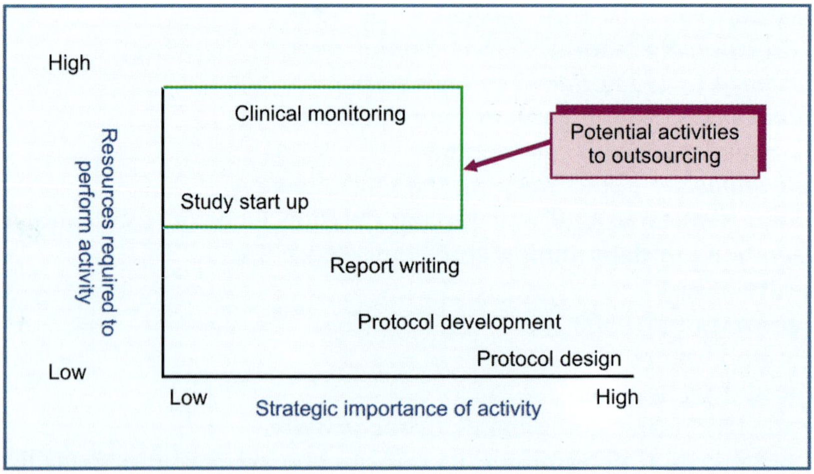

Fig. 14.1: Resources vs strategic importance: A clinical development example

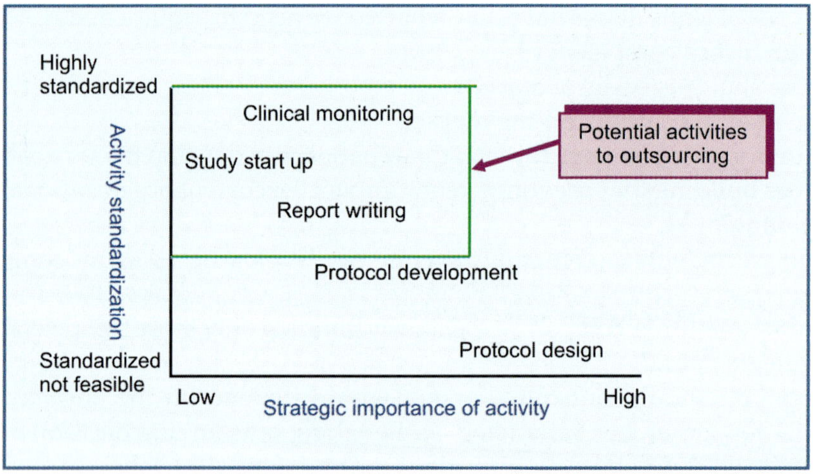

Fig. 14.2: Standardization vs Strategic importance: A clinical development example

Clinical study conduct and management includes a set of activities that require a high volume of resources, are strategically not very important and easier to standardize. These are sets of activities most often outsourced.

Important thing to remember is that here is no single 'right way.' Typically outsourcing strategies are indeed aligned to corporate strategies and they have to be different. Your corporate culture will also set certain limitation on what you outsource and on your decision-making processes. Your outsourcing strategy will (and should) be as individual as you are as a corporation (Fig. 14.3).

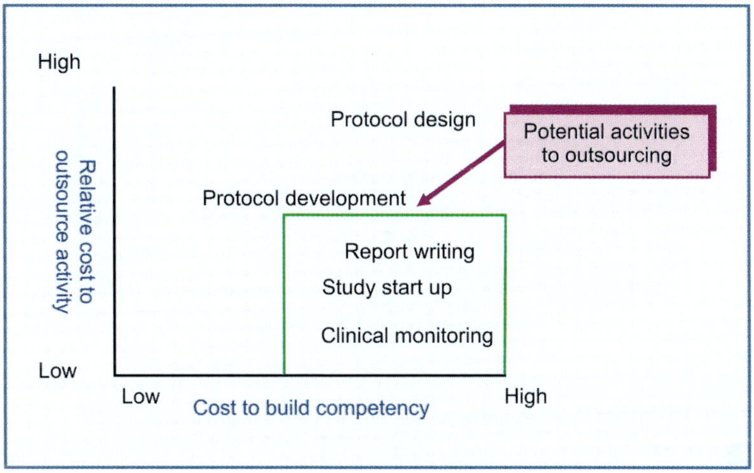

Fig. 14.3: Cost to outsource vs cost to build: A clinical development example

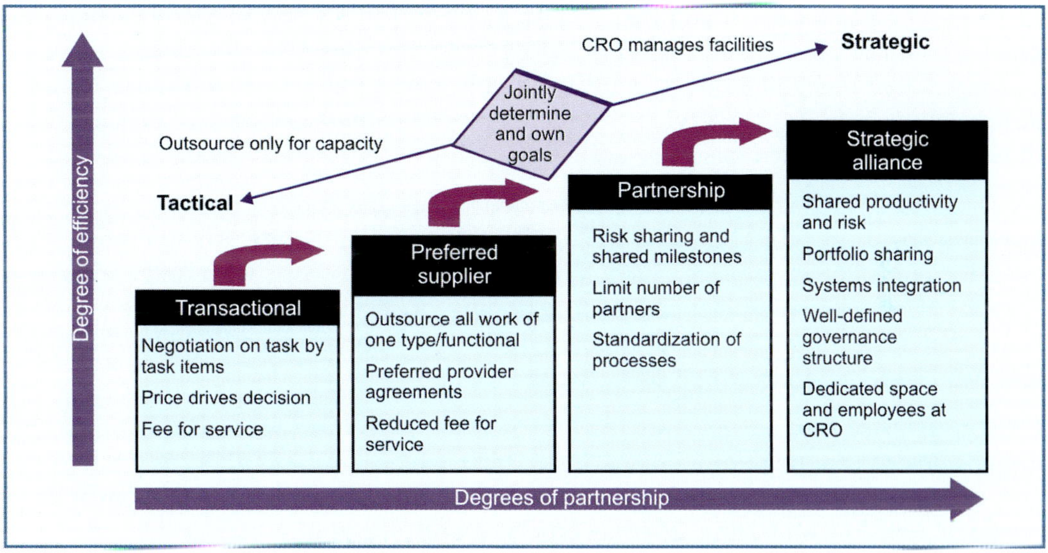

Fig. 14.4: Outsourcing: An evolving concept
(Source: Allan Wood's presentation on "Collaborative Partnerships," Covance)

OUTSOURCING STRATEGY

Outsourcing in clinical research ranges from strategic to tactical. Typically strategic outsourcing is long term, well-planned, identifies specific value additions and is based on a careful evaluation of company's core competence. The range of relationships is summarized in Figure 14.4.

Tactical outsourcing is generally a short-term arrangement, opportunistic, unplanned and based on singular targets of cost saving or capacity management.

Type of contract — Tactical → Strategic

- Fixed price
- Fee for service
- Time and materials
- Fixed unit price—task-based
- Fixed unit price—milestone/deliverable-based
- Risk sharing

Fig. 14.5: Type of contract

Types of contracts that companies use are a reflection of their outsourcing strategy. The major types of contracts used are summarized in Figure 14.5.

Fixed Price Contracts: These contracts determine the price for completion of project upfront and clearly defined scope of work. They must have a mechanism for changes in scope and are typically paid according to predefined payment schedules. From a sponsors perspective the final price is known and payments are for results. There is a great amount of pressure on the service providers to deliver. The down side of such a contract is that renegotiation is almost inevitable; such contracts do not make for long term relationships. From a service provider perspective there is incentive to be efficient though the price quoted has to be accurate.

Fee for Service: Such contracts are open-ended where the sponsor is billed according to hours spent on project and FTE (Full Time Equivalence) rate. This is most often used for consultancy projects. Such contracts are easy to work with and can help a sponsor benefit from efficiencies in functioning of service providers. The problem being that such contracts are notoriously difficult to control, encourage inefficiencies and can create an atmosphere of mistrust.

Fixed unit price-task based: Sponsor and service provider agree definitions and dimensions of task (e.g., monitoring visit, database design) and allocate price to the task unit. Sponsor pays according to number of units completed. For a sponsor such contracts help in comparing internal activities with those of a service provider and are easier to manage, though there is generally a long drawn out process of negotiation to agree on definitions of tasks.

Fixed unit price-milestone/deliverable based: Sponsor and service provider agree definitions of milestone (e.g. agreed number of investigators initiated, patients entered, database locked, etc.) Sponsor pays when milestone achieved. Such contracts are beneficial to both sponsors and service providers, sponsors pay for results. These provide an incentive for service providers to improve their efficiencies.

Risk sharing: Sponsor and service provider agree on objective. Service provider assumes some predefined risk and is rewarded when the risk pays off – e.g., Royalties Bonus on registration. These are the most progressive types of contracts and take outsourcing to level of a partnership. The sponsor manages risk by sharing it with the service provider and requires a level of trust between the parties.

Evolution of Outsourcing in Clinical Research

Clinical research outsourcing began in the 1980's as a capacity management response to a volatile supply and demand as it provided easier access to resources and removed risks associated with captive infrastructure. This fuelled the growth of the CROs (Contract Research Organizations) in the 1980s.

As competition drove profit improvement in supply chain, the service providers became increasingly productive and cost effective, cost reduction then came in as a benefit to the sponsors. This led to a shift in value premise for the CROs in the 1990s.

In the current decade shareholder value driver has forced companies to focus on core competencies and this has seen emergence of newer models of partnership in clinical research arena.

The current acute pricing pressure in response to global market dynamics presents the next opportunity in developing strategic partnerships.

Outsourcing Models in Other Industries

It is quite insight full to take a look at a context from a mature outsourcing model in engineering space.

This is an excerpt from "Source - Engineering Management journal of the Institution of Electrical Engineers in England"

- Outsourcing entails using external providers to perform recurrent, normally internal, activities or to facilitate profound change.
- Providers assume specific authority and deliver defined services, over specified periods, under agreed pricing regimes.
- The primary driver underlying outsourcing is the incessant need to improve competitiveness and to achieve peak performance by using best-in-breed providers in any activity that is amenable to external fulfillment, and is non-core and not a specialism of the customer.

A gap analysis between this context and clinical research outsourcing is revealing!

Currently in clinical research most outsourcing relationships are tactical, allow limited control over projects to service providers, and are focused around cost effectiveness.

New Outsourcing Models in Clinical Research Industry

Wyeth-Accenture partnership, The Alliance for Clinical Data Excellence:

This outsourcing model links clinical data management (CDM) Business Process Outsourcing with up-front Accenture consulting to re-engineer clinical development. This has involved an up-front investment by Accenture and promises to provide significant cost savings to Wyeth over 10-year contract. The contract has service level agreements (SLA's) with bonuses and penalties.

OUTSOURCING PROCESS

The form of outsourcing may differ based on your outsourcing strategy, but the outsourcing process essentially remains the same. It is important before you begin that you are very clear on your project requirements, internal requirements, expectations from your service provider and the type of contract you need to implement.

Request for Proposals (RFP) Process

Once you have established the project requirements it is essential that you prepare a budget estimate and confirm availability of funds within your organization. The company operation procedures and policies may guide you in this regard. For preparing an estimate you may look at historical data from your own organization or discuss ballpark figures with some service providers.

The next step is to prepare a request for proposal. This is a critical aspect of outsourcing process, the more candid you are about sharing information and expectations, the more reliable the proposals you receive will be.

Depending on the type of outsourcing and the services sourced the following forms an indicative list of documents/information that should be part of the RFP package:

1. Purpose of the RFP
2. Responsibilities of service provider
3. RFP process
4. Milestones
5. Selection criteria for service provider
6. RFP deliverables (includes your expectation from the proposal)
   a. Company information
   b. Experience in relevant activity/therapeutic area
   c. Resumes of key personnel
   d. Proposed business terms and fees
7. Project overview
   a. Project dimensions (sites/patients/ CRF pages)
   b. SOPs to be followed (CRO/sponsor)
   c. Expected timelines
   d. Assumptions
8. Protocol/synopsis
9. Task ownership Matrix in a RACI format detailing the activities/tasks proposed to be transferred.

A budget bid grid is a useful tool to include in the RFP package, a simple table as to how you expect the proposal to be structured.

Selecting a Service Provider

Selecting Service Providers for RFP Process

It is important to maintain a database of service providers with a detailed prospectus of services offered. Select the service providers that have capacity and capability to manage and execute the services required. It is a good practice to maintain a log of experience with various service providers with details of issues faced for future reference.

Before sending out the RFP package, it is essential to have a confidentiality agreement in place. The confidentiality agreement should be drawn up in consultation with a lawyer to ensure that the organizations rights are respected.

Understanding a Proposal

Once the RFP package has been sent and proposals have been received, the next task is to evaluate the proposals. It is important to understand that different service providers use different formats for proposals and may also have differing terminology for the same tasks.

Essentially following are the elements of the service charges by providers:

Direct Costs: These include operational hours by e.g., project manager, CRA, data manager etc., depending on their qualification, and the cost associated. Usually all the tasks are detailed along with number of hours of the particular resource deployed and cost per hour.

Alternatively, service providers may assign fixed costs based on tasks defined in the TOM of the RFP.

Indirect Costs (Passthrough Expenses): These include investigator/hospital fees, telephone, unexpected expenses for certain procedures not in the protocol, CRF printing, courier/shipping, travel etc.

Few important things to note at this stage are:

i. It is essential that you ask the service providers to give you an estimate of passthrough costs, which would be paid at actuals. A broad comparison across service providers would help you make a realistic estimate.

ii. The travel and hotel costs for a substantial cost of such a project, it is important to explore if the service provider has regional presence i.e. people deployed in various cities. This can bring about a huge cost saving for the organization. Depending on where your sites are located if it is possible to eliminate or minimize air travel costs, you can trim a clinical trial monitoring and management cost by atleast 30 percent.

iii. Please note that a handling charge may be applied by the CRO for all indirect expenses!

Service provider takes the risks if the indirect costs are fixed. In short, well predictable studies the risk is smaller than in longer and unpredictable studies with more probable changes. This is something that the sponsor and service provider has to mutually agree upon.

Key Financial Terms

These are some key financial terms one comes across while evaluating proposals and negotiating contracts.

a. *Cash Flow:* Measure of the actual cash generated by a business rather than the accounting profit.
b. *Cash Neutral (negative/positive):* Equitable balance between income and expenditure.
c. *Up Front Payment:* Often requested as standard practice on contract signature.
d. *Profit/Operating Margins*: A ratio used to measure a company's pricing strategy and operating efficiency and is a measurement of what proportion of a company's revenue is left after paying for variable costs such as wages etc.
e. *Accruals:* By using accruals a company can measure what it owes (liabilities) and what cash revenue it expects to receive, i.e. by matching revenues to expenses when the transaction occurs rather than when the payment is made.
f. *Revenue Recognition:* Revenue is what companies report in their financial statements and thus influence the perceived value of the company to the external market. A company can recognize revenue when it is earned. Some companies cannot recognize revenue until a final contract is signed some accept an LOI.
g. *Working Capital:* Measures how much in liquid assets a company has available to build its business. Companies who have a positive working capital can expand and grow, where companies with a negative working capital may lack the necessary funds to grow.
h. *Sarbanes – Oxley Act 2002*: Effective since 2004, came as a result of the large corporate financial scandals. All publicly traded companies trading in the US are required to submit an annual report of the effectiveness of their internal accounting processes.

Negotiating and Contracting

Once all the proposals have been evaluated a comparison grid should be made of all the key elements that were previously identified to rank the proposals. This is an important step for management approval of the project internally.

Service Provider "Due Diligence"

Conducting a due diligence visit to the service provider is essential. The timing of visit can be at the RFP stage or anytime before final selection.

Visit to the CRO site should cover as many of the following areas as required under the scope of project:

Facilities
Check that the facilities are of suitable size, construction, and / or design to meet the requirements of the outsourced clinical trial activities.
Check that access to/security of the facility is adequately controlled (e.g.) • Limited access • Locked doors, keycard access • Intrusion protection • Escorts provided Check that fire detection/protection is available to maintain both facility and records (e.g.) • Smoke/Fire alarms, fire suppression • Facility wide, archive, computer rooms Check that alternate power is available to critical equipment/systems in the event of a short term/ long term power outage – IT systems, analytical systems Check that appropriate environmental monitoring and controls are in place for temperature/humidity sensitive areas –IT systems, archives Check that there is a business continuity plan in place to describe processes to be undertaken in the event of a disaster or other high potential risk that leaves the vendor unable to carry out their function within their existing facility.
Organization and Personnel Check that a record of the qualifications, and experience are available for each individual working on contracted functions. Check that a job description is available that defines the scope and requirements of the position for each individual working on contracted functions. Check that staff meet the qualification described in the job descriptions, contracts or other defined requirements. Check that personnel have been trained sufficiently on SOPs, appropriate regulations and project or function specific requirements. Check that organizational charts or other documentation are available to clearly identify and attribute staff performing trial specific functions to the data and or functions they are performing Check organizational charts are properly version controlled, and that both current and historical copies are available. Check that sufficient number or staff is assigned to perform the contracted function. Check that the organization has not been identified by a regulatory agency/agencies as having significant deficiencies. If so, Check these deficiencies have been adequately addressed and will not impact sponsor study processes.
SOPs Check that current/updated SOPs/written procedures were utilized. Check that processes are fully defined in written procedures. Check that management approves written procedures. Check that written procedures are available for the tasks performed.

SOP Management

Check that historical versions of written procedures are adequately maintained.

Check that SOP distribution practices are adequate and SOPs are available for review.

Check that SOP format and/or content is consistent with relevant standards.

Check that SOP revision practices are in place and adequate.

Check that SOP version control practices are in place and adequate.

Check that deviation from SOP are documented.

Check that SOPs are in compliance with external requirements.

Quality Systems

Check that quality control/quality assurance practices are adequate and available for review.

Check that quality control documentation is adequate and available for review.

Check that quality assurance is independent of the function being evaluated.

Check that escalation processes are available to describe actions when quality issues are identified.

Record Retention and Archive

Check that there is adequate environmental control and/or monitoring of the archive.

Check that access to the archive is limited.

Check that there is adequate tracking of documents removed from/placed in the archive.

Check that the vendor has evaluated any off-site archives.

Check that the vendor's record retention period is sufficient.

Project Management

Check that delegation of authority and responsibility was adequately defined.

Check that correspondence (i.e., letters, meeting notes, telephone contacts) adequately document relevant communications pertaining to the conduct of the study.

Data Acquisition/Transfer

Check that the electronic data transfer was adequately secured by encryption, VPN, or dedicated connection.

Check that there are adequate quality control measures and/or validation around data acquisition or transfer.

Data Management/Biometrics Addendum

Check that there are sufficient data entry processes/controls in place.

Check that there are sufficient data query and tracking process in place and that queries are being adequately resolved.

Check that there is adequate database maintenance processes in place to include programming updates to validation checks, documenting and testing changes, amendments to standard reports and system maintenance.

Check that adequately controlled edit check processes are in place.

Check that there are sufficient database QC measures in place.

Check that there is an adequate process for final database audits.

Check that there are agreed upon mechanisms for database/dataset transfers to sponsor.

Check that there are documented statistical programming controls in place.

Check that there is adequate documented statistical planning.

Creating a Good Contract

A contract is a good tool to manage risks in a clinical trial. Clinical development projects are seldom predictable and face various risks, some of them may be:

- The study may be cancelled
- The study can be prematurely terminated
- Patient recruitment may not be as expected
- Study timelines may not be met
- Low quality data
- Misunderstanding in responsibilities/ procedures
- Misunderstanding in payment schedule /milestones
- Compound may be out licensed during the study phase
- The study may be postponed
- Acquisitions/mergers
- Higher dropout rate than expected
- Higher amount of screening failures than expected
- Higher turnover of (key) staff than expected
- Inflation in long term studies
- Cost overruns
- Breach of confidentiality
- Under qualified staff

Most of these risks can be eliminated or mitigated by using a good contract template which would include:

- Definition of the contracting party (global CRO or affiliate, investigator or institution)
- Definition of terms (to ensure mutual understanding!)
- Definition of the study, protocol that will be used with its amendments (essential part of the contract!)
- Investigational product
- Definition of the service, responsibilities of both contracting parties and timelines in detail
- The fee and payment schedule
- Commencement and completion of the service, timing and possible delays
- Ownership of data, study results and publication policy
- Confidentiality

- Sponsor's right to monitor/audit the study, inspections
- Warranties
- Indemnity by the sponsor
- Termination of the contract
- Liability
- Material supply/equipments provide by sponsor
- Governing law and disputes
- Notices and contact persons
- Amendments
- Force majeure
- Conflict of interest
- Performance guarantee and insurance
- Termination (if the project/study will be terminated for strategic or administrative reasons)
- Assignments and relationship with CRO affiliates and (independent) subcontractors
- Names of the key team members (project manager, lead monitor)

It is good to work with a lawyer to prepare a contract template; it is best if the lawyer you work with is dedicated/specialized in clinical trials.

MANAGING OUTSOURCED PROJECTS

Well the ink on the contract is now dry and outsourced project is now ready to kick off!

There are a few fundamentals to successful service provider management. Communication is essential and should be open, honest, appropriate and two way. It is important to understand the service provider's perspective. Set clear expectations as well as contract scope as early as possible. Always identify and resolve root causes of issues not just symptoms.

Right at the out set prepare a good oversight plan that would identify key people on both sides. From the service providers end identify.

- *Operations Manager:* Day to day operational management
- *Contract Manager/Business Development Manager:* Financial / legal management.

The oversight document should clearly state expectations, this is not a project scope, it should state the obvious and inspire mutual trust and respect.

Key elements of an oversight plan would include:

- Budget / financial management
- Risk assessments and contingency planning
- Proactive management and issue resolution
- Shared commitment to achieving study objectives
- Explicitly measure performance versus expectations.

Also draw up a communication plan including,

- Kick off meeting
- Operational management meeting
- Business review meeting
- Project close out meeting.

A Kick-Off meeting is very important to transfer the project from "bid teams" to "delivery teams," it is essential to have right attendance. Get the senior management with project responsibility, business development/negotiation leads and operational teams including key functional representation (Lead CRA/Data Manager/Statistician as appropriate).

At this meeting re-iterate project aims and expectations, walk through "operating manuals" to ensure buy-in /understanding, get clarity on functional aspects- SAE flow, data flow, lab manual etc. Clarify communication plan, issue escalation, contingency plans etc. and agree metrics, performance indicators and feedback loops.

Operational Management Team should meet monthly and review day-to-day program/operational management over-sight, discuss program/study/timelines/milestones, ongoing assessment of performance metrics, issue diagnosis and resolution.

Business Management Team should be held quarterly specially if you are in a long term relationship with a service provider.

Project closeout meeting is a good tool to review project with focus on learning/improvement, contract deliverables, metrics and performance indicators. Again it is essential to have right attendance especially senior management with project responsibility, negotiation leads, and operational teams including key functional representation. This should feed into service provider reselection and process improvements.

MANAGING PARTNERS

The four most common problems in managing partners are:

Communication Problems

Communication problems can be of different kinds, from different interpretations of functions to failure to indicate what is really important. It is important to communicate what are the priorities.

Service Provider Over Promising

In a competitive market a service provider will try to show that it is offering good value for money. Unfortunately this can lead a service provider to agree to do things which it cannot deliver within the time and budget constraints.

Micromanagement by the Sponsor

This can be a nightmare situation with the sponsor team unwilling to let go, as they fear their baby will not be looked after! It is important to remember that if CRO project managers spend a lot of their time on the sponsor's perceived need to know every detail, it can take their time and focus away from actually doing the work, and that can have a major impact on the relationship between the teams.

Scope-creep

The continuous small changes in scope add a burden to the project. It is important to handle such situations with care as they can spoil the relationship between sponsor and service provider.

Managing outsourced projects is as much about managing relationships as it is about managing projects.

15

Biostatistics in Clinical Trials

Suresh Bowalekar

INTRODUCTION

New drug discovery process is an information intensive, very tedious, long, yet inevitable process. It consists of series of activities like identifying diseases, target compounds and planning and conducting investigations and experiments. Target compounds go through a series of tests, investigations or experiments in animals before they are tested in human beings. Experiments carried out in human beings with the target compounds are called as Clinical Trials. Clinical trials are conducted in a specific order and categorized into phases. Usually the first stage of experiments in humans is carried out to generate preliminary information on the chemical action, safe dose level and safety of the indicated drug. All such experiments are termed as Phase I trials. Different phases of clinical trials are explained below (Table 15.1).

Each phase of trial consists of experiments designed to test a specific aspect/ objective. Data generated in each phase are analyzed statistically using statistically valid methods, techniques or tests to draw a meaningful conclusion. Conclusion/s derived in any phase are used as guideline to decide whether or not to move over to next phase.

Very often a problem or some novel finding is encountered by a scientist (chemists or pharmacist) in the pharmaceutical or chemical laboratory or by a practicing medical professional in the clinic during clinical practice. The problem or novel finding is expressed in simple language, and then gets articulated as clinical question. To obtain solution to problem or to support or refute the newer finding experiment is planned to collect data. Statistician before setting up experiment converts the clinical question in to a statistical question. Thereafter, entire process of clearly defining objective, designing study, collecting and summarizing relevant data, analysis of data and arriving at statistical solution gets completed. The statistical solution is then converted

Table 15.1: Different phases of clinical trials	
Phase	*Details / definition*
Phase I	First stage of testing usually in healthy subjects to get preliminary information on chemical action, safe dose level and safety of indicated drug
Phase II	Second stage of testing carried out in subjects having disease or condition of interest, to get preliminary information on efficacy and safety of indicated drug
Phase I/II	Trial have features of both Phase I and Phase II carried out to get information on efficacy and safety of indicated drug
Phase III	Third and final stage of testing before submitting New Drug Application (NDA). These trials are also called as registration trials as data and results of data analysis are used to get product registered for marketing. These experiments are carried out with an objective of assessing dosage effects, safety and efficacy
Phase II/III	A trial having some features of both Phase II and Phase III
Phase IV	This is fourth stage of testing. It is carried out, if required, after the approval of NDA, under real world conditions may be to compare efficacy and safety of some existing drug
PMS studies	Drugs approved for marketing, remain under surveillance for adverse/serious adverse effects, are required to undergo Post Marketing Surveillance Studies. PMS studies involve systematic collection of reports of adverse events in large No. of patients

into clinical knowledge, which is used in clinical practice. In case the clinical knowledge leads to further question, cycle of events gets repeated. This relationship is depicted in Figure 15.1 below.

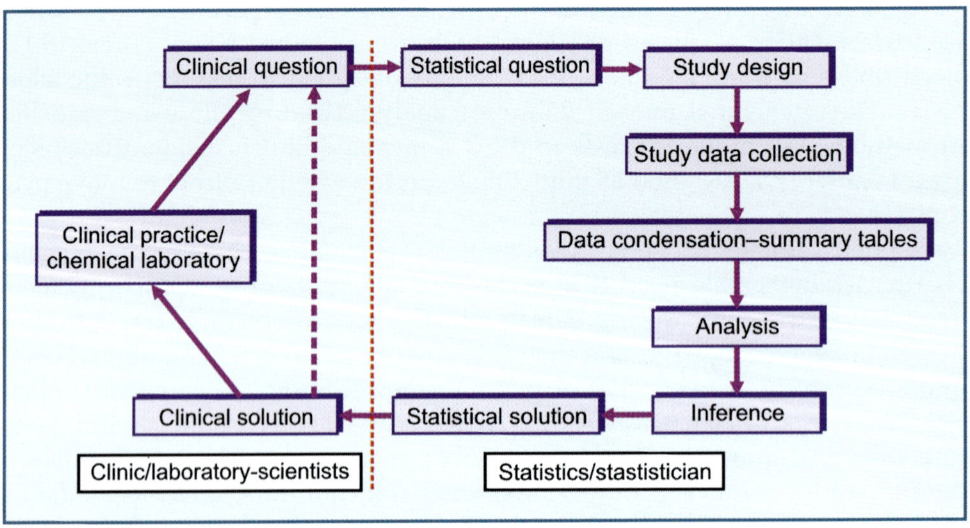

Fig. 15.1: Relation between medicine and statistics

Some topics related to Statistical Principles and Methodology are included within ICH (International Conference on Harmonization) under Code E9 which need consideration while planning scientific experiment are listed below:

- General–Basics for any experiment
- Sample selection–Selection criteria for including/excluding subjects
- Study design–Experimental design most appropriate to the study objective
- Randomization–Allocation of subjects to experimental group
- Blinding–Care to avoid bias
- Scales of measurements–Bringing in some objectivity
- Statistical inference–Level of significance, power of test
- Sample size–Number of subjects required
- Statistical tests–Identification of most suitable test.

A clinical trial is planned scientifically. A document, which describes the process of conducting clinical trial, is prepared prior to commencement of the trial. This document is called a clinical trial protocol or clinical study protocol. The format of the study protocol or clinical trial protocol has scientifically evolved over a period of time.

This protocol describes clearly all methods in various sections to ensure conduct of study to be scientific. These sections are also called elements of protocol. Listed below are some elements important from statisticians' point of view:

- Introduction – An account of background information and rationale for study
- Study objective
- Ethical and regulatory consideration
- Study design
- Study population
    - Sample size
    - Selection and withdrawal of patients/study subjects
    - Study procedures–An account of materials and methods
- Randomization
- Blinding
- Adverse events–An account of definition of adverse events, serious adverse events (SAE) reconciliation
- Drug supplies–An account of study drugs, labeling, storage
- Assessments–Efficacy and safety
- Efficacy criteria
- Data management
- Statistical analysis–Statistical methods.

In view of the above, it is clear that Statisticians and Clinicians who work together in the process of development of new drug need to establish healthy communication with each other. Lack of understanding of technical/scientific language used by statisticians and clinicians is often the cause of communication gap. Each side must try to improve understanding of viewpoints of other side. Statistician must try to understand basics of medicine and clinician must try to get familiarized with basics of statistics. Thus the main or primary role of Statistician in clinical trials is to get acquainted with medical viewpoint so as to provide services listed below:

To provide guidance in interpretation of published/unpublished results of studies carried in the past, use findings in the published/unpublished material to identify study design compliant to study objectives and to suitably define/redefine study end-points for evaluation of efficacy and safety.

An attempt is made in the following pages to explain basics principles in statistics in order to:

- Make researchers/scientists aware of what to expect from statistician and
- Make statistician aware of how to provide right kind of guidance or assistance to sponsors of clinical trials.

GENERAL CONSIDERATIONS

Irrespective of field of application, the experiment of any kind requires that due consideration be given to three aspects, namely clarity, comparability and generalisability. Prior to carrying out any experiment, sufficient time is spent on information gathering from different sources including literature and assessing the accuracy and reliability of information gathered. Based on the utility of the information, a plan of the experiment (called as protocol in clinical trials) is prepared. Then tasks like conducting experiment, collecting data, analysis of data, interpretation of results and preparation of report are completed as per the plan. Each task is performed keeping in mind three aspects listed above.

Relevance of these three aspects to clinical trials is discussed below:

Clinical trial process begins with task of preparing protocol and format to record relevant data (usually called as Case Report Form or Case Record Form or CRF).

Clarity

Statistician should try to:

- Understand the background of the experiment and then study published / unpublished studies in the past and brings in clarity in the section on "Introduction" in protocol
- Clearly spell out objective of the study. In case of the experiments, which try to test many things at a time, the objective should be split in to primary objective and the secondary objective. This splitting will be useful in estimation of sample size. Generally the sample size is estimated on the basis of information related to primary objective
- Identify appropriate study design which is compliant to the objective of the study as well as type of subjects planned to be included in the study

In short ensure clarity at each stage of experiment.

Comparability

In an experiment designed to compare efficacy of two compounds in certain type of patients then two groups of patients receiving two different compounds (drugs) must be comparable in terms of relevant factors. For example if in one group there are elderly patients and the second group there are youngsters then it is likely that young patients may show better response than the elderly patients. Statistician and clinician jointly have to decide about the composition of subjects to be included and ensure that as far as possible they are comparable. Statisticians always advocate, "Compare apples with apples". Under such a situation statistician advises/should advise the scientist to first select patients satisfying certain criteria like age group, height, weight and then use statistical technique of randomization to allocate this selected group of patients in to two treatment groups. This planning or precaution taken in the beginning will help researcher to attribute the observed differences, if any, in the outcome variable or end-points to the drug alone and not to other factors.

Generalisability

It is not feasible to carry out experiment in entire population due to many administrative reasons, and time lines. So testing or experiment is done in a small group of subjects called "sample" and results are extrapolated to whole population. Statistics helps in providing techniques and tools to provide estimates of the extent of confidence (certainty) with which results in sample could be generalized to entire population.

STUDY OBJECTIVE–FIRST ELEMENT IN PROTOCOL

Statistician and the researcher (scientist) should jointly articulate the objective of the study. The objective of study is a very important statement. Many dimensions of the study like design of the study, sample size, method of allocation of subjects to treatment etc depend on the objective of the study. The objective should be clearly defined. For example, a clinician while treating patients of hypertension with a drug 'x' finds that a subset of hypertensive patients with baldness has reported hair growth in addition to control of hypertension. This is an accidental finding giving an idea to the clinician that drug "x" can be used in treating patients suffering from hair loss. Enthused with this finding, clinician may hurriedly plan a study to evaluate effectiveness of drug x in hair growth in bald hypertensive patients. Actually, clinician may be interested in testing whether or not the drug x is useful in hair growth in bald subjects not necessarily with hypertension. In such cases statistician has to understand what exactly the researcher wants to study - usefulness of drug x in bald subjects without hypertension or in bald subjects with hypertension. Suppose clinician feels that the drug x is useful in growing hairs in subjects who are bald as well as hypertensive and not in bald subjects without hypertension. In this case the statistician should guide him to carry out comparative study in which the objective can be "to assess usefulness of drug x in hair growth of bald subjects with hypertension and compare the same with that of bald subjects without hypertension".

STUDY DESIGN – SECOND ELEMENT IN PROTOCOL

As mentioned in the previous section the choice of study design depends on many factors some of which are:

- Hypothesis to be tested (back ground/a priori information)
- Variability within, between subjects
- Variability within study sites and between sites.

Sound study design enhances the power of test/experiment. So, careful choice of suitable study design is very important. Listed below are some commonly used experimental designs:

Parallel Group Design

In this design, first a homogenous group of subjects is selected using suitable selection criteria and then subjects from this group are randomly allocated to two or more treatment groups. Homogenous group will restrict the variability within and between subjects. The design is shown in Figure 15.2.

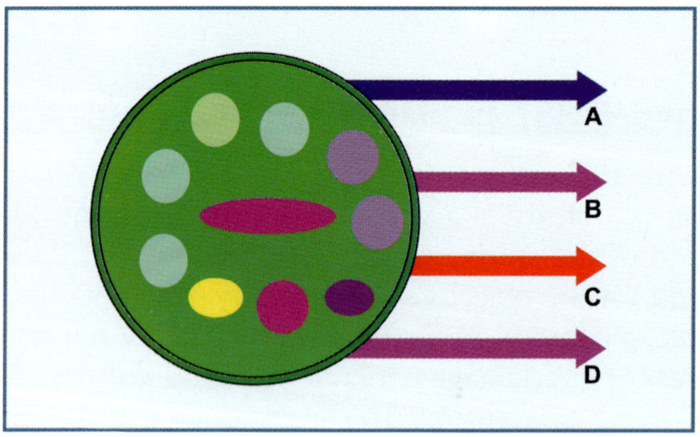

Fig. 15.2: Parallel group

Matched Pairs

In the above example the subjects to be assigned to two or more groups are matched to reduce overall variability. However in certain experiments matching of relevant factors like age severity of disease is required to be exactly matched and then assigned randomly to two groups. Thus, first a set of many pairs of subjects matched with respect to certain factors are identified and then each matched pair is randomly assigned to two groups. Such a design is called as "Matched Pairs" design and is depicted in Figure 15.3.

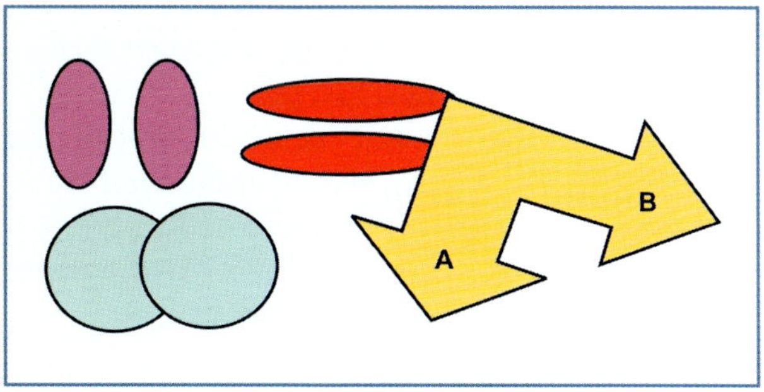

Fig. 15.3: Matched pairs

Crossover Designs

In this study design each subject is treated with two or more treatments successively in random order. Before switching over to next treatment each subject is brought back to original status of the disease prevailing at the time of commencement of the first treatment. The time lapsed between stoppages of the previous treatment and achieving original severity status in an individual is called as "Wash out" period. The duration of "wash out period" is determined scientifically. Patients suffering from arthritis and hypertension remain under control as long as they are under some treatment and revert back to original status after withdrawal of the previous treatment. The disease statuses revert back to original status as soon as the treatment is stopped.

Introduction of "wash-out period" between two successive treatments prevents the effect of treatment given in first period, from having any impact on the response to treatment given in the second period. This impact, if exists, is called as "period effect" or "treatment-period interaction". The pictorial representation of crossover design is given in Figure 15.4.

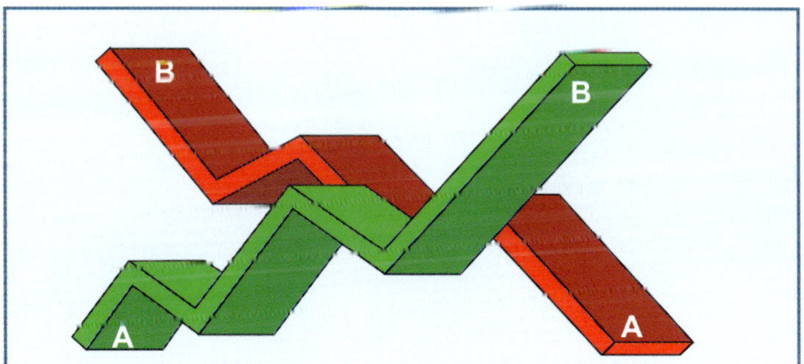

Fig. 15.4: Cross over design

Specific designs under crossover designs are:

Two-Treatment, Two-Period Crossover Design

In a study involving two treatments in which each subject receives both treatments, an even number of subjects are selected and half of them are assigned to first treatment (A) and the rest half to the other treatment (B) in the first period. After a washout period as planned the subjects receiving treatment A or B in the first period are treated with treatment B or A respectively in the second period. This design is very often used in Bio-equivalence studies, comparison of two anti-hypertensive agents. See Table 15.2 for treatment assignment under this design.

Table 15.2: Two treatment, two-period crossover design

Subject No.	*Period 1*		*Period 2*
1	A		B
2	A		B
3	B		A
4	A	Washout Period	B
5	B		A
6	B		A

Two-Treatment, Four-Period or Switchover Design

Like in previous design the patients are randomly assigned to two treatments and thereafter two treatments are given alternately for more than two periods. Switch over designs are used in diseases that are associated with periodic conditions. In females some diseases are associated with menstrual cycles. These menstrual cycles may be ovulatory or non-ovulatory. If any study is restricted to only two cycles it is likely that one or both menstrual cycles in some females are non-ovulatory. So in order to have exposure to ovulatory as well as non-ovulatory cycles, more than two periods are included in the study design. Table 15.3 for presentation of two-treatment four-period crossover or switchover design.

Table 15.3: Two-treatment, four-period crossover design/switchover design

	Period@			
Subject No.	1	2	3	4
1	A	B	A	B
2	B	A	B	A
3	B	A	B	A
4	A	B	A	B
5	A	B	A	B

@ = Include washout period after each treatment period

Latin Square Design

In a study where three or more treatments are involved with a condition that each subject is required to be exposed to all treatments in different sequences. Such designs are used in bio-equivalence studies and agricultural experiments. In this design with three treatments, total number of subjects (generally in multiples of three) is randomly assigned to three treatment groups in period one. The treatment in 2nd and 3rd periods is given in cyclic order (namely A to B, B to C or C to A). Table 15.4 represents such a design.

Table 15.4: Latin square design

Subject No.	*Period 1@*	*Period 2@*	*Period 3*
1	A	B	C
2	C	A	B
3	B	C	A
4	B	C	A
5	A	B	C
6	C	A	B

@ = include washout period after each treatment period

Graeco Latin Square Design

This design is used when effect of treatments and factors are required to be studied simultaneously in cases where number of treatments and number of factors is exactly the same. In this design subjects are assigned to different combinations of treatment and factor in period 1. For example, if A, B and C are treatments and x, y and z are factors and combinations available are treatment A with factor x (Ax), B with factor y (By) and C with factor z (Cz) then corresponding design in Graeco Latin Square will appear as shown in Table 15.5. This design is mostly used in agricultural experiments and some times to identify drug – drug or drug – food interactions.

Table 15.5: Graeco Latin square design

Subject No.	*Period 1@*	*Period 2@*	*Period 3*
1	Ax	By	Cz
2	Cz	Ax	By
3	By	Cz	Ax
4	By	Cz	Ax
5	Ax	By	Cz
6	Cz	Ax	By

@ = include Washout period after each treatment period

Balanced Incomplete Block Design (BIBD)

In bio-equivalence (BE) studies involving more than three treatments, simple three-treatment, three-period crossover design can actually be used. BE studies, carried out with this design will need withdrawal of blood samples in each period. Thus over three periods, total volume of blood sample withdrawn from each subject exceeds ethically permitted upper limit posing ethical issues. So a study is carried out using another statistically valid design in which each subject is expected to receive atleast two out of three or more than three treatments. This design shown in Figure 15.7 is known as Balanced Incomplete Block Design or BIBD. As per this design if there are four treatments A, B, C and D, six possible pairs of treatments can be formed namely, AB, AC, AD, BC, BD and CD. Subjects are first assigned randomly to six pairs treatments, then remaining subjects are assigned randomly to exactly opposite pairs. Table 15.6 shows assignment of six subjects in BIB design. Next six subjects will be assigned randomly to exactly opposite combinations.

Table 15.6: Balance incomplete block design (BIBD)- four treatments and two periods

Subject No.	*Period 1@*	*Period 2@*
1	A	B
2	C	D
3	B	C
4	A	D
5	A	C
6	B	D

@ = include washout period after each treatment period

Factorial Design

This design is used to assess simultaneously the effects of main treatments and one or several other factors. In a specific case of two treatments A and B if one wishes to assess simultaneously the effects in subjects who are:

- Given neither A (A=0) nor B (B=0),
- Given A alone (A=1) and not B (B=0),
- Given B alone (B=1) and not A (A=0) and
- Given both A (A=1) and B (B=1).

The subjects can be assigned to one of the above four groups as shown in Figure 15.5. Such design is specifically used to assess drug – drug interaction.

RANDOMIZATION–THIRD ELEMENT IN PROTOCOL

In experiments involving two or more treatments subjects are assigned to one of many treatments. In absence of any guidelines on allocation of subjects, in an

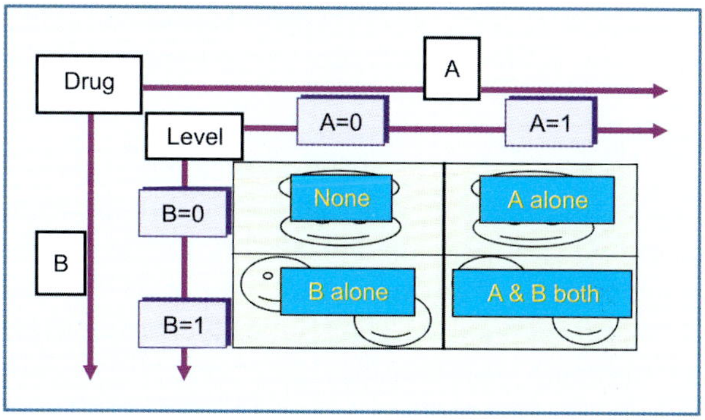

Fig. 15.5: Factorial design – 2 by 2 type (two treatments: A and B, two levels: 0 and 1)

experiment involving two treatments, one may treat first 50 percent of subjects with one treatment and the rest 50 percent of subjects afterwards with the other treatment. This process of allocation of subjects to treatments is likely to create imbalance in respect of some of the factors leading to unrealistic conclusion. Such an allocation is also likely to give rise to bias in assessments of effect of treatment. Hence, the subjects are randomly assigned to treatments. Random assignment does not mean haphazard assignment. Random assignment means probability of each subject to either treatment is equal and no one can predict in advance to treatment to which next subject will get assigned. In actual practice first subjects satisfying selection criteria (inclusion/exclusion criteria) as defined in the protocol are identified. These subjects are then assigned to different treatment groups using random tables generated using appropriate randomization techniques. Randomization results in assignments, consistent with the laws of probability upon which all statistical tests are based.

Randomization Techniques

Simple Randomization

As shown in Figure 15.6, all subjects meeting selection criteria are assigned to one of

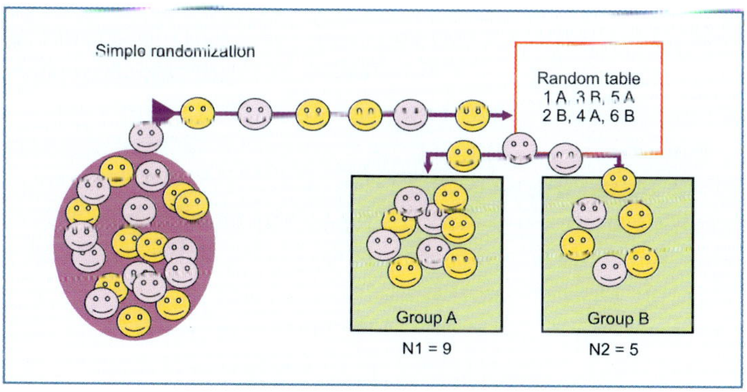

Fig. 15.6: Simple randomization

two treatments as per a pre-designed randomization schedule generated using "ballots drawn from hats", random tables or advance computerized techniques.

Stratified Randomization

Sometimes researcher is interested in assessing/comparing response to treatments in subjects classified in two groups (called as strata) on the basis of some predefined factor. This a priori knowledge of formation of two strata demands classification or stratification of subjects into two strata. Then subjects from each stratum are assigned randomly two treatments using valid randomization schedule. Schematic of the process of randomization in a study designed to assess the response to treatments in males and females independently is shown in Figure 15.7.

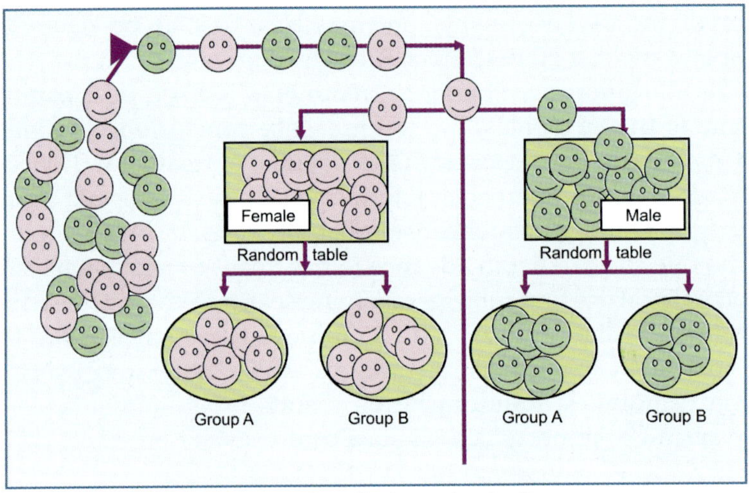

Fig. 15.7: Stratified randomization

Factorial (Balanced) Randomization

There are certain experiments in which objective is to compare responses in subjects classified in to different groups based on two or more factors. One such example is comparison of response pattern with two treatments in depressed as well as non-depressed male and female subjects. The process of randomization of the entire group of subjects satisfying selection criteria into two treatment groups is termed as factorial randomization. The process is depicted in Figure 15.8. It involves following steps:

- Identify subjects satisfying selection criteria
- Classify subjects as males and females based on factor *Sex*
- Further classify both male and female subjects as depressed and non-depressed based on the factor *Disease Status*
- Randomize subjects from each type (Male depressed, Male non–depressed, female depressed and female non–depressed) in to two treatment groups using pre-designed randomization schedule.

BLINDING – FOURTH ELEMENT IN PROTOCOL

In experiments, more specifically in clinical trials if a researcher (investigator) knows which treatment is given to which subject, there is likelihood of bias creeping in while assessment of response by investigator. Bias can also creep in while describing

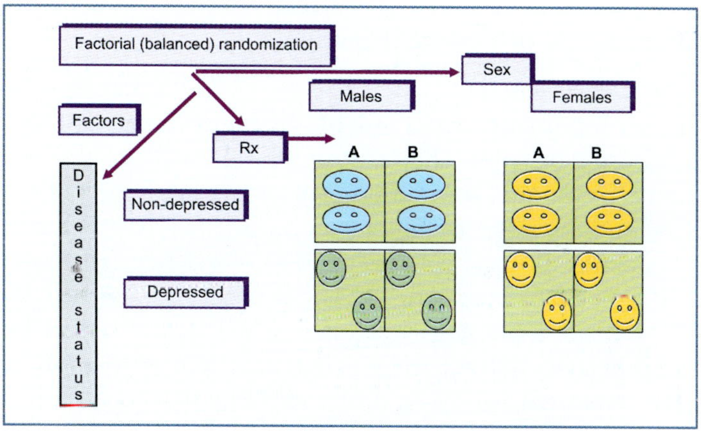

Fig. 15.8: Factorial (Balanced) randomization

response to investigator in case participating subjects know the treatment given. For example if there are two treatments–one well established and the other relatively new. Then investigator while recording responses of subjects may get biased towards established treatment. So also subjects receiving well established treatment may psychologically feel better with it. Blinding is a technique that helps preventing influence of biases of such kind (Fig. 15.9).

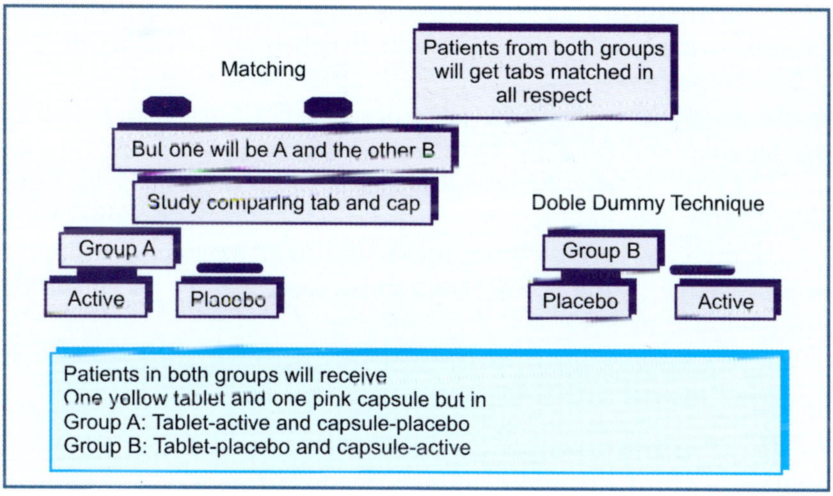

Fig. 15.9: Blinding techniques

Types of studies classified on the basis of status of blinding:
- Open–No blinding, investigator subjects are aware of treatments.
- Single Blind–One party, either researcher (investigator) or subjects is aware of assigned treatments
- Double Blind–Neither investigator nor subjects are aware of treatments
- Triple Blind–In addition to investigator and subjects, statistician or laboratory technician is not aware of treatments assigned.

Methods of achieving double blinding:
- Matching: if two treatments are available in the form of tablets then matching both tablets in terms of color, shape, strength, texture etc.
- Double Dummy Technique: some times out of two treatments one is available as capsule (say A) and the other as tablet (say B). In such cases all subjects are given 1 tablet and 1 capsule. But subjects assigned to A will have real capsule containing A and 1 tablet (placebo) matching B. The subject assigned to B will have real tablet B and a capsule matching A. Thus one will know which real treatment is given to which subjects. Subjects or investigators will only know that all subjects are given same treatment – 1 tablet and 1 capsule.

SAMPLE SIZE – FIFTH ELEMENT IN PROTOCOL

Measurements Scales

In all experiments data is collected. This data is expressed as numbers (Quantitative data) or as categories. The measurement scale is very important aspect for a statistician and appropriate consideration must be given to this aspect while designing an experiment.

Three types of measurement scales are:

i. Interval scale–scale in which the difference between two adjacent marks is always equal (Regular scale).

ii. Nominal scale–which categories/classifies observations in to broad categories like Big, Medium and Small or Excellent, Good, Fair and Poor.

iii. Ordinal/Ranking Scale–which places items to be measured in ascending or descending order and assigns rank or order on the basis of value.

Figure 15.10 presents various types scales and their inter-relationship.

A prior knowledge of the scales used/to be used is very useful in identifying most appropriate test for analysis.

Statistical Significance

Statistically, it is advisable to start planning experiment with some hypothesis. Set up a null hypothesis, which in simple language is hypothesis of no difference. Then gather the information or data via well-planned experiment to create evidence to

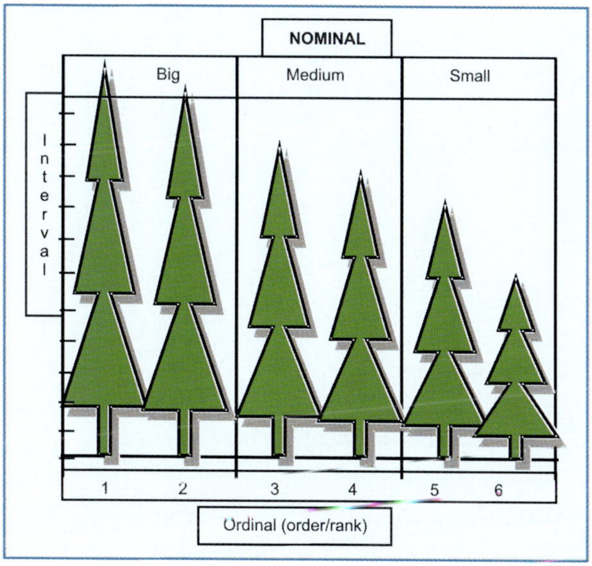

Fig. 15.10: Types of data and scales of measurement

prove or disprove the "null hypothesis." The process explained above is called as "Testing of Hypothesis."

If data and test give verdict in favor of rejecting true null hypothesis then it results in error called as type I error and the probability of committing rejecting true null hypothesis is called as " Level of significance". Figure 15.11 presents an example of type I error.

Similarly error can occur if one accepts false null hypothesis. (Fig. 15.12). This type of error is called as type II error. The probability of accepting false null hypothesis is called as beta (β). Generally (1 - β) expressed as percentage is used as parameter to measure "Power of Test".

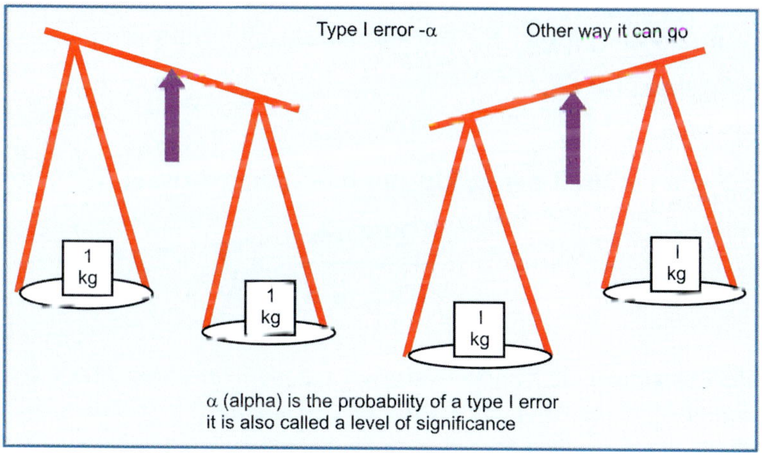

Fig. 15.11: Type I error (α) or level of significance (α)

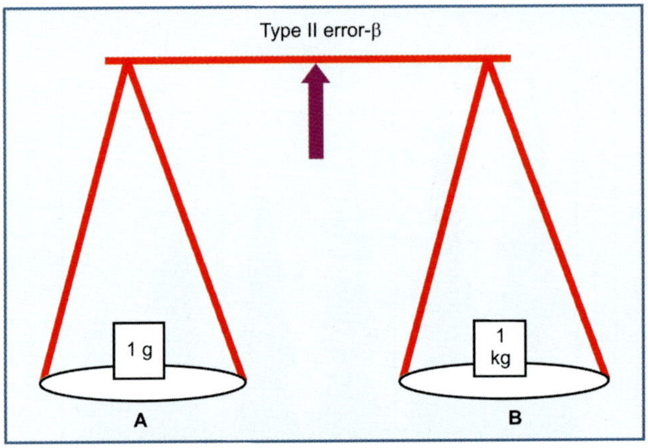

β (beta) is the probability of a Type II error
(1-β) expressed as % is POWER OF TEST

Fig. 15.12: Type II Error (β) or Power of Test (1 - β)

Sample Size

Statisticians are always for inclusion of large number of subjects. But the cost, time and ethical issues in this field of application advocate use of minimum number of subjects enough to create evidence or otherwise to reject or accept null hypothesis.

Scientific method of estimating sample size requires following information:

- Type of response – continuous, nominal, ranking scale
- Expected difference in response between two treatments – Delta (Δ)
- For categorical variable – success rate
- For continuous variable–Sample standard deviation (σ)
- Level of significance – (α)
- Power of test– (1–β) percent where β is probability of mistake of accepting false null hypothesis.

Depending on the design of study, nature of variable and measurement scale there are various formulae developed for the estimation of sample size.

Sample Size Formula for Qu

antitative Response

Number of subjects required per group can be estimated using following formula:

$$\text{N per Group} = \frac{2\,(\text{SD})^2}{(\text{Diff. or } \Delta)^2} \times (Z_\alpha + Z_\beta)^2$$

Where,

SD = estimated standard deviation – know or based on some other study

Diff = Δ = expected difference between two treatment considered as clinically important

Z_α = Z value from statistical tables corresponding to level of significance (α)

Z_β = Z value from statistical tables corresponding to (β the probability of type II)

For 2 sided tests, corresponding to $\alpha = 0.05$ and $\beta = 0.20$

Z_α = Corresponding to level of significance (0.05) = 1.96
Z_β = Corresponding to ($\beta = 0.20$ the probability of type II) = 0.842

Example: Estimate number of subjects required to detect a difference 0.25 between mean levels of creatinine with 2 – sided level of significance as 0.05 and power of test equal to 80 percent. The estimated value of standard deviation of creatinine is 0.51 units.

Given Data:
α = Level of significance = 0.05
β = Probability of type II error = 0.20

Type of test = 2 – sided
Δ = Difference = 0.25
σ = Standard Deviation = 0.51

For 2-sided tests, corresponding to $\alpha = 0.05$ and $\beta = 0.20$

Z_α = Corresponding to level of significance (0.05) = 1.96
Z_β = Corresponding to ($\beta = 0.20$ the probability of type II) = 0.842

Hence, using

$$\text{N per Group} = \frac{2\,(\text{SD})^2}{(\text{Diff. or D})^2} \times (Z_\alpha + Z_\beta)^2$$

N per group works out to 65.3 ≅ 66 per group

Sample Size Formula for Qualitative (Binary) Data

Number of subjects required per group can be estimated using following formula:

$$N = \frac{(2 \times \text{Joint Success Rate} \times \text{Joint Failure rate})}{(\text{Diff})^2} \times (Z_\alpha + Z_\beta)^2$$

Example: How many subjects will be required in each group in a study designed to detect that new treatment is more useful than the well established treatment. The existing drug has a success rate of 30 percent which new drug is expected to reach to 60 percent. Use 2– sided tests, level of significance of 0.05 and power of 80 percent.

Given Data:
P1 = Success rate of existing drug = 30/100 = 30%
P2 = Success rate of new drug = 60/100 = 60%

α = Level of significance = 0.05
β = Probability of type II error = 0.20

Type of test = 2 – sided
Δ = Difference = 30%

For 2 sided tests, corresponding to α = 0.05 and β = 0.20
Z_α = Corresponding to level of significance (0.05) = 1.96
Z_β = Corresponding to (β = 0.20 the probability of type II) = 0.842

Joint Success Rate = Total No. of successes / Total No. of subjects = 90 / 200 = 45%
Joint Failure Rate = (1- Joint Success rate) = 55%

Hence using following expression

$$N = \frac{(2 \text{ x Joint Success Rate} \times \text{Joint Failure rate})}{(\text{Diff})^2} \times (Z_\alpha + Z_\beta)^2$$

$$\text{Thus, } N = \frac{(2 \times 45 \times 55)}{(30)^2} \times (1.96 + 0.842)^2$$

= 43 subjects per group

More complex formulae are used for sample size estimation in complex designs.

CHOICE OF MOST SUITABLE STATISTICAL TESTS

One needs to consider many aspects before selecting the most suitable test. The important considerations are:

- Type of variable–qualitative or quantitative,
- Measurement scale–Ratio, Interval, Categorical, Nominal, Ranking
- Assumptions–matching of assumption listed while developing test with the experimental situation.

Broadly statistical tests are classified into two groups – Parametric and Non-parametric.

Tests whose models specify certain conditions about parameters of the population from which the study sample is drawn are called as parametric tests. Provided other assumptions are fulfilled the data measured on interval or ratio scale are analyzed using parametric methods/tests.

If the model of test does not specify conditions about the parameters of population from which the sample is drawn, a non-parametric statistical test is used. Non – parametric tests are also called as "distribution free" tests. Data measured on nominal or ordinal scale are subjected to non-parametric tests.

Table 15.7 gives guidelines based on the type of measurement scale for identifying most suitable test:

Table 15.7 Guidelines for selecting suitable test

Measurement Scale	*Tests*
Dichotomous (Yes, No) (Success, Failure)	Chi-square (χ^2) test Fisher's Exact Probability Test (FEPT) for small numbers
Nominal - Categories (Excellent, Good, Fair, Poor) (Mild, Moderate, Severe)	Chi-square (χ^2) test
Ordinal – Ranking	Mann Whitney Test, Wilcoxon Rank Sum Test, Kruskal Wallis Test, Friedman Two Way ANOVA for more than two groups
Grouped Censored Survivals	Log Rank Test
Continuous Scale two different groups Before and after measurements	 Students t-test – Unpaired Students t-test - Paired
Continuous ScaleMore than two groups	Analysis of Variance (ANOVA)

There are many tests besides a few listed above but can be studied and applied for complex designs.

It is very important to note that no statistical design or test can rescue the poorly conducted experiment. Utmost care needs to be taken to monitor entire conduct of the study appropriately involving right kind of professional at right time throughout the experimentation.

Always remember what Sir Ronald Fisher – the father of modern statistics said.

"To call in the statistician after the experiment is done may be no more than asking him to perform a post-mortem examination : he may be able to say what the experiment died off".

SUGGESTED READING

1. Anello C. "Statistical Issues in Comparative Clinical Trials," Drug Inf., 1983;17: 55
2. Armitage P. Statistical Methods in Medical Research. New York : Willy and Sons, 1973.
3. Buncher CR and Tsay, J.Y. Statistics in the Pharmaceutical Industry New York : Marcel Dekker 1981.
4. FDA guidelines: http://www.fda.gov/cder/regulatory/default.html.
5. Fienberg S.E. The Analysis of Cross-Classified Categorical Data, 2nd edn., Cambridge, Massachusetts: MIT Press 1980.
6. Freiman J.A., Chalmers T.C. Smith, H. et al. "The importance of Beta, the Type II Error and Sample Size in the Design and Interpretation of the Randomised Controlled Trial,"New England Journal of Medicine, 1978;299.
7. Hill AB. Principles of Medical Statistics, 9th edn, London : The Lancet 1971.

8. Hill A.E. Nunn A.J., Fox W. " Matching the Quality of Agents Employed in Double-Blind Controlled Clinical Trials," Lancet I: 1976;352.
9. Hills M, Armitage P. "The Two-Period Cross-Over Clinical Trial", British Journal of Clinical Pharmacology, 1979;8: 7.
10. ICH: http://www.ifpma.org/ich.html.
11. Peto R.M., Pike M.C., Armitage P, et al. "Design and Analysis of Randomised Clinical Trials Requiring Prolonged Observation of Each Patient", British Journal of Cancer, 1976;34:585.
12. Pockok S.J. "Allocation of Patients to Treatment in Clinical Trials," Biometrics, 1979;35:183.

16

Bioequivalence Studies in Drug Development

Satish Bhatia

INTRODUCTION

With mounting international pressure to cut down healthcare costs, the generic drug industry came into prominence in the early 1990s. Notwithstanding the GMP-controlled manufacture of the active ingredient and the formulation, a key determinant of a generic product's quality lies in a GCP-controlled bioequivalence study in healthy human volunteers to assess the product's performance vis-à-vis the innovator product. It is imperative for the generic product to be equivalent and not inferior or superior to the original product.

Bioequivalence studies are a series of comparative tests designed to establish equivalence between the test and reference (innovator) products. If a test and reference products are found to be bioequivalent then it is reasonable to expect that the test product will also be therapeutically effective i.e., the test and reference are therapeutically equivalent. The majority of bioequivalence studies are pharmacokinetic studies carried out using healthy volunteers. The underlying rationale is that if two products have the same active ingredient, in the same dosage form and in the same strength, then they are likely to produce similar systemic exposure and hence similar therapeutic effect. Pharmacodynamic studies are only considered appropriate when a pharmacokinetic approach is not possible and a suitably validated pharmacodynamic model is available. Clinical studies are considered an unethical and expensive approach to demonstrating bioequivalence since the product's safety and efficacy have been demonstrated in protracted trials before launch by the innovator. *In vitro* dissolution studies are complementary to a bioequivalence study and are usually the first studies performed.

The concept of pharmacokinetic bioequivalence and the logistics involved in its testing would be the subject of this chapter.

DEFINITIONS

Pharmaceutical Equivalents

Medicinal products are pharmaceutical equivalents if they contain the same amount of the same active substance(s) in the same dosage forms that meet the same or comparable standards.

Pharmaceutical equivalence does not necessarily imply bioequivalence as differences in the excipients and/or the manufacturing process can lead to faster or slower dissolution and/or absorption.

Pharmaceutical Alternatives

Medicinal products are pharmaceutical alternatives if they contain the same therapeutic moiety but differ in chemical form of that moiety or in the dosage form or strength. The therapeutic moiety may be used in the form of salts, esters, etc.

Bioavailability

Bioavailability is defined as "the rate and extent to which the active ingredient or active moiety is absorbed from a drug product and becomes available at the site of action. For drug products that are not intended to be absorbed into the bloodstream, bioavailability may be assessed by measurements intended to reflect the rate and extent to which the active ingredient or active moiety becomes available at the site of action."

Bioequivalence

Bioequivalence is defined as "the absence of a significant difference in the rate and extent to which the active ingredient or active moiety in pharmaceutical equivalents or pharmaceutical alternatives becomes available at the site of drug action when administered at the same molar dose under similar conditions in an appropriately designed study."

Essentially Similar Products

"A proprietary medicinal product will be regarded as essentially similar to another product if it has the same qualitative and quantitative composition in terms of active principles (substances), and the pharmaceutical form is the same and, where necessary, bioequivalence with the first product has been demonstrated by appropriate bioavailability studies carried out."

Pharmaceutical products essentially similar to an "innovator" product are usually designated as "generics" or "branded generics." A product is an "innovator" product if its marketing authorization has been obtained on the basis of a dossier with full documentation.

Therapeutic Equivalents

A medicinal product is therapeutically equivalent with another product if it contains the same active substance or therapeutic moiety and, clinically shows the same efficacy and safety as that product, whose efficacy and safety has been established.

In practice evidence of bioequivalence is generally the most appropriate proof to substantiate therapeutic equivalence between medicinal products, which are pharmaceutical equivalents or alternatives, provided they contain excipients generally recognized as safe and carry the same labeling for use. However, in some cases where different rates of absorption are observed the products – though not bioequivalent–can be judged therapeutically equivalent since the differences in absorption rate are not of therapeutic relevance.

It is, however, important to point out that bioequivalence may not necessarily dictate therapeutic equivalence since excipients may raise safety questions; therefore excipients should be well-known and safe.

When is a Bioequivalence Study Needed ?

Bioequivalence studies may be required in a number of circumstances:

- To establish links ("bridging") between different formulations used during the development of a new product (e.g., clinical trial formulation(s) and the to-be-marketed product).
- To demonstrate the therapeutic equivalence of a generic product and the reference (innovator) product.
- To support line extensions of a product (e.g., development of a modified release form of a product, approved as an immediate release formulation).
- To support certain post approval changes (variations) in approved products (e.g., a major change in the method of manufacture).

When is a Bioequivalence Study Not Needed ?

Bioequivalence studies may not be required under the following circumstances:

- The product is a simple solution intended only for intravenous administration or a gas for inhalation.
- Products for local use (after oral, nasal, ocular, dermal, rectal, vaginal, etc application) intended to act without systemic absorption. This does not exclude the potential need for safety studies in case of unintended partial absorption. However, to prove therapeutic equivalence clinical or pharmacodynamic studies are required.

ELEMENTS OF A BIOEQUIVALENCE STUDY

- *Clinical*
  - Study protocol
  - Informed consent form
  - IEC/Regulatory approval
  - Subject selection
  - Dosing
  - Blood sampling and monitoring of vitals
- *Bioanalytical*
  - Bioanalytical method development and validation
  - Analyses of clinical samples
  - Pharmacokinetic and statistical analyses
  - Quality assurance
  - Final report.

Clinical Logistics

Study Protocol

The bioequivalence study protocol should describe the objectives, design, methodology, statistical considerations and organization of a clinical study. The protocols also contain the history for the clinical study and its rationale. Another source of information for preparing a clinical protocol is the International Conference on Harmonization (ICH). According to the ICH, the sections that may be contained in a protocol are:

- *General information*
  - Protocol title, number and date;
  - Confidentiality paragraph;
  - Name and address of the sponsor and monitor (in the event he is not the sponsor);
  - Name and address of the clinical laboratories;
  - Names and titles of the investigators and co-investigators.
- *Information on the study design*
  - Study type and design;
  - Primary and secondary objectives;
  - Description of the randomization and blinding procedures;
  - Study treatments and dosages regimen, including package and label information;
  - Washout period.
- *Information on study population*
  - Number of subjects;
  - Duration of subject participation;
  - Informed consent form;
  - Maintenance of the randomization codes and procedures for code break (double-blind study);

- *Selection and discontinuation*
  - Inclusion criteria;
  - Exclusion criteria;
  - Subject discontinuation criteria;
  - When and how to discontinue;
  - Type of data to be collected;
  - Subject replacement;
  - Discontinued subject follow-up;
  - Subject treatment;
  - Names of all products, doses, dose escalation, administration routes, treatment
  - Period and follow-up period;
  - Allowed and forbidden treatments/ medications, before and during the study;
  - Compliance monitoring methods
- *Efficacy and safety evaluations*
  - Specification of the efficacy and safety parameters;
  - Methods and time points to evaluate, record and analyze these parameters;
  - Procedures for the recording and reporting of adverse events and intercurrent illnesses;
  - Type and duration of subject follow-up after the occurrence of an adverse event;
- *Conduction of the study*
  - Monitoring frequencies;
  - Audits;
  - Data and records maintenance;
  - Publication policy;
  - Procedures to monitor subject compliance.
- *Others:*
  - Clinical laboratory parameters;
  - Concomitant therapy;
  - Documentation of investigator's approval and date (signature page);
  - Funding and insurance;
  - Direct access;
  - Ethics.

All documents requested for the protocol are essential tools for the ethical appraisal by the ethics committee. Among them, special attention should be given to the Informed Consent Form (ICF) to be signed by the research volunteer.

Informed Consent Form

Informed consent form encompasses all aspects related to the ICF, to which the investigator should give attention when preparing it. Special attention should be given to the obtaining process of the ICF that, in addition to being just the process of obtaining a signature, is a real educational process for the research subject. The informed consent form should provide study subject with all the information required for his/ her decision to participate in the research. The study subject should be free to make questions, clarifying any doubt that he may have, as well as have an adequate time to reflect on his participation. The informed consent form should also:

- Meet ICH-GCP/ Declaration of Helsinki requirements;
- Be approved by an Ethics Committee before its use;
- Be revised whenever any new information arises;
- Be written in accessible language for the study subject;
- Not lead the subject to waive any of his legal rights;
- A copy of the signed informed consent form should be given to the subject;
- State that the study involves research;
- State that the participation of the subject in the study is voluntary;
- Provide the rationale, objectives and procedures that will be used in the research, including all invasive procedures;
- State the possible discomforts and risks and the expected benefits. In the event there is no clinical benefit intended for the subject, he should be aware of this fact;
- Existent alternative methods, as well as their potential benefits and risks;
- The responsibilities of the subject participating in the study;
- Experimental aspects of the study;
- The follow-up and assistance manner;
- The expected duration of the participation of the subject in the study;
- The approximate number of subjects involved in the study;
- The assurance of clarifications on the methodology, before and after the course of the research, informing the possibility of inclusion in a control or placebo group and the likelihood inclusion in each arm;
- The person to be contacted in the event of additional clarifications regarding the study and rights of the subjects involved. Who to be contacted in the event of fortuitous damages arisen from the research;
- Compensation manner from the expenses arisen from the participation in the research;
- Indemnification manners in the event of fortuitous damages arisen from the research;
- That monitor(s), auditor(s), Ethics Committee and regulatory authorities will be granted direct access to the source medical records of the subject in order to check clinical study procedures and/or their data, without violating their confidentiality concerning applicable laws and/or rules and that, when signing the Informed Consent Form, the subject or his legal representative authorize this access;
- The records that identify the subject will be kept confidential in accordance with the applicable laws and rules, not becoming of public use. In the event the study results are published, the identity of the subject will be confidentially kept;
- The subject or his legal representative will be informed in the event any new information that may be relevant for the subject's decision arises, regarding his/ her participation in the study.

Study Design

Comparative bioavailability studies should be designed so as to reduce possible sources of variation, which are not directly related to the drug products under test. Ideally the only potential source of variation in a bioequivalence study should be actual differences in the drug products. The conditions, under which the study is performed, including human subjects themselves, should be standardized as far as possible.

Following are the commonly used designs:

a. 2 × 2 *Crossover Design:* This is a conventional not replicated design with two formulations (Reference R and Test T), two periods, two sequences. Each individual is randomly assigned to RT or TR sequence in two dosage periods. That is, individuals assigned to RT (TR) sequence receive formulation R (T) in the first dosage period and formulation T (R) in the second dosage period. Dosage periods are separated by enough time for the drug received in the first period to be fully metabolized and/or eliminated from the body when the second dosage period starts.

b. 3 × 3 *Crossover Design:* This is a not replicated design with three formulations, three periods, three sequences. Each individual is randomly assigned to ABR or BRA or RAB sequence in three dosage periods. That is, individuals receive the formulation according to randomization schedule. Dosage periods are separated by enough time for the drug received in the first period to be fully metabolized and/or eliminated from the body when the second dosage period starts and same way for third period.

c. *Replicated Crossover Design:* This design is recommended for bioequivalence studies of formulations with modified-release dosage or highly variable products (intra-individual variation coefficient = 30%), including the quick-release, and modified-release ones and other oral administration products. The same test and reference formulation batches shall be used for this design for replicated administration. The periods shall be sufficiently spaced (washout) to assure non existence of carryover effects.

- Four-sequence and two-period design (Balaam's design)
- Two-sequence and four-period design
- Four-sequence and four-period design
- Two-sequence and three-period design

The most common design for a crossover trial is the well known TR/RT trial. It tells that one splits the entire sample of subjects randomly into two groups. In the first period 50 percent volunteers receive T and 50 percent volunteers receive R. In the second period the order is reversed.

The study shall be designed in such a way that the effects of formulation can be distinguished from other factors. If two formulations are compared, a randomized two-period, two-sequence crossover study is considered the design of choice. An adequate washout period between periods is needed to avoid drug carryover effects.

Replicate studies, although not mandated, offer the advantage of providing a comparison of intra-subject variances for the test and reference products.

All facets of the study are to be tightly controlled. The full characteristics, including lot numbers and expiry dates of the test and reference products, shall be known. Normally subjects fast for 10 hours prior to product administration. Normally, the highest safe strength/dose of the test or reference product will be administered at the start of an experimental day with about 8 ounces (240 ml) of water. Further fluid will be withheld for about 2 hours; standardized meals are to be permitted beginning at four hours after drug administration. All subsequent meals will be carefully standardized according to a fixed schedule.

For most drugs, subjects shall not be permitted to recline until at least two hours after product ingestion. Physical activity and posture is to be standardized to limit variable effects on gastrointestinal blood flow and motility. Blood samples (about 12 to 18, including a pre-dose sample) shall be drawn at appropriate, specified, and carefully recorded times (to capture increasing and decreasing concentrations during the absorption, distribution and elimination phases). The collections are to continue for about three terminal drug half-lives in order to capture at least 80 percent of the total area. At least three to four samples need to be obtained from the terminal log-linear phase to derive an acceptable estimate of the terminal constant from linear regression. For long half-life drugs, a truncated AUC (e.g., up to 72 hours) is generally considered adequate.

Blood samples or the harvested plasma/serum shall be analyzed for the administered drug or metabolites by means of a validated analytical method.

Subjects

Bioavailability studies generally will be performed with healthy volunteers. If feasible, taking into account reproduction toxicology, they should belong to both sexes and be between 18 and 55 years old. In the case of genetic polymorphism in clearance it is wise to take this into consideration in selecting subjects.

The volunteers should provide a history of their health status; undergo physical examination, ECG, Chest X-ray and laboratory investigations for liver and kidney function and for absence of infectious diseases and drugs.

To minimize intra- and inter-individual variation subjects should be standardized as much as possible and acceptable. They should preferably be fasting at least during the night before administration of the products or they should take a standard meal at a specified time before the treatment. Time and preferably composition of meals taken after the treatment should be standardized. Because fluid intake may profoundly influence gastric passage, it should be strictly standardized and specified. The subjects should not take other medicines during a suitable period before and during the study. They should preferably abstain from food and drinks, which may interact with circulatory, gastro intestinal, liver or renal function (e.g., alcoholic or xanthine containing beverages). Preferably they should be non-smokers. If smokers are included they should be identified as such. In some cases (e.g., study of high clearance substances) even posture or physical activity may have to be standardized.

Sample Size

The number of subjects required is determined by the error variance associated with each of the pharmacokinetic parameters of primary interest (e.g. AUC, C_{max}) as estimated from a pilot experiment, from previous studies or from published data, by the coverage probability of the confidence interval from relative bioavailability, by the expected deviation from the reference product compatible with bioequivalence and by the required power. The clinical and analytical standards imposed may also influence the statistical determined number of subjects. However, the minimum number of subjects should not be smaller than twelve and the number of recruited subjects should always be justified.

Randomization

Randomization is the process by which subjects are assigned randomly and is used to decrease the effect of one's own biases in assigning subjects to therapy groups, ensures unbiasedness and this allows valid statistical inferences to be drawn from the resulting clinical trial data. In bioequivalence trials generally 50 percent of the subjects are to be administered formulation T in the first period and 50 percent formulation R to guarantee balanced design. Whether the subjects receive T or R depends on chance.

Volunteer Recruitment and Selection

Volunteers may spontaneously come to a bioavailability/bioequivalence clinical center or be recruited by advertisements, provided that these are previously approved by an Ethics Committee. After being informed on the nature of the study and signing the informed consent form, the volunteer should be submitted to medical evaluation and complementary exams, according to the legislation in force and the research protocol. The entire volunteer recruitment and selection should be duly described, known and followed by all professionals involved.

Volunteer Hospitalization and Discharge

The volunteer selected for a bioavailability/bioequivalence assay should be hospitalized the night before starting the study, being reevaluated by a physician at the time of admission, preferably at the clinical unit, where they will have their vital signs (pulse, blood pressure and temperature) evaluated to reduce a possible interference that may occur in the pharmacokinetics of the drug to be given, due to the ingestion of alcoholic beverages, sleep deprivation or intense physical activity within the hours previous to the study, as well as identifying occurrences of possible exclusion factors between selection and hospitalization.

The procedures regarding volunteer hospitalization should be standardized in a specific document and followed by those in charge of admission and release. The equipment used in the evaluation and pre-hospitalization sphygmomanometer, stethoscope and thermometer should be in good use conditions. It is recommended that when admitted, the volunteer receives written information of the events to be carried out during the confinement period, with, at least, the scheduled times for the drug administration, meals, blood sampling and release. After the end of the drug administration and biologic material collection phases foreseen by the protocol, the volunteers shall be mandatorily subject of a new medical evaluation and complementary exams foreseen by the study protocol for diagnose of possible intercurrences that may have been caused by the participation in the clinical study.

Administration of the Drug and Biological Material Collection

The volunteers should fast for at least 10 hours before drug administration. Immediately before the start of the drug administration, a peripheral vein should be catheterized and maintained for the period required in order to blood sampling. Sampling should be carried out according to the pharmacokinetic profile of the drug to be studied and protocol, the first collection (baseline collection) being mandatorily performed before the drug is administered. All drug administration, sample collection, preparation and storage procedures should be recorded in a specific document, with an identification of the person in charge of it. The time points determined by the protocol for sample collection should be strictly followed and any deviation shall be recorded.

The drug should be given as described in the protocol under medical supervision, by a nurse, pharmacist or a qualified professional. A physician should supervise the volunteers during the hours after the administration of the drug, in a period enough to assure medical support to fortuitous adverse events. Vital signs from volunteers should be controlled during all confinement period. Complementary measures should be taken in the event the protocol determines them. Fortuitous intercurrences should be duly documented. The clinical unit should keep an on-duty physician during the entire hospitalization period, who should be aware of the performance of a bioavailability/ bioequivalence study, if not directly involved on it. In this case, the physician in charge of the clinical step should be easy to locate and available for the resolution of possible intercurrences. The occurrence of adverse events, their intensity, as well as the measures taken for their reversion, should be duly recorded in an adequate document, with the identification and signature of the person in charge for the assistance of the volunteer, as well as the principal researcher. The occurrence of severe adverse events should be documented and reported to the competent authorities. During the hospitalization period, the diet of the volunteers should be supervised by a nutritionist, and defined to not interfere with drug analysis and pharmacokinetics.

Bioanalytical Logistics

Bioanalytical chemistry is the qualitative and quantitative analysis of drug substances in biological fluids (mainly plasma and urine) or tissue. It plays a significant role in the evaluation and interpretation of bioavailability, bioequivalence and pharmacokinetic data. The main analytical phases that comprise bioanalytical services are method development, method validation and sample analysis (method application).

Pharmacokinetic and bioequivalence studies require very precise and accurate assay methods that are well-validated to quantify drugs in biological samples. The assay methods have to be sensitive enough to determine the biological sample concentration of the drug and/or its metabolite(s) for a period of about five elimination half-lives after dosage of the drug. The assay methods also have to be very selective to ensure reliable data, free from interference of endogenous compounds and possible metabolites in the biological samples. In addition, methods have to be as robust and cost effective as possible, making of particular importance to bioequivalent studies.

The bioanalytical part of bioequivalence trials should be conducted according to the applicable principles of Good Laboratory Practice (GLP).

Method Development

A bioanalytical method is a set of all of the procedures involved in the collection, processing, storing and analysis of a biological matrix for an analyte. Analytical methods employed for quantitative determination of drugs and their metabolites in biological fluids are the key determinants in generating reproducible and reliable data that in turn are used in the evaluation and interpretation of bioavailability, bioequivalency and pharmacokinetics.

Method development involves evaluation and optimization of the various stages of sample preparation, chromatographic separation, detection and quantification. To start these work an extensive literature survey, reading work done on the same or similar analyte and summarizing main starting points for future work is of primary importance. Based on the information from this survey, the following can be done.

- The choice of instrument that is suitable for the analysis of your analyte of interest. This includes the choice of the column associated with your instrument of choice, the detector, the mobile phase in the high performance liquid chromatography (HPLC), and the choice of carrier in gas chromatography (GC).
- Choice of internal standard, which is suitable for your study. It must have similar chromatographic properties to your analyte.
- Choice of extraction procedure, which is time economical, gives the highest possible recovery without interference at the elution time of the analyte of interest and has acceptable accuracy and precision.

Method Validation

The bioanalytical methods used to determine the active moiety and/or its biotransformation product(s) in plasma, serum, blood or urine or any other suitable matrix must be well characterized, fully validated and documented to yield reliable results that can be satisfactorily interpreted. The main objective of method validation is to demonstrate the reliability of a particular method for the quantitative determination of an analyte(s) concentration in a specific biological matrix. The characteristics of a bioanalytical method essential to ensure the acceptability of the performance and the reliability of analytical results are: (1) stability of the stock solutions and of the analyte(s) in the biological matrix under processing conditions and during the entire period of storage; (2) specificity; (3) accuracy; (4) precision (5) limit of quantification, and (6) response function.

The validation of a bioanalytical method should comprise two distinct phases: (1) the prestudy phase in which the compliance of the assay with the six characteristics listed above is verified and (2) the study phase itself in which the validated bioanalytical method is applied to the actual analysis of samples from the biostudy mainly in order to confirm the stability, accuracy and precision.

A calibration curve should be generated for each analyte in each analytical run and it should be used to calculate the concentration of the analyte in the unknown samples in the run. A number of separately prepared Quality Control samples should be analyzed with processed test samples at intervals based on the total number of samples. In addition, it is necessary to validate the method of processing and handling the biological samples.

All procedures should be performed according to pre-established Standard Operating Procedures (SOPs). All relevant procedures and formulae used to validate the bioanalytical method should be submitted and discussed. Any modification of the bioanalytical method before and during analysis of study specimens may require adequate revalidation; all modifications should be reported and the scope of revalidation justified.

Pharmacokinetic Parameters

In the in-vivo bioequivalence study these characteristics are determined by measuring the following parameters:

i. Area under the plasma concentration time curve (AUC) because it describes the total number of drug molecules of the drug present in plasma, thereby informing the researchers on the extent of the release.
ii. The maximum plasma concentration (C_{max}) because it is linked to the speed of the release.
iii. The time at which maximum plasma concentration is reached (T_{max}) because it is linked to the speed of the release.
iv. The elimination half-life $T_{1/2}$, because it is linked to the elimination of the drug. $T_{1/2}$ is obtained by calculation of K_{el} the elimination constant.

Figure 16.1 is a typical example of a plasma concentration time profile of a drug with test and reference. One can distinguish an absorption and elimination phase. When the mass absorbed equals the mass eliminated, C_{max} is present. Before C_{max} is reached (before T_{max}) the absorption is higher than the elimination, after T_{max} the situation is reversed.

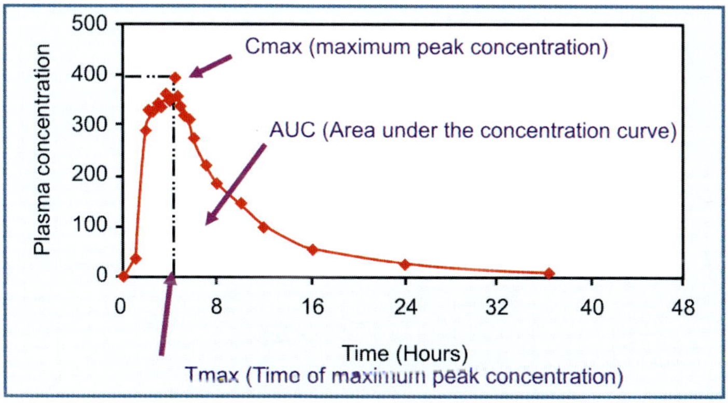

Fig. 16.1: Nontransformed plasma concentration time curve, showing C_{max}, T_{max} and AUC

A log transformation of the measured plasma concentrations will provide a straight line during the elimination phase, later on it is used to calculate the elimination half-life (Fig. 16.2).

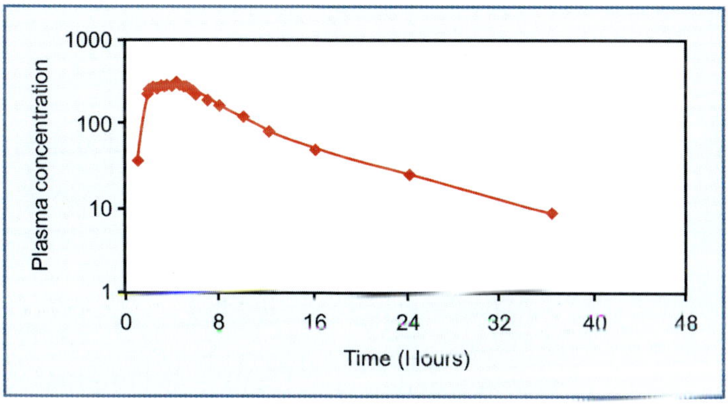

Fig. 16.2: An ln-transformed plasma concentration time curve, showing a linear elimination phase

C_{max}: Maximum measured plasma concentration over the time span specified.

T_{max}: Time of the maximum measured plasma concentration.

K_{el}: Apparent first-order terminal elimination rate constant calculated from a semi-log plot of the plasma concentration versus time curve. The parameter calculated by linear least-square regression analysis using the maximum number of points in the terminal log-linear phase (e.g., three or more non-zero plasma concentrations).

The calculation of K_{el} is an essential part of any bioequivalence study. Elimination is a first order process and a natural log (ln) transformation makes it possible to draw a straight line through the elimination phase. The slope of the regression line is now equivalent to K_{el} or the elimination constant (Figure 16.3).

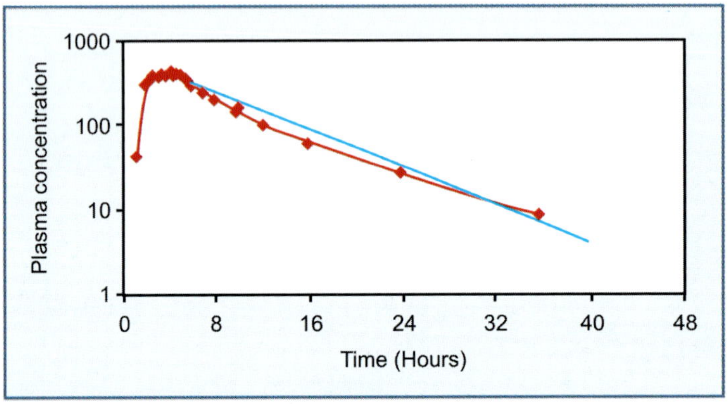

Fig. 16.3: Ln-transformed plasma concentration time curve, showing a regression line through the elimination phase. The slope of the regression line represents the elimination constant

The apparent first-order terminal elimination half-life calculated as $0.693/K_{el}$.

$$T_{½} = \frac{0.693}{K_{el}}$$

Equation 1 Calculation of $T_{1/2}$

$T_{1/2}$: The apparent first-order terminal elimination half-life calculated as $0.693/K_{el}$.

AUC_{0-t}: The area under the plasma concentration versus time curve, from time zero to the last measurable concentration, as calculated by the linear trapezoidal method.

$$AUC_{0-t} = \sum_{i=t}^{t} \left(\frac{C_i + C_{i-t}}{2} \right) (t_i - t_{i-t})$$

Equation 2 Calculation of the area under the plasma concentration time curve

AUC_{0-inf}: The area under the plasma concentration versus time curve, from time zero to Infinity. AUC_{0-inf} is calculated as the sum of AUC_{0-t} plus the ratio of the last measurable plasma concentration to the elimination rate constant using following equation:

$$AUC_{0-\infty} = AUC_{0-t} + \frac{C_{last}}{K_{el}}$$

Equation 3 Estimation of the $\mathbf{AUC_{0-inf}}$

Parameters for Sustained Release

Bioequivalence are also required for sustained release preparations, which release the drug over longer periods of time. The testing of these formulations is more difficult because the most important goal of these formulations is to obtain smooth steady-state plasma concentration time profile. It is, therefore, not surprising that the mean goal for sustained release preparations bioequivalence studies to show similarity of the steady-state plasma concentration profile.

The classical single dose parameters maintain their validity, but no longer describe the plasma concentration time profile adequately. New added parameters are the C_{min} and the percent peak through fluctuation. C_{min} describes the lowest plasma concentration just before the next dose is given and the peak through fluctuation the swing of the plasma concentration time profile between two administrations. The latter is calculated by percent fluctuation = $(C_{max} - C_{min})\ C_{average}$. The $C_{average}$ is the average plasma concentration over the dosing interval and it is calculated as AUC_{0-t} / τ, where τ = the dosing interval.

Statistical Analysis

Equivalence Limits

A test product is considered to be bioequivalent to a reference product if the 90 percent confidence interval for testing the following interval hypothesis on ln-transformed pharmacokinetic responses of AUC and C_{max} between the test and reference fall within 80-125 percent. Currently, the bioequivalence limits of 80-125 percent have been applied to almost all drug products.

In certain cases a wider interval may be acceptable. The interval must be prospectively defined for C_{max} e.g. 0.75 – 1.33 and justified addressing in particular any safety or efficacy concerns for patients switched between formulations.

Ratio Analysis

Ratio of means calculated using the least square means (test/reference) for log-transformed C_{max}, AUC_{0-t} and AUC_{0-inf}. Ratio of means expressed as a percentage of the least square means for the reference formulations.

Intrasubject Variability

Intrasubject variability within subjects for each pharmacokinetic parameter reflects the residual variability and calculated using mean square error (MSE). This is a major determinant for sample size, power and the width of the confidence interval for crossover studies.

Power Calculation

Power calculation at the 5 percent level of significance using the t-test (derived at the null hypothesis of no difference between the two formulations means for the ln-transformed data).

Software

The following regulatory approved validated software are needed for pharmacokinetic and statistical analysis:

i. Analyst 1.4.1, MDS Sciex
ii. LC-solution 1.1.2, Schimadzu
iii. WinNonlin 5.0.1, Pharsight Corporation 800 West El Camino Real, Suite 200, Mountain View, California 94040
iv. SAS 9.1.3, SAS Institute Inc., Cary, NC, USA.

Reporting of Results

The report of a bioavailability or a bioequivalence study should give the complete documentation of its protocol, conduct and evaluation complying with GCP rules and related EU and ICH E3 Guidelines. This implies that the authenticity of the whole of the report is attested by the signature of the principal investigator. The responsible investigator(s), if any, should sign for their respective sections of the report.

Names and affiliations of the responsible investigator(s), site of the study and period of its execution should be stated. The names and batch numbers of the products used in the study as well as the composition(s), finished product specifications and comparative dissolution profiles should be provided. In addition, the applicant should submit a signed statement confirming that the test product is the same as the one that is submitted for marketing authorization.

All results should be clearly presented and should include data from subjects who eventually dropped-out. Dropout and withdrawal of subjects should be fully documented and accounted for. The method used to derive the pharmacokinetic parameters from the raw data should be specified. The data used to estimate AUC should be reported. If pharmacokinetic models are used to evaluate the parameters, the model and computing procedure used should be justified. Deletion of data should be justified.

All individual subject data should be given and individual plasma concentration/ time curves presented in linear/linear and long/linear scale. The analytical report should include the results for all standard and quality control samples as well. A representative number of chromatograms or other raw data should be included covering the whole concentration range for all, standard and quality control samples as well as the specimens analyzed. The analytical validation report should be submitted as well.

The statistical report should be sufficiently detailed to enable the statistical analysis to be repeated, e.g. randomization scheme, demographic data, values of pharmacokinetic parameters for each subject, descriptive statistics for each formulation and period. A detailed ANOVA and/or nonparametric analysis, the point estimates and corresponding confidence intervals including the method of their estimation should also be included.

FACILITY

The following infrastructure is recommended for conducting bioequivalence studies:

Clinical

- A ward with at least 30-40 beds
- A pharmacy with provision for storing drug products as per prescribed conditions
- Phlebotomy stations (at least one for every six beds)
- Sample separation area with refrigerated centrifuges
- An ICU with crash cart and emergency resuscitation equipment
- Access to an accredited pathology laboratory
- Access to a radiology centre
- Dining and recreational facilities
- Sufficient number of toilets (at least one for every six beds)
- A volunteer data bank
- Access to IEC or IRB.

Bioanalytical

- Sample processing wet labs with fume hoods and facility for handling light-sensitive drugs
- An alcove with vibration-free table for weighing balances
- Instrumentation labs for sophisticated equipment like HPLCs and LCMS
- Room for air compressors and gas cylinders
- Store for solvents and reagents
- Sample store with freezers.

Information Technology
- Local Area Network with a server
- Firewalls with anti-spam server and anti-virus software.

General
- Biological waste segregation area
- Security access throughout the facility

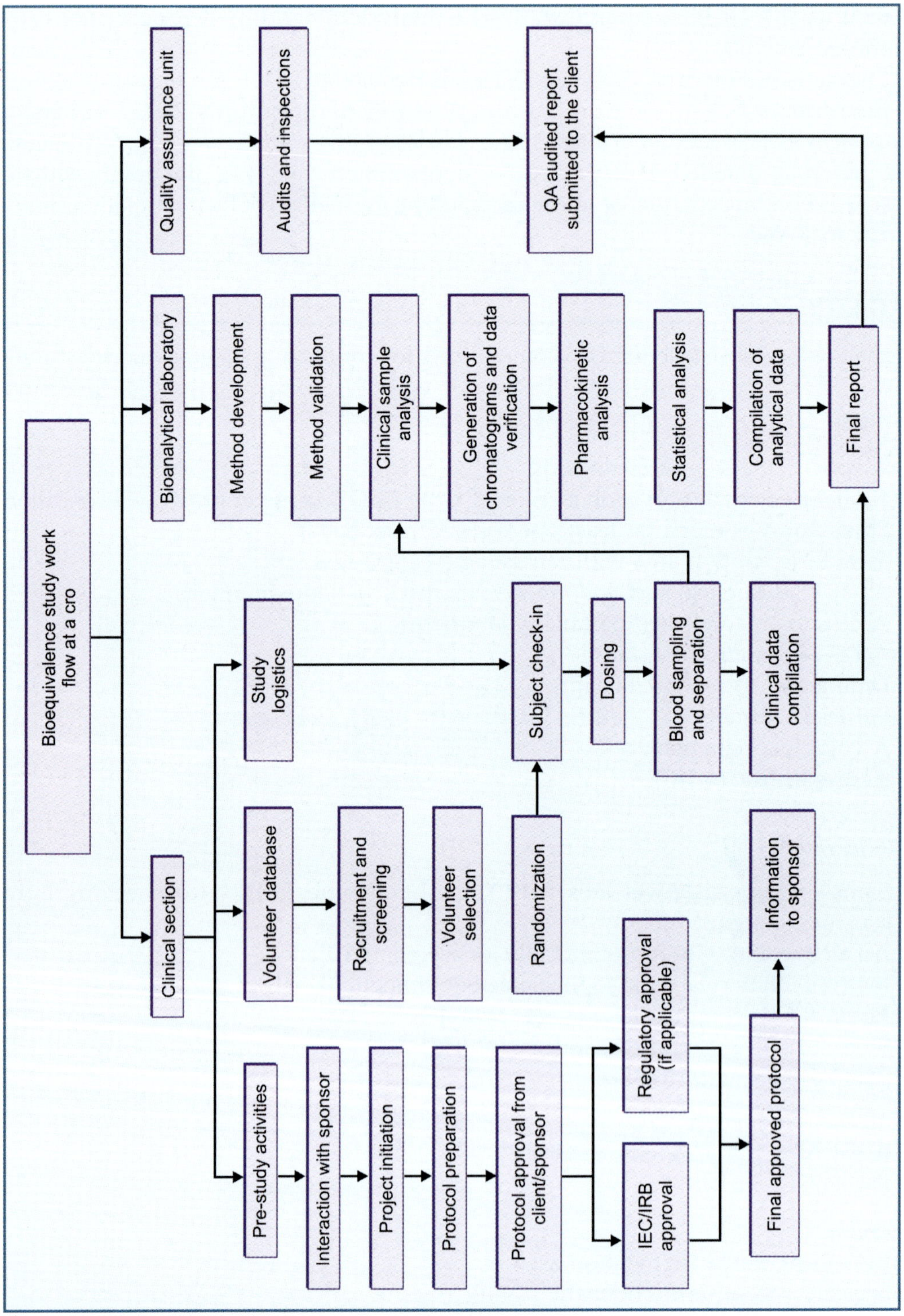

Flow chart 16.1: Schematics of a bioequivalence study work flow at a CRO

- Fireproof archives
- Disaster management back up
- Quality assurance
- Pharmacokinetic and statistical analyses and report writing
- Quality systems to show conformance to GCP and GLP for all operations.

WORK FLOW AT A BIOEQUIVALENCE CENTRE

Bioequivalence studies may be conducted by pharmaceutical companies within their R and D laboratories or at contract research organizations (CROs) equipped to do so. For a CRO, the work flow is the gamut of activities starting from the sponsor's query till the submission of the final report and a possible regulatory audit. The schematics of work flow are best summarized in Flow chart 16.1:

SUGGESTED READING

1. Abdou HM. Dissolution, Bioavailability and Bioequivalence. Easton: MACK Publishing Company; 1989.
2. Blanchard J, Sawchuk RJ, Brodie BB. Editors. Principles and Perspectives in Drug Bioavailability. Basel (Switzerland): S. Karger; 1979.
3. Chow S-C, Liu J-P. Design and Analysis of Bioavailability and Bio-equivalence Studies. New York: Marcel Dekker, Inc.; 1992.
4. EMEA (European Agency for the Evaluation of Medicinal Products), CPMP (Committee for Proprietary Medicinal Products). Note for guidance on the investigation of bioavailability and bioequivalence. 2001.
5. FDA (US. Food and Drug Administration), CDER (Center for Drug Evaluation and Research). Guidance for Industry: Bioavailability and bioequivalence for orally administered drug products—general considerations (Draft). 2002.
6. FDA (US. Food and Drug Administration), CDER (Center for Drug Evaluation and Research). Guidance for Industry: Food-effect bioavailability and fed bioequi-valence studies. 2002
7. Health Canada. Conduct and Analysis of Bioavailability and Bioequivalence Studies: Part A: Oral dosage formulations used for systemic effects (1992); Part B: Oral modified release formulations (1996); Report C: Report on bioavailability of oral dosage formulations, not in modified release form, or drugs used for systemic effects, having complicated or variable pharmacokinetics (1992);1992-96..
8. Marzo A. Clinical pharmacokinetic registration file for NDA and ANDA procedures. Pharm Res 1997;36:425-50.
9. Midha KK, Nagai T. Eds. Bioavailability, Bioequivalence and Pharmacokinetic Studies: FIP. Bio-International '96. Tokyo: Business Center for Academic Societies Japan, 1996.
10. Steinijans VW, Hauschke D. Update on the statistical analysis of bioequivalence studies. Int J Clin Pharmacol Ther Toxicol 1992;30(Suppl 1):S45-50.

17 Finance and Budgeting in Clinical Trials

Kiran Marthak

INTRODUCTION

With escalating pressures on research and development (R and D) cost-containment across the global pharmaceutical industry, there is increased focus on reducing the costs of clinical development, which comprises two-thirds of development costs. The additional problem of delayed development times is also affecting new drug introductions, losing incremental revenues. One of the major factors for this delay is an unsatisfactory patient recruitment rate. This dual challenge of accelerating clinical development and reducing costs has forced major pharma companies to look at alternative destinations for sourcing patients for their global studies.

Exploration on these lines would then take you to selected countries in Latin America, Eastern Europe, Commonwealth of Independent States (CIS) countries and Asia. Amongst the Asian countries, India stands out prominently due to its huge patient population, English-speaking doctors (many of whom are educated in Western countries) and a large pharmaceutical presence that has dominated the world markets due to cheap generics.

TYPES OF COSTS IN MEDICINAL DEVELOPMENT

Apart from the cost incurred in new medicine development i.e. Phases 1, 2 and 3 clinical developments, there are numerous other types of costs that are incurred during the process.

- Non-clinical studies: These are the cost which are including the toxicology programme.
- Administrative and patent costs: These are costs, which are substantial in the pursuit of NDA (New Drug Application).
- Patent costs: Patent costs can be considered as a part of the administrative costs. Most patents require periodic fees to maintain their viability.
- Marketing costs: Cost incurred for promotion and advertizing.

- Cost related to professional staff providing information about the product/company
- Manufacturing costs.
- Other support costs.

TRIAL ACTIVITY AND PERFORMANCE PARAMETERS

Clinical trial activity and performance is linked to various factors which are the inputs in a clinical trial process. The clinical trial planning process manages a number of inputs by project phase over time. These inputs (or influences) include protocol assumptions, fixed costs (central and site), patient retention and recruitment, and organizational targets. Each of these inputs provides data that drives clinical trial performance (Fig. 17.1).

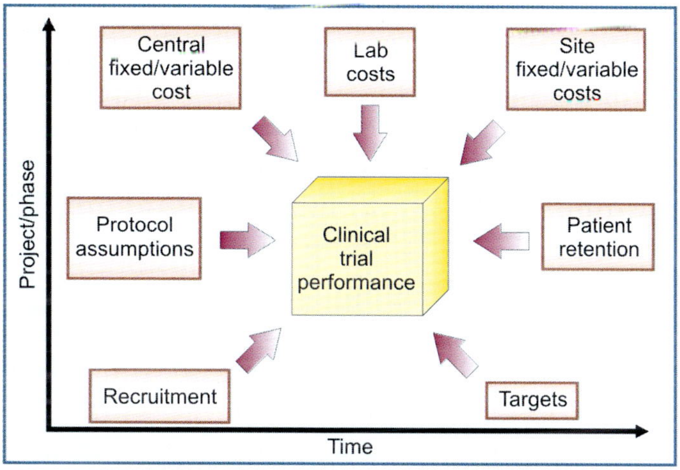

Fig. 17.1: Inputs to the planning process

Driver-based Approach to Planning Clinical Trials

Companies struggle to build an effective planning model based on Clinical Trial Management (CTM) systems along with tools like Microsoft Excel (Fig 17.2). Reasons for ineffective planning of a clinical trial could be the following:

- Data is difficult to access or understand
- Spreadsheets strain under the weight of complex calculations
- Input from various clinical trial managers, laboratories, CRO's and financial analysts come in different formats, at different times, or at irregular intervals.

Finance experts tend to agree that conventional planning, budgeting, and forecasting methods involve too much detail and too little focus on the key metrics that drive expenses. Driver-based planning is based on common components that typically underlie a given expense.

Driver Data for Clinical Trial Cost Measures can include

- Investigator fees
- Procedure cost
- Enrollment rate
- Investigator overhead cost
- Investigator fees (PP)
- Clinical lab fees (PP)
- Trial protocol
- Number of visits
- Patient retention percentage

Importance of the Driver Based Approach

- Facilitates communication across all stakeholders in the clinical trial process.
- Provides a standardized corporate rationale for clinical trial planning.
- Provides a consolidated view of clinical trials across the organization.
- Enables resources to be transferred to under-performing clinical trials to insure completion.
- Accommodates the input of thousands of field-level reps.
- Offers senior executives visibility into overall clinical trial spend.

Driver-based Forecasting Improves Accuracy

Protocol definition begins the process. Based on assumptions and fixed costs, enrollment drivers can be established to predict variables such as per patient costs that include investigator and lab fees.

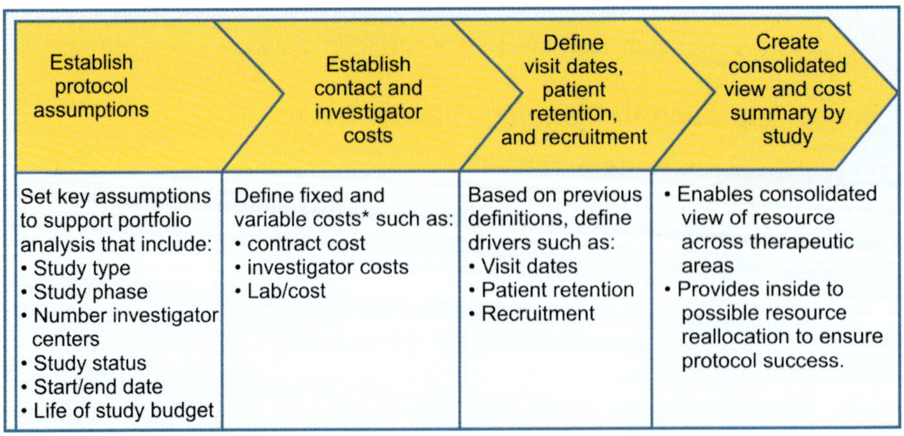

Fig. 17.2: Driver-based approach to planning clinical trials

"WHAT SHOULD BE BUDGETED FOR?"

Salaries

Types of staff:

Regular research staff	Specialist consultants
Cost in: Basic salary *And on-costs:* National Insurance Superannuation Increments/pay rises Institutional overheads	Usually need to budget for an agreed rate

Materials and Consumables

Stationery

Consider the numbers of questionnaires or data collection schedules required throughout the life of the project. Postal questionnaires often need reminders sent and copies of the original questionnaire. Budget for invitations, information sheets and general correspondence. The project may require a commissioned logo featured on correspondence.

Printing

Costs of above stationery are eligible as a direct cost but must be project specific and identifiable in an audit trail.

Postage

Consider the amount of general correspondence, number of mailings, including follow-ups and reminders. Budget for stamped addressed envelopes or pre-paid envelopes (more cost effective—no payment for non-responders). Postage costs are eligible as a direct cost but must be project specific and identifiable in an audit trail.

Travel

Include researcher to participant visits and *vice versa*; site meetings required to set up and run the project. Some funders will allow conference expenses associated with the project.

Tests

Include clinical and laboratory tests.

Equipment

Include monitoring instruments, computing equipment and software, desks, chairs, renting room space.

Telephone Costs

Communications office staff will advise on recommended standard rates for telephone calls and associated costs. Depending on the type of research undertaken, if telephone costs are particularly high, they should be included as a direct cost.

Space and any Special Environments

These can be costly and need careful budgeting.

Miscellaneous

Includes staff training, advertisements for staff and recruitment costs (travel etc.) and equipment running costs.

Non-commercial Research Costs

Patient care costs associated with research and development.

Research Team and Associated Costs

Include collaborators (funders will require an appropriate skill mix and that staff have necessary expertise, e.g. statisticians; overseer and/or steering committee made up of senior staff and lay or consumer representatives); day-to-day project manager/coordinator (requires wide experience including keeping up to date with the literature, planning and implementing the study, establishing communication with sites and other researchers, co-ordinating the data collection, undertaking data analysis, and writing reports); research assistants (responsible for data collection, professional interviewing, or technical support including processing samples); administrative staff, support staff, consultants, data monitoring committee and research governance monitoring.

Always round up and allow some leeway for unforeseen events

Recruitment Issues: Staff

A need to consider costs involved in:

- Development of job descriptions and job description outlines
- Advertisements
- Interviewing.

Study Design Costs

- Sample selection - size of sample will have knock-on effects elsewhere e.g. if your sample consists of individuals with a rare condition, this may involve a large number of sites, recruiting a small number of patients in each. If your sample consists of a common condition, all participants may be identified in one site.
- Randomization - it is important to have a robust procedure of randomization. This needs to be set up in advance, and should be discussed with a statistician when the project is being planned.
- There may be charge by Pharmacy
- Costs of intervention - some projects may require researchers to organize an evaluation of the intervention.
  Assign responsibility for these items and allow sufficient time for completion.

Data Collection, Management and Storage Issues

- Measuring outcomes - there are many validated tools available but permissions may need to be sought, and sometimes a fee paid to use these tools. If you are developing your own measurement tools this may involve statistical reliability and validity testing.
- Non - English speaking issues - does provision need to be made for translations or interpreters?

Data management and analysis issues

- Statistical advice before you start
- Equipment (hardware and software) should be available.
- Data entry and checking
- On-going statistical and computing support
- Administrative assistance (for example, for transcribing).
- Data analysis and writing up of findings

Other/Miscellaneous costs: Dissemination Costs

Dissemination may involve:

- Individual feedback
- Local workshops
- A report for the funding body
- A report to the Ethics Committee(s)
- Academic and health services related conferences and meetings
- Journal articles
- Dissemination through websites
- Dissemination through the press. This may result from the presentation of findings at conferences or through journals.

Time-tabling

Sample Research Planning For A Clinical Trial Spread Over A Time Frame of 3 Years.

Nature of Trial: Rct

Number of Trial Sites: 3

Calculation of Clinical Trial Costs

- Patient-based (Fig. 17.3)
- Protocol-based
- CT cost-based on methods used
- Sample headings which are used to track financial expenses for clinical trials in a project.

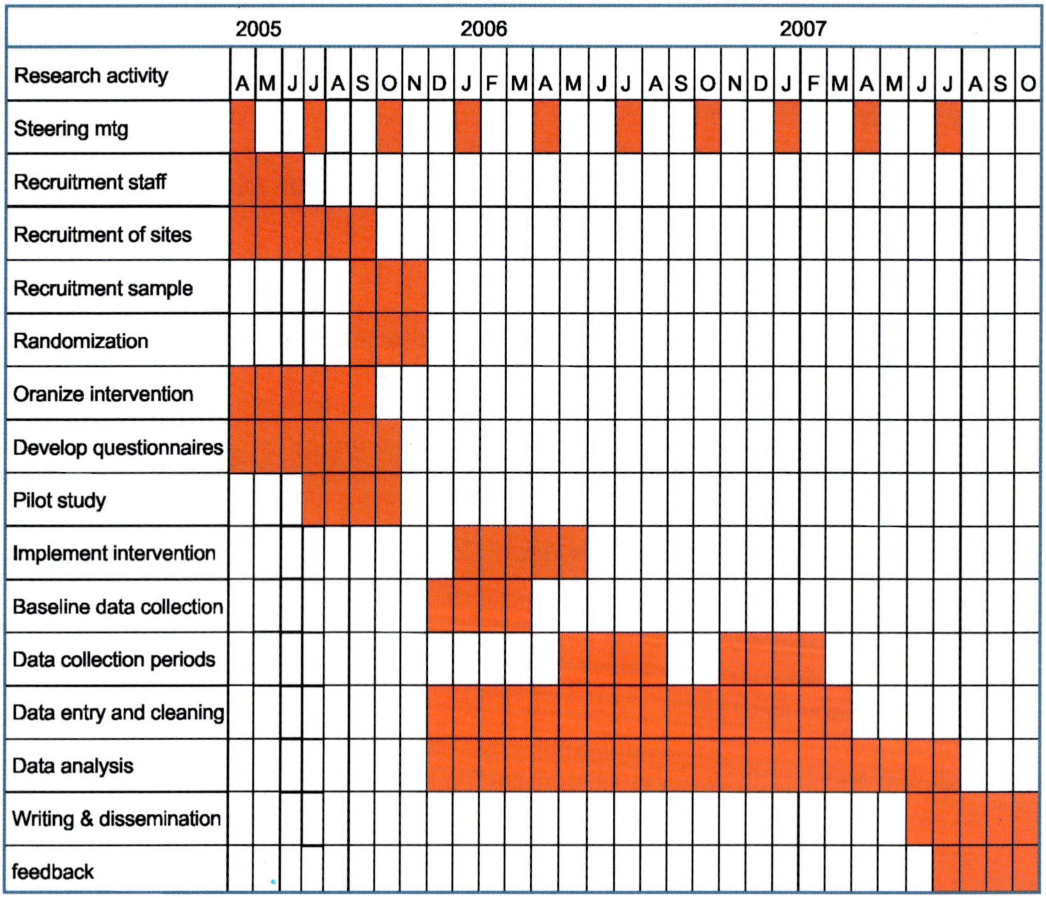

Fig. 17.3: Patient-based costing sheet

Sample costing sheet; patient-based costing sheet

A	Examinations		Cost per patient
	Initial patient history and physical examinations		
	Abbreviated physical examinations	No of exams*cost per exam	
	Ophthalmologic examinations	No of exams*cost per exam	
	Other examinations	No of exams*cost per exam	
B	Laboratory		
	EKG 12 Lead		
	EKG Lead II(No of tests *cost per test)		
	Clinical chemistry	No of tests*cost per test	
	Hematology	No of tests*cost per test	
	Urinalysis	No of tests*cost per test	
	Other tests	No of tests*cost per test	
C	Efficacy examinations		
	Test 1	No of tests*cost per test	
	Test 2	No of tests*cost per test	
	Test 3	No of tests*cost per test	
D	Administration		Total cost per patient
	Nurse	(percent of fulltime*yearly/ monthly salary)/no of patients	
	Telephone; postage; miscellaneous	Total Cost/no of patients	
	University Overhead	Cost per patient=X% *cost per patient)	
	Total Cost of Trial=Number of patients *Total cost per patient		

Sample costing sheet; protocol-based costing sheet

A Item Cost per Item | Per Patient: Number of Tests, Costs | Total Cost

List each point of the protocol for which there is a charge

B Item Cost per Item | Part A of trial per patient: Number of Tests, Total Costs | Part B of Trial: Screen (n=x): No of tests, Total Cost; Trial (n=y): No of tests, Total Cost | Overall total cost

List each point of the protocol for which there is a charge and total each column

C Group of patients	No of patients per group	No of analyses per patient	Cost per analysis	Total cost per patient	Total Cost per group
1	A				
2	B				
3	C				
4	D				
5	E				
TOTAL					

Sample Costing Sheet: CT cost based on Methods Used-1

Sample costing sheet for CT calculation based on Methods used	
	Amount
A Microbiology Cultures. No of cultures per patient per week*A weeks*B $*C patients	
Pharmacy fees for dispensing medicines and collecting returns	
Salaries	
Research Nurse: A hours at B $ per hour*C patients	
Secretarial support	
Professional support	
Data analysis	
Subtotal	
Overhead (x %)	
Total	
Cost per patient	
B Equipments	
Individual patient costs	
Patient recruitment (includes advertizing costs)	
Patient Stipend (includes meals)	
ECG's	
Opthalmological examinations	
Technical support (includes computer fees)	
Medical Support	
Physical examination	
Clerical support	
Total cost per patient	
Total trial cost	
C Dr A at 25 degrees of time	
Dr B at 10 degrees of time	Total Cost=Salary +Benefits
Office supplies (copying, phone, typing, etc.)	
Professional travel to one meeting (each for Drs A and B)	
TOTAL	

Sample Costing Sheet: CT cost-based on Methods Used-2

Sample costing Sheet for CT calculation based on methods used
D Personnel
Anesthologists (n=A)*Days at Y $ per day
Recovery Room Nurses (n=B)*Days at Z $ per Day
EEG Technician (n=C)*Days at E $ per day
Research Coordinator H days at F $ per day
Secretarial assistance J Days at G $ per day
Operating room use of space and equipment*days at K $ per day
Operating room: Supplies and forecast
Pharmacy supplies
Laboratory procedures
Each listed, plus number of times performed
Times Cost Times no of patients
TOTAL COST PER TRIAL
TOTAL COST PER PATIENT
E Laboratory assistance
Itemize-No done per patient at cost in $
Clinical assessments
Itemize-cost per patient
Personnel costs
Research coordinator cost per patient
Secretary and clerical cost per patient
Estimated costs per patient prematurely discontinued
TOTAL
F Personnel costs (% Effort of each worker listed)
Trial admin costs (Each Aspect Listed)
Patient management
Lab experiments
ECG evaluations
Psychiatric consultations
Other aspects listed
TOTAL
TOTAL COST PER PATIENT

Sample Costing Sheet: CT Cost Based on Methods Used-3

Sample costing sheet for CT calculation based on methods used		
		Amount
I		
A	**Patients screened but not entered**	
	Initial visit, medical history and physical examination	
	Efficacy assessments	
	Research coordinator's fee	
	Laboratory fees	
	Patient fees for meals and transportation	
	TOTAL	
B	**Patients who complete screening and interim visits**	
	Initial visit, medical history and physical examination	
	Interim visit physical examination	
	Efficacy assessments (*2)	
	Research coordinator's fee (*2)	
	Laboratory fees (*2)	
	Patient fees for meals and transportation (*2)	
	TOTAL	
C	**Patients who complete the CT (3 visits)**	
	Initial visit, medical history and physical examination	
	Interim visit physical examination	
	Final visit physical examination	
	Efficacy assessments (*3)	
	Research coordinator's fee (*3)	
	Laboratory fees (*2)	
	Patient fees for meals and transportation (*3)	
	TOTAL	
Estimated no of (A) patients		
Estimated no of (B) patients		
Estimated no of (C) patients		
Estimated budget total=A+B+C		

Budgeting for Contingencies

Following are the significant features that should be included in the costing sheet to protect from situations, which could result in financial loss:

i. For termination of study prior to enrollment of the first patient-the site should be paid a percentage of the total budget to cover start-up costs, payable immediately after thirty-day written notice.

ii. Delay of study start up - How many times has this happened? Current thinking in this area would be to ask for an additional 5% of the total budget for the holdup, after a reasonable time period; (e.g. three months).

iii. Build in language to cover changes to the study that add extra work 3 - when amendments or CRF pages are added that increase workload. This is a way to keep a budget down, yet a site can receive payment for any additional functions.
iv. Bonus payments-, this is a way to increase the budget with less risk for the sponsor/CRO (e.g., an additional $ 500.00 per patient after ten patients enrolled).
v. Consider adding language to cover the possibility of an audit by the FDA - Most studies will not be audited, but investigators who have conducted pivotal studies, accrue the most patients on a trial, or have participated in several phases of the same study are more likely to be selected for an audit. If there is a possibility that the study will be subject to an FDA audit, the contract should include a contingency to cover the costs of audit preparation. If there was a notification that a study completed three to five years ago at your site was to be audited within the next two weeks, what would be involved in preparing for it? If one assumes that one person will need to work full time for ten days to prepare for the audit, request a contingency of about $3,000 to cover the cost of salary and overhead.

Trends in Budget and Payment Schedules

Due to the ever-growing business climate in the clinical trials industry today, there is an increasing effort on the part of clinical sites to ask for payment schedule terms that more genuinely meet their needs. A "typical" budget and payment schedule that sponsors have historically used (quarterly schedule - 25 percent at study initiation; 50 percent when the study is 1/2 complete; 75 percent at 3/4 study completion and 100 percent when all work is complete) to payment schedules that factor in the "real world" scenario of clinical trials.

Challenges to Clinical Trial Forecasting

Materiality and Understanding Drivers

Clinical trials represent the biggest direct spend component in most bio-pharma companies' R and D budgets. Executing large, global phase 3 clinical trials frequently cost more than $20 million. It is important to be able to understand, model, and consolidate project costs at the portfolio level to run what-if scenarios and analyses (Fig. 17.4). It is also important to understand the performance characteristics of particular sites or countries. Modeling performance data makes it easier to analyze the data and make more effective resource allocation decisions. For example: "*Per patient costs for running studies in Russia are low, but patient enrollment always undershoots and we end up spending more by adding additional centers. What would be the impact of running more of the study in France where costs are higher, but patient drops are lower?*"

Complexity and Process

Clinical trials managers are acutely aware of the difficulty inherent in producing robust, accurate, phased budgets and forecasts. Payments to investigators, which typically comprise 60-80 percent of trials costs, are often made without invoice, since investigators do not issue them. Without an invoice or purchase order, deriving an accurate and timely picture from accounting systems is problematic indeed.

Traditional Usage of Project Management Data

Bio-pharma R and D businesses are driven by projects. Traditional or clinical project management systems, whether home-grown or commercial, already contain the source data needed to build financial models. But traditional budgeting and finance applications are cost-center focused and do not take into account the multiyear project and portfolio management processes that are used to run the R and D business.

Volunteer Recruitment Factors Needed to be Taken Into Account

- Per patient per visit costs for investigator fees and labs.
- Planned drop percentages by visit by country.
- Visit occurrence relative to enrollment.

Financial Functionality of Project Management Systems

Commercial project management software solutions contain budgeting and forecasting as an afterthought and lack sufficient functionality to create and maintain a robust forecast.

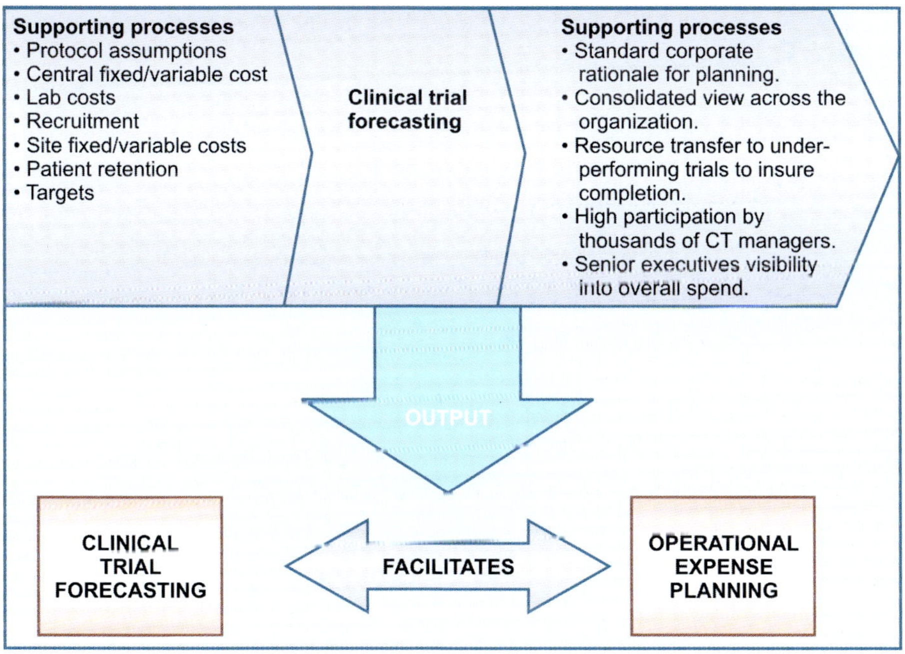

Fig. 17.4: Key output of clinical trial forecasting

Some common issues are:

- Inabilities to link-in and update the plan based on actual spend.
- Phasing based on a representative patient across all visits and not using the relative occurrence of the visits.
- Difficult integration with other financial forecasts to present a consolidated view of the overall department.
- Finance requirements such as accounting periods and foreign exchange rates are not typically supported.

Clinical trial forecasting requires the setting of protocol assumptions, tracking of central fixed and variable costs, lab costs, recruitment, site fixed and variable costs, while taking into account patient retention and protocol targets or goals. Such factors are all inputs to the clinical trial process. Clinical trial forecasting provides a standard rationale for trial planning and a consolidated view across all protocols which enables resource transfer where necessary, high participation by clinical trial managers, and executive visibility to overall spending. Ultimately, the forecasting process provides a pharmaceutical company an accurate prediction of clinical trial operating expenses.

18

Clinical Data Management

Babu S Nema, Shwetha Ramakrishnan

INTRODUCTION

All clinical trials are performed to answer certain questions about the efficacy and safety of a drug or device. The answers solely depend upon the quality of data, which are collected during the trial and submitted after the trial. The study data is an immense asset for the pharma and biotech companies. Probability of getting a drug or device being approved for marketing increases if the study data is in good shape. Hence data management plays a crucial role in ensuring the success of a trial. Adopting proper methods to manage the trial data helps in increasing the quality of data. Learning, practicing and improving upon these methods has lead to the creation of clinical data management as a subject.

Drug development encompasses stages such as formulation, toxicology and clinical trials. Clinical trial or a study in turn has various stages as depicted in Figure 18.1.

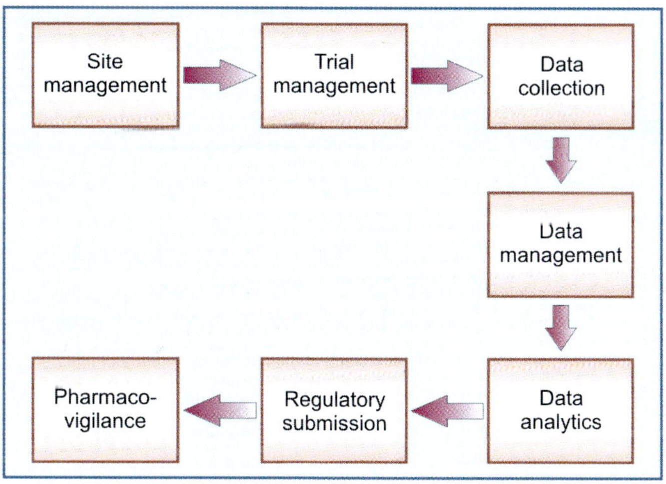

Fig. 18.1: Overview of clinical trial processes

However these may overlap. A study starts with an objective, which gets translated to a protocol, proceeds with identification of sites and management of the trial. Actual process of data management is initiated with the collection of data.

HISTORY OF CLINICAL DATA MANAGEMENT

Clinical data management (CDM) has evolved from a data entry process into a diverse process referred to as "provide clean data in a useable format in a timely manner", "provide a database fit for use" or "ensure data are clean and database is ready to lock".

Though clinical data management had to be done with whatever data was being collected for clinical trials from its earliest days, the processes were given a major focus in the early 1970s, when the Public Health Service recognized the need for good practices in clinical data management. With the advent of electronically transmitted clinical trial data, the standardized practices and procedures developed further. Regulatory requirements have advanced the necessity of clinical data management as a science.

Quality of the trial data is much more critical as pharma companies invest vast amounts of money in drug research. It is also vital for regulatory submission and approval. Hence CDM has grown from a mere data entry process to a technology based science.

OVERVIEW OF CLINICAL DATA MANAGEMENT

Clinical data management consists of processes such as trial data acquisition, validation, integration, database administration, backup, security and quality assurance. The locked database undergoes a statistical analysis after which it is ready to be submitted to the regulatory authority for approval. Processes used to support the clinical data must be clearly defined and documented. Documents supporting CDM activities include protocol, standard operating procedures (SOPs) (Fig. 18.2).

DATA MANAGEMENT PLAN

Before starting with the data management processes, a data management plan (DMP) must be put in place. DMP helps to proactively assess and plan for the study-specific data management processes (Fig. 18.3). The DMP serves as the backbone of overall quality system of data management (DM) and outlines:

- How and when each step of the CDM process must be carried out
- What documents are to be created and finalized
- Defines the data management tasks, responsibilities, deliverables and timelines
- Which SOPs or guidelines will apply to the various processes
- What document or output to collect or produce
- What level of quality must be achieved

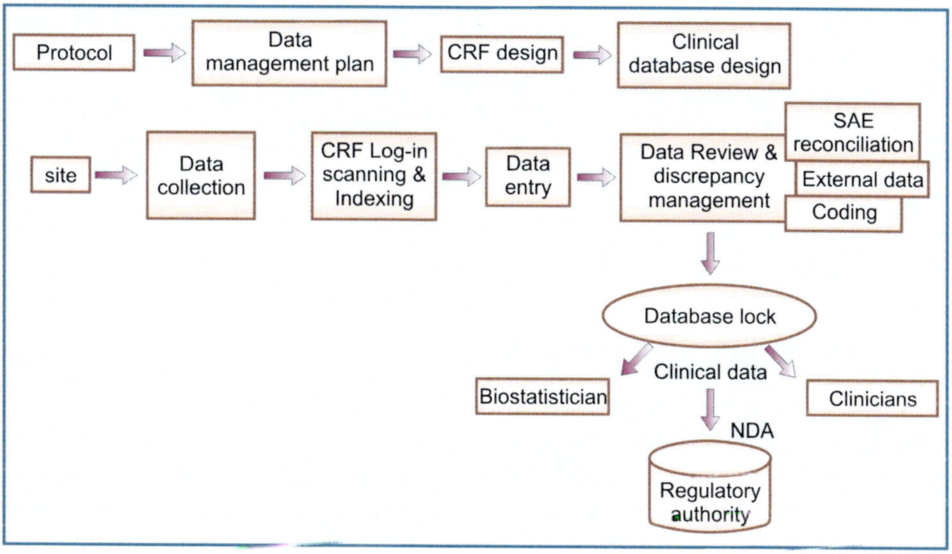

Fig. 18.2: Overview of CDM process

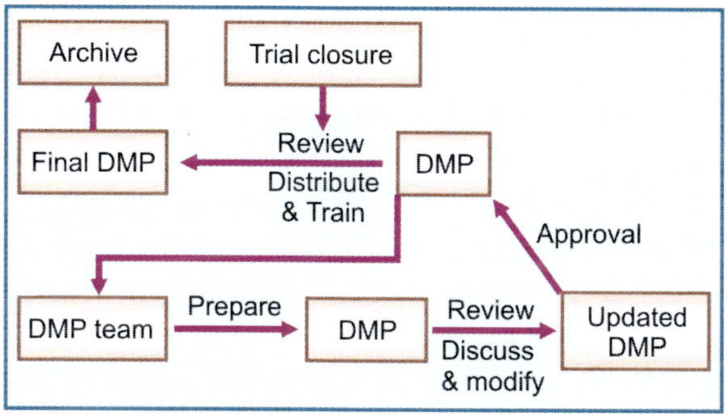

Fig. 18.3: An outline of the development and review process of a DMP

Preparation, review and finalization of the DMP involves participation from sponsor, lead data managers, project managers, biostatisticians, database programmers, lead clinical research associates (CRAs), project directors, medical monitors and clinical scientists.

Some of the key elements included in a typical DMP include:

- Trial work flow
- Study set-up/design
- Computing environment
- Database development and testing
- CRF management, including CRF flow and tracking
- Data capture, data entry and study specific guidelines
- Serious adverse event reconciliation

- Data validation procedures
- Coding procedures
- Lab data management
- Data transfer procedures
- Discrepancy management
- Reporting processes
- Study lock
- Quality audit

DATA CAPTURE AND COLLECTION

Data capture is a key concept in data management. This refers to procedures for gathering and recording data from or related to subjects in the study. It could either be paper-based or through electronic data capture (EDC). Promise of enhanced efficiency has led to increasing movement towards implementation of the electronic medical record and to computerized automation in general.

Paper CRF-based Study

Trial data are written on paper CRFs at the investigator sites. The study co-ordinator refers to "the source" (patient, patient's chart or other medical records, source document, etc.) and transcribes the data onto the paper CRF. This is just the first of many 'transcription' processes in clinical data management. These CRFs are periodically reviewed by CRAs to ensure that the data is valid and complete. A copy of the CRF is retained at the site, and additional copies are sent to the sponsor and the data management team where the data is entered into a database. Data editors then review the data in the database and identify any discrepancies in the data. These are resolved using a discrepancy clarification form (DCF), which is sent to the investigator at the site. After all the discrepancies are resolved, the data in the database is declared as "clean", at which point the database is locked. These paper CRFs have to be retained for up to 15 years at the sponsor and investigator sites.

Paper-based trials have their own disadvantages. The cost of printing and distributing CRFs is high. Enormous amount of time is spent in resolving simple data entry errors. Study performance information is not available to project managers in time for smooth conduct of trials. Repetition of tasks by different departments in regard to serious adverse event recording and reporting is common.

EDC-based Study

EDC is the capability to collect data electronically, without using paper CRFs. It could consist of both online and offline technologies. EDC is defined by the Clinical Data Interchange Standards Consortium (CDISC) as follows:

"Collecting or acquiring data as a permanent electronic record with or without a human interface (e.g., using data collection systems or applications that are modem-based, web-based, optical mark/character recognition, or involve audio text, interactive voice response, graphical interfaces, clinical laboratory interfaces, or touch screens). Note: 'Permanent' in the context of these definitions implies that any changes made to the electronic data are recorded via an audit trail."

Interactive voice response system (IVRS) consists of interactive speech or touch-pad menu-driven systems that take the caller through a series of prompts. Responses are entered through a telephonic keypad. This technology is typically used in areas such as patient randomization, adverse event reporting, trial supply management, patient visit tracking, assisting with study startup or collecting subject diary information.

Image recognition technology includes optical character recognition (OCR) and optical mark recognition (OMR). Here the data is captured from handwritten printed copies. Then the handwritten information is translated into electronic text documents. The image recognition software converts the scanned image to machine-readable and editable text.

Electronic CRFs (eCRFs) can be created as flexibly as if they were created on paper. When viewed on-screen, the eCRF appears as it would on paper. eCRF is a replacement for the entry of study data into paper CRFs. These eCRFs will have some form of built-in real-time data validation checks. The entered data is written directly to the central clinical database and is then immediately available for review to all study staff. This technology is also referred to as remote data entry (RDE) or remote data capture (RDC).

eCRFs have certain advantages over paper CRFs:

- Facilitates faster and more active management of the data gathering and processing workflow, thereby accelerating the transmission time of data to the sponsor.
- Automated data edit checks alert the site to possible errors in data entry.
- Ensures faster correction of issues and immediate site education, hence is cost saving.
- Ensures immediate viewing and review of the data by the sponsor and data management, hence online feedback is provided to the site immediately.

EDC has its own demerits. Primarily the reluctance of the investigators to use technology is a concern. As use of technology not only involves newer processes but also integration of other systems and groups, it requires higher planning and investment.

Data Privacy

The ICH Guideline for Good Clinical Practice (GCP) states, *"The confidentiality of records that could identify subjects should be protected, respecting the privacy and confidentiality rules in accordance with applicable regulatory requirement(s)."*

Adherence to sponsor's privacy policies is essential for maintenance of subject confidentiality. Security of all paper and electronic data has to be maintained. Paper CRFs are preferably stored in fireproof vaults with restricted access and all electronic data are protected with a password and firewall. Regulatory issues associated with patient data collection include finalization of error correction rules for CRFs using GCP, ensuring computer systems are 21 CFR Part 11 compliant and ensuring that all SOPs related to data management are in place and adhered to.

Investigator's training helps to generate better quality data thereby avoiding the generation of frequent queries. Detection of training issues by study monitors for common problems associated with CRFs and looking for recurring types of queries adds to improve the quality of the data.

CRF DESIGN

CRFs are instruments used to collect data from the clinical trials. They are designed to collect all data points specified in the protocol. CRFs standardize the collection of study data and also help in meeting the needs of medical, statistical, regulatory and data management personnel (Fig. 18.4 and 18.5). The CRFs are filled in by the investigator and then forwarded to the data management unit for entry and review.

In terms of design, well-designed CRFs should have the following features:

- Consistency across patients and sites
- Clear, concise and easy to fill questions
- Support data management activities
- Well designed headers
- Aid computerization of data
- Reliable and clean data for analysis
- Grouping of similar type of data together
- Collect raw data rather than calculated data
- Avoidance of long fields of free text
- Easy access of header information
- Legible font style and size
- Sufficient margins for binding and punching purposes

Some of the CRF essentials include study name/identifier, unique subject identifier, form name, page number, signature of person completing the form, date of form completion, instructions (when to complete, where to send) and numbering of items for easy reference. While designing a CRF, there are typically three types of question responses that can be incorporated:

- Open response: this typically involves free text, for example, adverse event (AE) text, medication text, medical history details, date/time, numeric lab values.
- Closed response: this typically consists of check boxes, multiple choice, etc.
- Combination response: this consists of a combination of both open and closed type responses. For example, on the medical history record, a question asking for

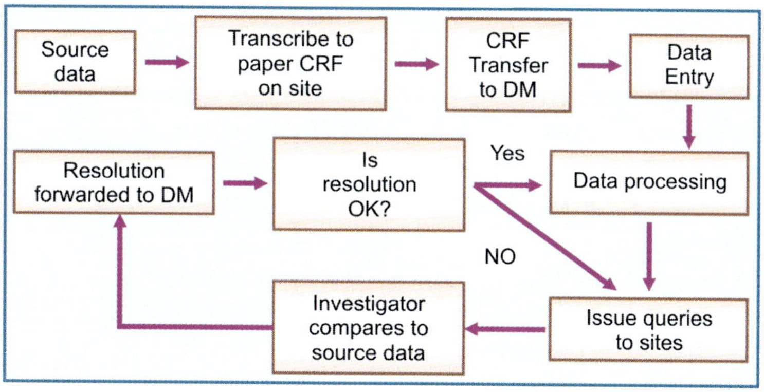

Fig. 18.4: Schematic representation of a typical paper-based process

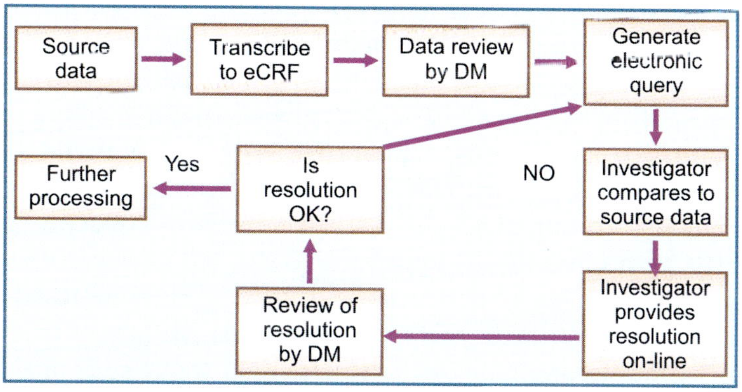

Fig. 18.5: Schematic representation of a typical eCRF process

specifying if any abnormality present, requires an answer yes or no (closed). If the answer is yes, then one is asked to specify details of the abnormality (open).

Before design finalization, a pilot is carried out with few 'dummy' CRFs to identify potential troublesome fields; accordingly training sessions are conducted for investigators and CRAs during study initiation. The CRF design review and finalization involves participation from the project data managers, statisticians, regulatory managers, medical monitors, lead CRAs and clinical scientists.

A set of CRF completion guidelines are finalized and documented in the DMP. This serves as a guideline to the investigators while filling in the CRFs and would typically consist of the following instructions:

- Read and follow all instructions carefully
- Write legibly on the form
- Use permanent ink on the forms
- Ensure all questions are answered and complete
- Write answers inside the space provided

- Submit original forms when necessary
- Use appropriate mechanisms for making corrections on the CRFs
- Check the forms before submission to the data management unit
- Ensure that patient ID information is correct
- Follow correct schedule/visits for forms submission
- Follow procedures for visits/examinations/tests that are not done and for unscheduled visits
- List abbreviations, if applicable
- Instructions for early terminators/study discontinuation
- Instructions for SAE reporting

CLINICAL DATABASE

A clinical data management system (CDMS) enhances the efficiency of the clinical trial process. Implementation of the CDMS involves planning and interaction of various teams. Design of CRF data flow into the system either manually or electronically is the first step. Subsequent steps are creating the global database, validation/derivation procedures, data extraction programs and reporting. One can also integrate dictionaries, AE reporting systems, EDC/RDC and CTMS with CDMS. It is essential to ensure that data is automatically transformed from a collection format to the reporting formats as needed by the sponsor and the regulatory authorities.

The main objective of database design is to capture and store clinical data accurately. The essential features of good design are ease of data capture, efficient creation of analysis data sets and accommodation of source data transfer formats.

CRF LOG-IN AND INVENTORY

The paper CRFs from site must be efficiently transmitted to the data management unit for entry and processing. Typical methods include faxing, mailing, scanning and in some cases hand delivery by the site monitor. Once the CRFs are received at the data management unit, each CRF page must be logged into the CDMS and each page gets inventoried into the CDMS. Tracking inventories are set up to detect missing pages and duplicate pages. When the CRFs are received as faxes or scanned images, some of the CDMSs can automatically store the images in a CRF image database. When paper CRFs are manually received, one can scan the CRF pages and store the images in CDMS. Subsequent processing steps may utilize images rather than paper.

Audit Trail

21 CFR Part 11 compliance requires that all persons accessing the clinical data management system must have electronic signatures of their own. All CDM personnel who access the database must have their unique electronic signature/user IDs. Any

modification, change, updation or deletion made in the database will be captured in the 'audit trail'. A well-designed audit trail captures details of the date and time of change, user ID of person making the change, original entry on database, final entry on database (changed value) and the reason for change.

DATA ENTRY

Data entry refers to the process of transferring data from the paper CRF to the database. This is also referred to as transcribing the data. Data entry results in creation of electronic data, which corresponds to the CRF data. Once data is entered into the database, it is reviewed and validated by the data editor. Emphasis for data entry is given on typing speed and typing skills, since this activity requires large amounts of data to be keyed into the database. Data entry consists of both double entry and single entry.

Double Entry

This involves entry of the same CRF page by two independent data entry personnel. The first data entry personnel keys in the data into the database. Later, a second independent data entry personnel keys in the same data. In case of a difference or discrepancy between the first and second entry, a 'pop up' box throws up, alerting the second data entry personnel to either key in what they see or to accept what the first data entry personnel has entered. Another option is to have a 'third' personnel review the differences/discrepancies and resolve them. Thus double data entry serves as a quality check in the data that is entered into the database.

Single Entry

This involves entry by single data entry personnel. This process is used when there are sufficient and extensive checks built into the database that would detect certain errors that might be missed out by the data entry personnel. Single data entry is extensively used in EDC and RDC systems, where the investigator and site personnel directly key in the data. This eliminates having data entry personnel within the data management unit. Once the data is keyed in directly at site, it is ready to be reviewed, edited and validated by the data editors.

The data entry could be of two types:

- Data entry is done locally at the site database and then transmitted periodically to the central database via internet or using a dialup line. Sometimes the data is also sent using other electronic media such as a CD, floppy or as a mail attachment.
- Data entry is done online directly into the central database via internet. Usually these systems are web-based and the data is available in real time for review.

DATA REVIEW AND VALIDATION

Once data entry is complete, the data is ready to be reviewed by the data editor. The data editor ensures that all discrepancies are addressed and resolved, and that the database is finally clean and ready to be locked. Discrepancies are any inconsistencies found in the clinical trial data that needs to be addressed. Discrepancies include incomplete data, illogical data, incorrect data and illegible data (Fig. 18.6).

Discrepancies could be checked either manually or through computer-generated checks (validations and edit checks) that are programmed into the database. System-programmed validations are designed before start of the data management activities, and these serve as checks or alerts to the data editor. The data editor ensures that all discrepancies and validations are addressed and resolved before locking the study.

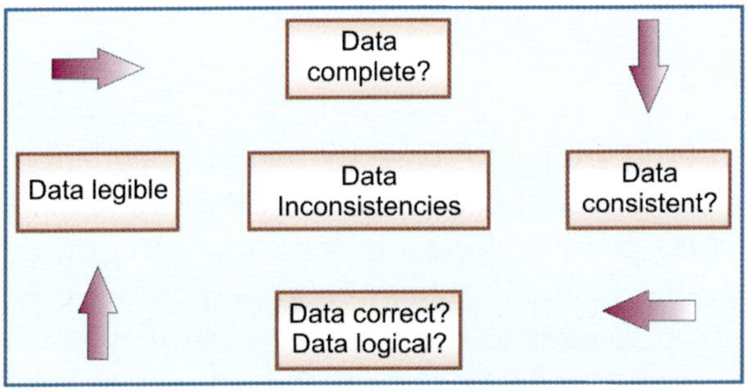

Fig. 18.6: Types of data inconsistencies

Data cleaning or validation refers to a collection of activities by data management, used to assure validity and accuracy of the clinical data. It comprises of both logical and statistical checks to detect impossible values due to data entry errors, coding and inconsistent data. The DMP and SOPs clearly defines the tasks, roles and responsibilities involved in cleaning a database.

There are various types of checks that must be performed and various types of data points and discrepancies that must be addressed during the process of review and cleaning (accordingly validations could be programmed for these discrepancies).

Point-by-Point Checks

This refers to cross checking between the CRF and the database for every data point. If the data editor performs this check, it serves as a second quality check apart from double data entry. Incorrect entries or entries missed out by data entry are corrected during this check. Special emphasis is given to dates, numerical values and header information, where there are likely to be more data entry misses.

Missing Data or Blank Field Checks

Missing data and blank fields must be queried for, unless indicated by the investigator as 'not done', 'not applicable' or 'not available'. It is better to program validations for missing data fields rather than review them manually. Examples of missing data include missing AE/medication term, missing start/stop dates, completely blank CRFs where none of the question responses are provided.

Data Consistency Checks

Checks are designed to identify potential data errors by checking corresponding events, sequence of dates, missing data (indicated as existing elsewhere), etc. Checks include cross checking between data points both across different CRFs and also within the same CRF.

Consider an example of inconsistent data across different CRF records: On the AE record, an AE is reported with action 'concomitant medication'; however on the concomitant medication record, there is no appropriate medication administered within the timeframe.

Consider the AE record where fever is reported with action 'concomitant medication':

Event	*Start Date*	*Stop Date*	*Action*	*Outcome*
Fever	13-Jun-2005	20-Jun-2005	Concomitant Medication	Resolved

Now consider the concomitant medication record where paracetamol is reported as follows:

Medication	*Start Date*	*Stop date*	*Outcome*
Paracetamol	21-Jun-2005	21-Jun-2005	Stopped

Here, paracetamol has not been given in the appropriate timeframe and hence this data is considered inconsistent.

Examples of inconsistent data across different fields, but within the same CRF include (a) an AE reported with a 'start date' but the outcome is reported as 'continuing/persisting' (b) stop date of a medication is greater than the visit date.

Consider another example of an antibiotics record versus a trial medication record Data consistency checks are to be reviewed both within a particular CRF and across different CRFs. Note the two sections/modules in the antibiotics record. The first section is designed to "report doses of antibiotics taken before intake of first dose of trial drug". The second section is designed to "report doses of antibiotics taken after intake of first dose of trial drug".

The first section of the antibiotics record is reported with the following details:

Antibiotic	*Dose*	*Route*	*Start Date*	*Stop Date*
Amoxicillin	6 mg	Oral	11-May-2001	14-May-2001

The second section of the antibiotics record is reported with the following details:

Antibiotic	*Dose*	*Route*	*Start Date*	*Stop Date*
Streptomycin	7 mg	IV	16-May-2001	17-May-2001

The trial medication record where the first dose of trial drug is reported with the following details:

Trial Medication	*Dosage*	*Route*	*Dosing Dates*
XX	50 mg	IV	15-May-2001

In this example, a cross-check of data between the two sections of the same antibiotic record and also between the antibiotic record and trial medication record shows that the data reported is logical and consistent.

Laboratory Data and Range Checks

Laboratory data has to be treated in a special manner, as they are different from all other CRF data. This data has to be interpreted with the help of reference ranges and must be expressed in the specified units for proper interpretation. This is much more important when data are combined from multiple studies. If the units are different they have to be converted to one common unit before interpretation. Hence the data has to be stored along with the original units in which they were captured. Linking the data with proper normal ranges is critical. Reference ranges may have to be taken from the study specific ranges or standard books when ranges are not available with the data.

Range validations are designed to identify statistical outliners, values that are outside normal variation of population under study and values that are physiologically impossible. An example of an 'out-of range' discrepancy is the reporting of hemoglobin value as 90 g/L, where the normal specified range as per the protocol is 110 – 160 g/L. While carrying out range checks, data editors need to ensure that appropriate range values and range units are applied for the particular test performed. For example, ranges for WBC types could be applied in units of either 'percentage' or 'absolute'. A granulocyte value could be reported in the unit of percentage, whereas the corresponding range could be applied in the absolute unit, hence the granulocyte value would most definitely be out of range.

Consider the following cross-check between the hematology record and AE record:

Hematology record

Hematology Test	Date	Result	Normal Range
WBC	05-Jan-2006	13,710 cells /µL/cu mm	4,300 - 10,800 cells/µL/cu mm

AE record

Event	Start Date	Stop Date	Outcome
Streptococcal	04-Jan-2006	07-Jan-2006	Resolved infection

In this case, a validation should ideally be programmed to flag a WBC 'out of range' discrepancy. The study guidelines may instruct the data editor to either query the site to confirm the correct value or to accept the discrepancy since an increase in WBC count is justified by streptococcal infection in the same time frame.

Discrete Value Group (DVG) Discrepancy Checks

DVG is a question where there is a fixed or expected set of responses. DVGs are built into the database in the form of drop-down options. An example of a DVG is the set of responses for the severity of an AE - 'mild', 'moderate', 'severe' and 'life-threatening'. However, if the severity is reported as 'not known', which is not part of this DVG, it constitutes a DVG discrepancy.

Another type of DVG discrepancy is a 'length' discrepancy. When the database is designed, each free text field is assigned a maximum number of characters that it will be allowed to accept when the data is keyed in. If the text reported exceeds the maximum number of characters, a length discrepancy is created, which needs to be addressed by the data editor.

Header Inconsistency Checks

Examples of discrepancies with the header information include (a) an incorrect visit date like 30-Feb-2005 (b) an incomplete visit date like 12-Jan, whereas the date is expected to be reported in the DD-MM-YYYY format (c) incomplete patient initials.

Missing Pages Checks and CRF Tracking

Details of transmittals and receipt processes of CRFs and DCFs are documented and maintained during all stages of the data management process. Missing and expected pages tracking systems are also planned and set up in the DMP. Tracking reports of missing pages have to be maintained to identify CRFs misrouted in-house as well as CRFs not sent from the site.

Protocol Violation Checks

Protocol adherence ought to be reviewed at all stages of data management. Violations found have to be queried. Special emphasis is given for reviewing primary safety and efficacy endpoints, adherence to inclusion and exclusion criteria, adherence to trial drug dosing regimen, study or drug termination specifications, etc.

Dates Out of Sequence Checks

Dates out of sequence refer to dates either in the header or the body of the CRF being inconsistent and out of sequence. Sequence of visits are reviewed and, if found to be out of sequence, will be either queried or corrected. Examples include (a) a record belonging to visit 4 has a visit date belonging to that of visit 2 (b) one of the records within a particular visit has a visit date that is out of sequence with the visit date of the other records of the same visit (c) the trial medication is to be taken on a 'daily' basis as per the protocol, however, the dosing details on one of the dates has not been reported in the trial medication record.

Example where one of the screening records is reported with an incorrect 'year', hence there is a screening visit date out of sequence:

Record Name	*Visit date*
Demography	20-Feb-2006
Med. History	20-Feb-2005
Inclusion Criteria	20-Feb-2006
AE	20-Feb-2006

Continuity of Data Checks

These are checks performed for ensuring continuity of events (AEs, medications, treatments/procedures, etc.) across the study and across visits. Overlapping start/stop dates are checked across visits.

For example, consider a scenario where the protocol states that AEs are to be reported in visits 1, 2 and 3. "Headache" is reported as follows:

Visit	*Start Date*	*Stop Date*	*Outcome*
1	01-Jan-2004	12-Jan-2004	Continues
2	01-Jan-2004	12-Jan-2004	Resolved
3	20-Jan-2004	20-Jan-2004	Resolved

There is an issue in visit 1 reporting, where the 'stop date' has been reported and the outcome is reported as 'continues'. There is also the issue of overlapping start/stop dates in visits 1 and 2. All such issues are queried and clarified with the investigators.

Coding Checks

All the data such as concomitant medications, adverse events, medical history, and diseases have to be substituted with a standard reference terminology. This is known as 'coding'. The reference terminology may come from sponsor specific dictionaries or other published dictionaries. The coding of data helps in grouping them under specific systems. Such groupings are required for summary analysis of these data. Coding is done before the database lock.

As an example, consider medications 'paracetamol' (generic name) and 'Crocin' (trade name) reported on the CRF. Both medications have the same active ingredient 'paracetamol' and hence must be considered as the 'same entity' for analysis purpose. Hence both terms must be coded to 'paracetamol', so that the safety and efficacy analysis during statistical analysis is not affected.

There are certain terms that cannot be directly coded without further clarification from site. For example, the adverse event "ulcers" requires a 'location' (gastric, duodenal, mouth, foot, etc.) in order to be coded. Hence this must be queried to the site in order to obtain the location of the ulcer.

Standard global dictionaries having their unique coding structures are used for coding terms collected in clinical trials. Different dictionaries follow different structures and different hierarchies based on the classification levels. However, there are many similarities among the dictionaries. There is a term or text (AE, medication, disease) that is often referred to as the "preferred term", and the related "code". In addition to terms and codes, dictionaries generally have auxiliary tables. For example, AE dictionaries have information on effected body systems and drug dictionaries may have additional information on the key ingredients. Some of the common standard dictionaries used are:

- *MedDRA*-Medical Dictionary for Regulatory Activities
- *COSTART* - Coding Symbols for a Thesaurus of Adverse Reaction Terms
- *WHO-DRL* - World Health Organization Drug Reference List
- *WHO-ART* - World Health Organization Adverse Reactions Terminology
- *ICD-9-CM* - International Classification of Diseases, Ninth Revision, Clinical Modification

Auto-encoding: most modern and advanced coding dictionaries heavily depend on auto-encoders rather than manual coding. Once data from the case report form has been entered and verified, the process of auto-encoding begins, where the text of the investigator term in the clinical trial database is compared to the text strings stored in the dictionary database. When an exact match occurs, the code from the term in the dictionary database is automatically entered into the clinical trial database, and the term is considered auto-encoded.

Auto-encoders help in handling synonyms, misspellings, word variations, etc. Auto-encoders may be built-in with CDMS or as stand-alone systems, Auto-encoders have numerous advantages over manual coding such as the ability to handle large numbers of terms and the ability to facilitate consistent coding, without having to rely on the manual re-evaluation of previously coded terms.

External Data Checks

During the conduct of a clinical trial, some data external to the CRFs, such as laboratory data, PK/PD data and device data (ECG, images, flowmetry, vital signs) are also collected.

Central labs are used to maintain 'uniformity' across the study and across the sites. External data from all the study sites is directly sent to a central lab, from where the vendors provide electronic transfer of computerized data into the sponsor's database. Electronic transfer of data helps in avoiding the transcription errors. At the time of data transfer one has to take care that all the variables are included, and are loaded onto the proper study/visit without affecting the blinding.

Data management tracks loading of incorrect subject number, incorrect visit number, incorrect study number, incorrect date/time of sample collection, incorrect date/time of examination, etc. Missing data such as missing collection date/time of blood sample, missing date/time of ECG, missing location of chest radiograph, missing systolic/diastolic blood pressure, missing microbiological culture transmittal ID, etc. are also tracked by data management. Incorrect and incomplete loading details are communicated to the centralized vendors so that the appropriate data can be subsequently 'reloaded'.

Duplicate Data Checks

This refers to duplicate data entries of a particular data value within a single CRF or across similar CRFs. Duplicate entries and duplicate records are generally deleted per guideline specifications. Examples of duplicate data include:

- Treatment 'physiotherapy' on '30-Aug-2001' reported twice on either the same treatment record or across two different treatment records.
- Both visit 4 and visit 10-blood chemistry CRFs (with different collection dates) are updated with same values for all tests performed. In this case, either the collection date on one of the CRFs is incorrect or the reported blood chemistry values in one of the CRFs are incorrect.
- Both 'primary' and 'additional' medical history CRFs at screening are reported with same details of abnormalities.

Textual Data Checks

All textual data are to be proofread and checked for spelling errors. Common examples of textual data include pre-existing conditions in medical history record, adverse events, medications/antibiotics, physical examination findings, etc.

SAE Reconciliation Checks

An adverse event is any undesirable experience associated with the use of a medicinal product in a patient. The event is considered as a serious adverse event (SAE) if it results in any of the following outcomes:

- Death
- Life-threatening illness
- Inpatient hospitalization or prolongation of existing hospitalization
- Persistent or significant disability/incapacity
  - Congenital anomaly/birth defect

Expedited reports are required by the regulatory agencies for certain SAEs. Accordingly the investigator submits the SAE report to the sponsor, and the SAE details are subsequently maintained in the SAE database. The SAE details from the clinical trials are also reported on the CRFs which are sent to data management. Before close of study, the data management staff must compare and reconcile the SAE data in the SAE database with that in the clinical trial database, to ensure that all SAEs were collected and reported properly (Fig. 18.7).

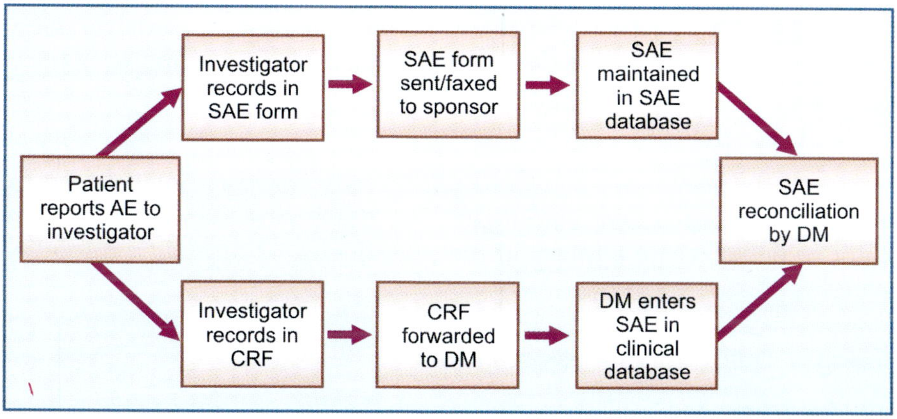

Fig. 18.7: Diagrammatic representation of SAE reconciliation

DISCREPANCY MANAGEMENT

A discrepancy is initially in an open or un-reviewed status. The data editor addresses the discrepancy and resolves it, based on the project-specific guidelines or standard guidelines (Fig. 18.8). There are various actions that can be taken to address a discrepancy:

Closing Discrepancy per Internal Correction

The data editor can 'internally' resolve and close out the issue without sending a query to the site. This action is applicable when the resolution is fairly 'obvious'. For example,

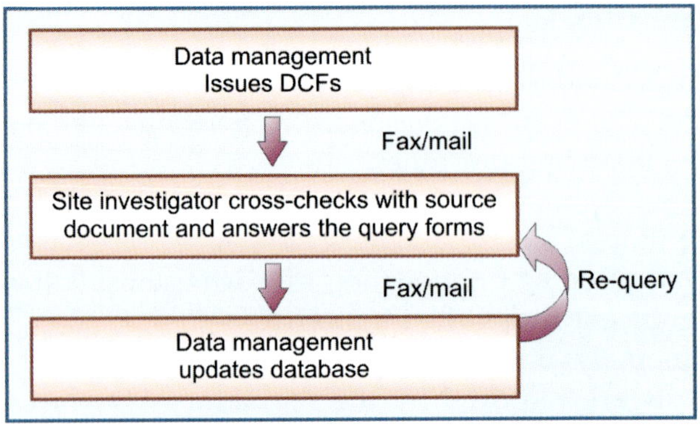

Fig. 18.8: Process of discrepancy management

a. A lab value 0.6 is out of range and an 'out of range' validation is generated. The data editor refers to the CRF and notices that the value is actually 6.6 and not 0.6, and that the value was incorrectly entered by data entry. In this case, the data editor could change the value in the database to 6.6.
b. A medication is reported as 'paracetamal'. This will not code and hence would throw up a coding validation. Since this seems to be very obviously a misspelling, the guidelines may allow the data editor to correct the spelling to 'paracetamol'.

Closing Discrepancy per Clinical Team

A discrepancy can sometimes be closed out directly based on instructions from the clinical scientist. Based on an ongoing review, the clinical scientist can instruct the data editor to either create a query to the investigator or provide a resolution for a discrepancy.

Generating a Query to the Investigator

The study guidelines can include instructions to the data editor to query a discrepancy in case it cannot be resolved per internal correction. Queries are generated on data clarification forms (DCFs), which are in turn sent to the respective sites. DCFs are also referred to as query forms, correction forms or discrepancy forms. DCF drafts can be auto-generated from a discrepancy management system and contain the query text templates.

The process of query management can be broadly classified into five steps.

Creating Queries

Queries for discrepancies are entered onto the DCF manually based on reports from the discrepancy management system, or the system may create them automatically. A DCF should ideally contain queries belonging to the same patient and to the same site.

A DCF would typically consist of the following entities:
- Study number/ID
- Site number
- Patient number
- Investigator name
- Date of generation
- Unique DCF ID
- Query text
- Space for the query resolution (to be filled by investigator)
- Date and signature of investigator

In the case of RDC systems, queries are entered directly into the database. The investigator answers the queries online and the responses are then available to the data editor.

Sending Queries

DCFs are delivered to site via fax, paper mail, in person or by e-mail. In the case of RDC systems, the queries are immediately accessible to the investigator who can view the queries and provide resolutions online.

Tracking Queries

The data editor tracks the flow of queries between self and the site. Following up on delayed responses and misrouted DCFs is important.

Resolving queries

Once the DCF is received back from a site the responses are integrated into the database. Common types of resolutions include retaining the queried value as the correct value, replacing the incorrect value with the correct one provided by the investigator, updating a missing response provided by the investigator.

Re-querying

Re-queries are needed when the investigators do not provide a response or provide an incorrect/inconsistent/incomplete response or provide the same response to a query.

Query Writing

Good query writing is extremely important so that the investigator can fully understand and comprehend the query and hence would in turn provide the correct response. This helps in avoiding re-queries and reduces the turn-around time for query integration into the database.

General tips for query writing include having a thorough understanding of the guidelines and protocol, stating the problem in a simple way, being precise and to the point while wording the query text, using proper punctuation and grammatically correct sentences, and avoiding repetition of words in the query text.

DATABASE CLOSURE

Database closure is done to prevent unauthorized or inadvertent changes to the database once the final analysis of the data has begun. This process is referred to as 'soft-locking' the database. This is done after completion of last patient last visit. (LPLV). Database lock is critical in randomized trials to ensure the integrity of the randomization process (as the blind has been broken). Database closure is done when all the discrepancies and validations are resolved, all edit checks are completed, all missing data/external data are in-house, all terms are coded, all lab ranges are applied and SAEs reconciled. In other words it is done once the database is cleaned completely (Fig. 18.9).

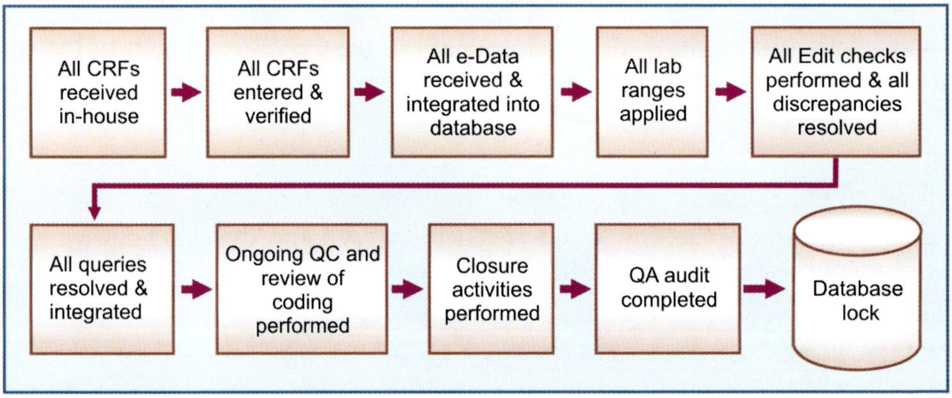

Fig. 18.9: Diagrammatic representation of database lock

In order to safeguard the integrity of the data well-defined procedures for the database closure have to be documented and followed. A database can be unlocked with special user access in case there is a necessity of making further updates or modifications to the database. In such cases, the change control procedures must be clearly defined and documented. Change control procedures include notifying the study team, clearly defining the changes being made, specifying the reasons for the changes and documenting the dates when the changes are made. Database closure is followed by final analyses, which lead to conclusions on the trial and for the regulatory submissions.

QUALITY ASSURANCE AND QUALITY CONTROL (QA/QC)

QA/QC audits are done periodically – on an ongoing basis as well as at or after the end of the study. QA audits are systematic and independent examinations of trial-related activities and documents to ensure that the CDM related activities and processes were conducted and completed, and that the data were accurately recorded, analyzed, documented and reported according to the protocol, SOPs, GCP and applicable regulatory requirements.

Errors or findings are mismatches found between the CRF and the database during a review. They could be due to incorrect transcriptions, incorrect data processing (at the level of data entry or data validation) and incorrect query integration. The error rate or quality index (QI) is calculated as number of findings against the number of fields in the database. The acceptable error rate is pre-determined by the sponsor and is documented early on in the DMP. For example, a sponsor may require a quality index of 99.9 percent, whereas another sponsor may require a quality index of 99.5 percent.

The sample size for audit should be statistically appropriate and could vary from sponsor to sponsor. For example, some audits could use a 10 percent random sample where the system can randomly auto generate 10 percent of the total enrollment for analysis. Some other audits could involve a 100 percent sampling of all safety and efficacy end points.

Interim analysis may be done at regular time intervals for an ongoing study, if specified in the protocol. The analysis may be done monthly, quarterly, biannually, annually, etc. depending on the study duration. The analysis could also be done either on specified modules in the study like safety modules or efficacy modules, or on all modules. Findings from the analysis give a clear picture if the study is on track. Decisions are taken on the proceedings of the trial and, if needed, amendments to the protocol are made in order to ensure successful completion of the trial. If major deviations are found against the protocol or the expected results, the data is assessed as a whole to evaluate the quality of the study and decide if the study should proceed as planned. Analyzing findings on a periodic basis helps in making appropriate rectifications to the database early on in the study. Accordingly training is provided to the data management staff so that the findings and errors are not repeated for the rest of the incoming data.

Final analysis is done after completion of LPLV. This analysis collates the data from all the interim analyses as well as the data analyzed after the last interim, and gives a combined result of all the data modules. The final analysis gives a collective conclusion about the safety and efficacy of the trial drug, which would be part of regulatory submissions.

DATA STORAGE AND ARCHIVAL

All trial related paper documents including CRFs and/or electronic files must be stored in a secure and controlled place. It is good to scan all paper documents so that they can be archived in an electronic form. Open formats such as CDISC or PDF are recommended for storage.

Information regarding all clinical data, database design specifications, external data, structural metadata, coding dictionaries, lab ranges, audit trail, listings for edit checks and derived data, discrepancy management logs, queries, program codes, PDF formats of CRFs, data management plan, validation documentation, regulatory documentation, documentation/memos of deviations from SOPs and other working procedures, are stored in a central document library and should be included in a clinical data archive.

RECENT ADVANCES IN CDM

Clinical trial systems to conduct clinical trials electronically has become a necessity today to increase the time to market as well as decrease the cost of trials. The various technologies utilized include EDC systems, adverse event reporting systems (AERS), OCR, OMR, IVRS, etc. These and many other technologies are providing number of benefits in the conduct of the clinical trial. Technology enables advances in trial design, faster data entry, more efficient communications between participants, and improved process management, collection of clinical endpoint data directly from the patients (Fig. 18.10).

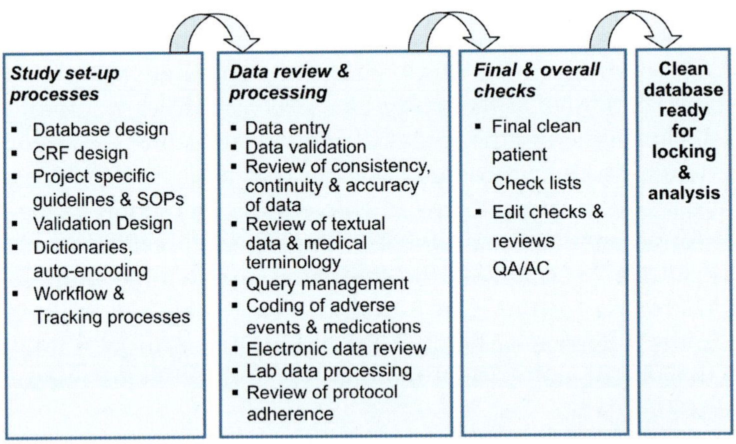

Fig. 18.10: Overview of processes in clinical data management

Technology can also help in the design of a clinical trial especially in the randomization process. It is possible to design a trial that is automatically modified as it progresses through an adaptive trial design. Continuous monitoring of a critical variable from EDC data can automatically adjust the sample size of a trial for the power that is desired.

EDC decreases paper handling, improves data clarification process, provides validations at the time of data entry, provides real time access to data, allows for remote monitoring, speeds up regulatory agency submissions, and lessens the number of CDM resources required to process the data. EDC data can be integrated by loading of SAS datasets or transport files into a data repository that becomes the source for study analysis and reporting. EDC systems can also be integrated with

IVR systems, electronic patient diaries, labs, EKGs and AERS. With lab integration investigators can also look at lab data on-line.

Smart pens are available which enables patients fill out a form, and then use the pen itself to transmit the recorded data via a cradle to the database. Discrepancies in the data are shown to the site, which can correct them against the paper copy. The pen also creates an exact copy of the CRF to be saved online.

Electronic devices such as personal digital assistants (PDAs), palm pilots are very efficient in capturing data from subjects. These typically work in an offline mode and are slowly replacing paper-based subject diaries. These devices can also display metrics or tracking statuses to monitor patient schedules and compliance with alerts to record the data as per the protocol. Some can even help collection of various parameters such as measurement of pain, etc.

Biometric devices provide another way of data collection. Electronic spirometers can record the time, date, and measurements of home-administered pulmonary function tests. Some devices can simultaneously record numerous physiological variables.

Data are stored in the memory of the clinical data systems or on paper, microfiche, computer tape, computer disk, optical laser disk, or smart cards. Data may be transmitted through hard-wired direct connections, disks, audiotape or videotape broadcast, microwave fibreoptic links. Retrieval of data can be done by automated prompts, query, search programs. The output may be in a typed format, an audio format, or a visual format (e.g., pictures, graphs and tables).

Number of technologies are available to help better communication between sites and sponsors which can help achieve higher quality data in a shorter period of time. Trial portals are available where start-up and other documents can be downloaded, completed and can be shared with the sponsor. In addition, these portals can be used for live investigator training, site personnel training, and for investigator meetings. Monitors can send edit checks and protocol changes to the trial sites via the portal. Monitors can conduct protocol-compliance checks by examining the data being collected and fully manage trial processes from their home or office via these web portals. They can also query sites and generate data-correction forms in real-time. Sites can be graphically shown their recruitment, time from query to response, queries per page, and many other metrics. These reports will allow the site to understand areas that need improvement, or areas in which they excel. Over all, much less efforts are spent reviewing and managing queries which helps to increase study capacities and smooth conduct of multicenter studies.

Desktop productivity tools have been integrated with ERP systems to enable process functions and data to be available through familiar desktop applications. They provide access to tasks such as time management, budget monitoring, and organization management from a desktop. Globalization management systems are available to accelerate capturing, authoring, managing, and distributing content across multiple formats and languages.

To avoid the problem of clinical trials generating mountains of paperwork, FDA is promoting eSourcing. This involves capturing clinical data electronically at the source meaning in the patient diaries and eCRFs. FDA is also encouraging completely paperless submissions of clinical trial results. As a method of eSourcing investigators can record all trial data in their laptops and the same can be synchronized daily with central servers.

Integrated data capture and management systems with lab data integration, integrated dictionary coding, and translation tools provide for better reporting. Some systems can help generate the extracts for analysis in analytical tools and also help in generating submission files exactly as requested by FDA. Web-based tools for safety research with search engine, querying, access to information sources—including FDA and WHO datasets, help manage and analyze data efficiently. FDA has collaborated with private vendors for electronic review tools, which provide quicker access to key information.

DATA STANDARDS

Data standards are being developed to overcome the problems of data integration from different systems. Data structure (variable names, variable types, and labels), screen layout/paper CRF module, completion instructions, monitoring guidelines, standard reports, tables, listings, laboratory data, global libraries are all being standardized. Clinical Data Interchange Standards Consortium (**CDISC**) is at present leading the way. There are currently over 60 companies that are members of CDISC, and many companies are starting to adopt the CDISC models, even down to the variable name.

Apart from data management personnel, the senior management, clinicians, statisticians, medical writers, auditors, regulatory affairs, IT support and central labs contribute to these data standards development. Standards have become necessity of the day because of the rapidly increasing number of drugs in development and global submissions.

SUGGESTED READING

1. Colleen M Cox. Planning the Data Management Process for a Clinial Trial, Technology and Data Management. Monitor, September 2005.
2. Louis Pozzo, Glen de Vries. Applied Clinical Trials Oct 5 2005.
3. Paul Bliecher. Applied Clinical Trials, Apr 1, 2005.
4. Rebecca Daniels Kush. eClinical Trials – Planning and Implementation, Thomson CenterWatch. 2003.
5. Rondel, R. Varley, S. Webb, C. Clinical Data Management. New York, NY: John Wiley and Sons LTD. 2000.
6. Society for Clinical Data Management. Good Clinical Data Management Practices Version 3. September 2003.
7. Spilker B. Schoenfelder, J. Data Collection Forms in Clinical Trials. New York, NY: Raven Press. 1991.
8. Susanne Prokscha. Practical Guide to Clinical Data Management, CRC Press LLC. 1999.
9. The Rough Guide to Electronic Data Capture, ENGAGE. i3 Pharma Resourcing. Issue 7, Oct 05.

19

Clinical Trials for Herbal Drugs and Traditional Medicines

CK Katiyar, SP Yadav

INTRODUCTION

The World Health Organization (WHO) estimates that 4 billion people (i.e. Approx. 80 % of the world population) use herbal medicine for some aspect of primary health care (Farnsworth et al., 1985). Herbal medicine is a major component in all indigenous traditional medicine and is a common element in Ayurvedic, homeopathic, naturopathic, traditional oriental, and Native American Indian medicine and herbal medicine is the most common form of alternative/traditional medicine (Brody 1998).

Worldwide, the botanical pharmacopoeia contains tens of thousands of plants used for medicinal purposes. Hundreds, perhaps thousands, of definitive texts, monographs, and tomes on herbal remedies exist. But most of this information is outside current databases and remains unavailable to physicians, researchers, and consumers.

During the last decade, use of traditional herbal medicine has expanded globally and has gained popularity. Traditional herbal medicine has not only been continuously in use for primary health care by the poor in developing countries, but has also been used in countries where conventional medicine is predominant in the national health care system. With the tremendous expansion in the use of traditional medicine worldwide, safety and efficacy as well as quality control of herbal and traditional medicines have become important concerns for both health authorities and the public and the medicines with insufficient evidence of safety are not justifiable because such products carry serious health hazards. This has necessitated a move from traditionally followed qualitative observations to the current concepts of quantitative research (Katiyar CK, 2006).

Globally, herbal remedies have been researched under rigorous controls and have been approved by the governments of technologically advanced nations. The scientific validation is good to excellent, and the history of clinical use is even stronger. Many phytomedicines have been used by thousands of physicians in their practices and are consumed under medical supervision by tens of millions of people. Much modern-day medicine is directly or indirectly derived from plant sources, so it would be foolish to conclude that plants offer no further potential for the treatment or cure of major diseases.

Hence, they can significantly contribute to the strategies for reducing the burden of sickness and death and there is a huge potential of herbal medicine development into standardized phytomedicines. However, the impact of scientific research into such medicines in respect of product development is still disproportionately low.

In developed countries, a resurgence of interest in herbal medicines has resulted from the preference of many consumers for products of natural origin. In addition, manufactured herbal medicines often follow in the wake of migrants from countries where traditional medicines play an important role. In both developed and developing countries, consumers and health care providers need to be supplied with up-to-date and authoritative information on the beneficial properties, and possible harmful effects, of all herbal medicines.

The status of herbal research and product development in India is largely unsatisfactory; however, after the 'WHO' emphasis to motivate the herbal or traditional medicine research, there is growing concern in this area (Annan, 2003; Hassan, 2002; Angell and Kassier, 2004). At the same time, Indian traditional medical knowledge and the medicinal plant resources are vanishing under the influence of modern medicine and axed plant habitat. Moreover the situation further worsened largely due to lack of adequate research funding, poor laboratory and human capacities among several other reasons.

Some of the scientists feel that current approach to medical use of herbal or traditional medicine without subjecting them to some rigorous scientific evaluation like their western counterparts is irrational. These scientists argue that there cannot be two kinds of medicines – one alternative (traditional) and the other conventional.

Let us understand that herbal medicines are different from synthetic ones in several aspects. Some of them are given below while others shall be discussed elsewhere in this chapter.

- Plants are polypharmacy themselves with active principles frequently unknown
- Standardization, stability and quality control are feasible but not easy
- The availability and quality of raw materials are frequently problematic
- Well-controlled double-blind clinical and toxicological studies to prove their efficacy and safety are rare
- Empirical use in folk medicine is a very important characteristic
- They have a wide range of therapeutic use and are suitable for chronic treatments
- The occurrence of undesirable side effects seems to be less frequent with herbal medicines, but few well-controlled randomized clinical trials have revealed that they also exist

- Most of the time they are used in holistic manner along with various restrictions on diet and deeds, especially when prescribed by a traditional medicine physician. In such cases, though, more often than not, single drug (single or poly herbal) is seldom prescribed
- They usually cost less than synthetic drugs

Since the present day scientists are trained in contemporary science and western medicine and these scientists have very limited knowledge on the traditional/ herbal medicines; they advocate a particular way of looking at herbal drugs, which includes the quality control, the toxicity, the proven efficacy through clinical trial using double blind placebo controlled methodology followed by post marketing surveillance with a view to monitor the adverse drug reactions. This approach was advocated by those countries, which do not have a rich tradition of healthcare like ayurveda or Chinese medicine. On the other hand, many advocates for the use of herbal traditional medicines argue that the current universal scientific procedures are simply not applicable to remedies that are already accepted and used by some communities based on their long history of use because traditional herbal medicines did not evolve from fundamental or basic science. Rather, they rely on traditional method of knowledge transfer from generation to generation. There is no doubt that the situation with herbal traditional medicines research offers a great opportunity to develop new strategies for the exploitation of these valuable resources.

The Table 19.1 given below explains the comparison between the need of Clinical Trials for contemporary medicines and traditional medicines.

The objective of clinical trial itself, therefore, becomes radically different for both new chemical entity and a traditional medicine herbal product. Before designing a clinical trial protocol for a traditional medicine herbal product, it must be understood that the purpose of trial should ideally be to elicit any side-effects rather than finding the efficacy, since these traditional medicine herbal products are already in human use for centuries. Let us not forget that traditional use for centuries provides much better parameter of efficacy evaluation than a clinical trial conducted for few days to few months on a representative population, that too in controlled manner. Probably

Table 19.1: Factors necessitating a clinical trial

	Why Clinical Trial	
Parameters	*Contemporary medicine (New drug)*	*Traditional medicine*
Dose	Unknown	Known
Duration	Unknown	Known
Indication	Unknown	Known
Side-effect profile	Unknown	Unknown

this is the reason why there have been no cases of withdrawal of the herbal products from the market in contrast to certain classes of synthetic drugs internationally.

Various practices of traditional medicine have been developed in different cultures in different regions without a parallel development of international standards and appropriate methods for evaluating traditional medicine. Therefore, the argument may not be so much of the need or otherwise for rigorous scientific studies. Rather this issue has more to do with the strategies used in establishing the scientific validity of herbal traditional medicines. It has more to do with the procedural, ethical and methodological issues involved in the research on herbal medicines. The challenges posed by the application of the universal ethical guidelines to the research and development of herbal traditional medicines have not been properly addressed.

Definitions and Classification

Traditional medicines are also known as complementary medicines, alternative medicines, herbal medicines, nutraceuticals, dietary supplements and more recently cosmaceuticals internationally. Additionally they are also christened as ayurvedic medicines, chinese medicines, kempo medicines, etc. depending upon their country of origin.

According to Therapeutics Goods Administration of Australia (TGA, 2006) complementary medicines comprise traditional medicines, including traditional Chinese medicines, Ayurvedic medicines and other indigenous medicines (Fig. 19.1).

In India Ayurvedic, Unani, Homoeopathic, Siddha systems of medicine are quite popular and are licensed accordingly. Their products contain herbs, minerals, metals, animal origin products and marine products. Recent years have witnessed introduction of European herbal products also in Indian markets, they however, are sold as dietary supplements. Herbal medicines, therefore, can also be categorized in Indian context as in Figure 19.2.

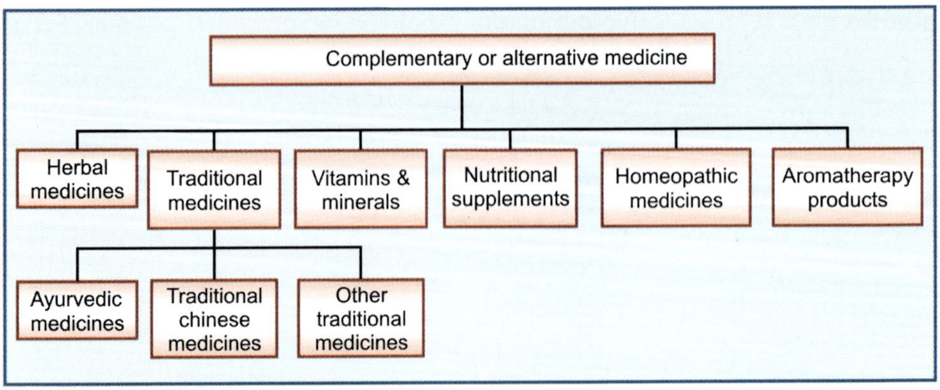

Fig. 19.1: Classification of complementary medicines according to TGA

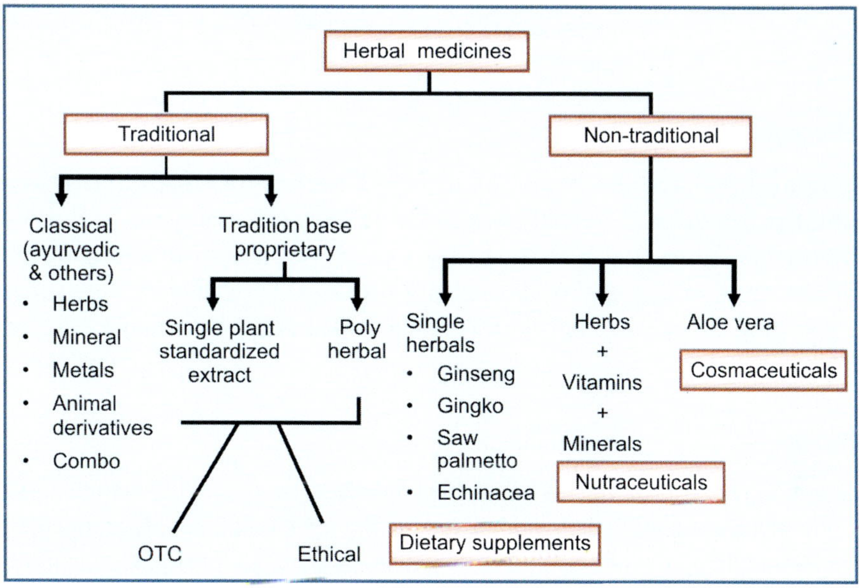

Fig. 19.2: Categories of marketed herbal medicines in India

World Health Organization (WHO, 2000) have specified the definitions of crude herbs, processed herb and finished herbal products, besides traditional medicines. All the related definitions are reproduced below.

Traditional Medicine

Traditional medicine has a long history. "It is the sum total of the knowledge, skills and practices based on the theories, beliefs and experiences indigenous to different cultures, whether explicable or not, used in the maintenance of health, as well as in the prevention, diagnosis, improvement or treatment of physical and mental illnesses." The term complementary and alternative medicine is used in some countries to refer to a broad set of health care practices that are not part of the country's own tradition and are not integrated into the dominant health care system.

Herbs

Herbs include crude plant material such as leaves, flowers, fruit, seed, stems, wood, bark, roots, rhizomes or other plant parts, which may be entire, fragmented or powdered.

Herbal Materials

Herbal materials include, in addition to herbs, fresh juices, gums, fixed oils, essential oils, resins and dry powders of herbs. In some countries, these materials may be processed by various local procedures, such as steaming, roasting, or stir-baking with honey, alcoholic beverages or other materials.

Herbal Preparations

Herbal preparations are the basis for finished herbal products and may include comminuted or powdered herbal materials, or extracts, tinctures and fatty oils of herbal materials. They are produced by extraction, fractionation, purification, concentration, or other physical or biological processes. They also include preparations made by steeping or heating herbal materials in alcoholic beverages and/or honey, or in other materials.

Herbal Medicines

WHO defines herbal medicines as "Finished, labelled medicinal products that contain as active ingredients aerial or underground parts of plants, or other plant material, or combinations thereof, whether in the crude state or as plant preparations. Plant material includes juices, gums, fatty oils, essential oils, and any other substances of this nature. Herbal medicines may contain excipients in addition to the active ingredients. Medicines containing plant material combined with chemically defined active substances, including chemically defined, isolated constituents of plants are not considered to be herbal medicines." Exceptionally, in some countries herbal medicines may also contain, by tradition, natural organic or inorganic active ingredients, which are not of plant origin.

Traditional Use of Herbal Medicines

Herbal medicines include herbs, herbal materials, herbal preparations and finished herbal products that contain as active ingredients parts of plants, or other plant materials, or combinations. Traditional use of herbal medicines refers to the long historical use of these medicines. Their use is well established and widely acknowledged to be safe and effective, and may be accepted by national authorities.

Finished Herbal Products

Finished herbal products consist of herbal preparations made from one or more herbs. If more than one herb is used, the term mixture herbal product can also be used. Finished herbal products and mixture herbal products may contain excipients in addition to the active ingredients. However, finished products or mixture products to which chemically defined active substances have been added, including synthetic compounds and/or isolated constituents from herbal materials, are not considered to be herbal.

Therapeutic Activity

Therapeutic activity refers to the successful prevention, diagnosis and treatment of physical and mental illnesses; improvement of symptoms of illnesses; as well as beneficial alteration or regulation of the physical and mental status of the body.

Active Ingredients

Active ingredients refer to ingredients of herbal medicines with therapeutic activity. In herbal medicines where the active ingredients have been identified, the preparation of these medicines should be standardized to contain a defined amount of the active ingredients, if adequate analytical methods are available. In cases where it is not possible to identify the active ingredients, the whole herbal medicine may be considered as one active ingredient.

HISTORICAL ASPECTS

Physical evidence of use of herbal remedies goes back some 60,000 years to a burial site of a Neanderthal man uncovered in 1960 (Solecki, 1975). In a cave in northern Iraq, scientists found what appeared to be ordinary human bones. An analysis of the soil around the bones revealed extraordinary quantities of plant pollen that could not have been introduced accidentally at the burial site. Someone in the small cave community had consciously gathered eight species of plants to surround the dead man. Seven of these are medicinal plants still used throughout the herbal world (Bensky and Gamble, 1993). All cultures have long folk medicine histories that include the use of plants. Egyptian, Indian and Chinese traditional medicines are considered as oldest system of medicine of the world. Ayurveda, the science of life, prevention and longevity is the oldest and most holistic or comprehensive Indian medical system. The first comprehensive documented treatise on Ayurveda is available in the form of *Charak Samhita*, which is almost 3000 yrs old (*Charak Samhita*, 2005). Sushruta was an ancient Indian surgeon (who was possibly born in 7th century BC) and is the author of the book *Sushruta Samhita*, in which he describes over 120 surgical instruments, 300 surgical procedures and classifies human surgery in 8 categories. Chinese traditional medicines also have the history of thousand of years; however, reliable historical records are not available before 722 BC. Three thousand year ago on Oracle bones (tortoise shells and animals bone) from the shell dynasty (1766 to 1122 BC) records of illnesses, medicines and treatments were found inscribed in China. Acupuncture have been used as a therapeutic method in China for all over 2000 years ago. The earliest Chinese text, the *Huang Ti Nei Jing Su Wen Ling Shu'* (The Yellow Emperor's Classic of Internal Medicine), is ascribed to the 2nd and 1st centuries BC.

Even in ancient cultures, people methodically and scientifically collected information on herbs and developed well-defined herbal pharmacopeias. Indeed, well into the 20th century much of the pharmacopeia of scientific medicine was derived from the herbal lore of native peoples. Many drugs, including atropine, quinine, strychnine, aspirin, vincristine, taxol, metformin, and ergotamine, etc. are of herbal origin. About one-quarter of the prescription drugs dispensed by community pharmacies in the United States contain at least one active ingredient derived from plant material (Farnsworth and Morris, 1976).

The past decade has seen a significant increase in the use of herbal medicines. As a result of WHO's promotion of traditional medicine, countries have been seeking the assistance of WHO in identifying safe and effective herbal medicines for use in national health care systems. In 1991, the Director General of WHO, in a report to the Forty-fourth World Health Assembly, emphasized the great importance of medicinal plants to the health of individuals and communities. Earlier, in 1978, the Thirty-first World Health Assembly (WHA) had adopted a resolution (WHA31.33) that called on the Director General to compile and periodically update a therapeutic classification of medicinal plants, related to the therapeutic classification of all drugs; subsequently, resolution of WHA40.33, adopted in 1987, urged member states to ensure quality control of drugs derived from traditional plant remedies by using modern techniques and applying suitable standards and good manufacturing practices; and resolution WHA42.43, of 1989, urged member states to introduce measures for the regulation and control of medicinal plant products and for the establishment and maintenance of suitable standards. Moreover, the International Conference on Primary Health Care, held in Alma-Ata, USSR, in 1978, recommended, inter alia, the accommodation of proven traditional remedies in national drug policies and regulatory measures.

REGULATION OF HERBAL/TRADITIONAL MEDICINES

The regulation and legislation on traditional herbal medicines varies from country to country (WHO, 2005). Their review draws the attention to the fact that safety and efficacy do not form the mandatory requirements in most of the countries. This may be due to the fact of long traditional usage, or other ethnic or cultural diversities.

Several regulatory models for herbal medicines currently exist, including prescription drugs, over-the-counter drugs, traditional medicines and dietary supplements, nutraceuticals (WHO, 2005). WHO, therefore, emphasizes the need to establish global and/or regional regulatory mechanisms for regulating herbal drugs. According to a global survey undertaken by WHO in 141 member states enquiring about the laws controlling traditional/conventional alternative medicines 54 countries (38%) confirmed having laws or regulations while 84 countries (60%) did not have any law to control traditional/conventional alternative medicines.

WHO initiative for regulation of traditional medicine were based on the recommendation of a workshop on the regulation of herbal medicines by The Fourth International Conference of Drug Regulatory Authorities, held in Tokyo in 1986, and another workshop on the same subject held as part of the Fifth International

Conference of Drug Regulatory Authorities, held in Paris in 1986. Both workshops confined their considerations to the commercial exploitation of traditional medicines through over-the-counter labeled products. The Paris meeting concluded that the World Health Organization should consider preparing model guidelines containing basic elements of legislation designed to assist those countries wishing to develop appropriate legislation and registration.

The objective of these guidelines, therefore, is to define basic criteria for the evaluation of quality, safety, and efficacy of herbal medicines and thereby to assist national regulatory authorities, scientific organizations, and manufacturers to undertake an assessment of the documentation/submission/dossiers in respect of such products. As a general rule in this assessment, traditional experience means that long-term use as well as the medical, historical and ethnological background of those products shall be taken into account. The definition of long-term use may vary according to the country but should be at least several decades. Therefore, the assessment should take into account a description in the medical/pharmaceutical literature or similar sources, or a documentation of knowledge on the application of a herbal medicine without a clearly defined time limitation. Marketing authorizations of similar products should be taken into account.

These efforts concentrate on herbal medicines, but might at a later stage be the basis for the assessment of other traditional medicines not covered by these guidelines. In the meantime, it is up to the national authorities to adapt the guidelines for assessment of traditional medicines and other herbal drugs.

Prolonged and apparently uneventful use of a substance usually offers testimony of its safety. In a few instances, however, investigation of the potential toxicity of naturally occurring substances widely used as ingredients in these preparations has revealed previously unsuspected potential for systematic toxicity, carcinogenicity and teratogenicity. Regulatory authorities need to be quickly and reliably informed of these findings. They should also have the authority to respond promptly to such alerts, either by withdrawing or varying the licenses of registered products containing suspect substance, or by rescheduling the substance to limit their use to medical prescription.

WHO has emphasized on four aspects of herbal medicines viz. quality, safety, efficacy and affordability. Keeping these basic factors in view, regulatory guidelines can be formulated by the member countries.

A summary of the regulatory agencies and processes related to herbal drugs of some selected countries is presented below.

Australia

Therapeutic Good Act (TGA, 1990) Working Party established by the Australian Parliament reviews the natural and nutritional supplements quality, safety, efficacy and labeling of herbal and related products. In Australia, complementary medicines referred for medicinal products containing herbs, vitamins, minerals, and nutritional supplements, homoeopathic medicines and certain aromatherapy products. These are regulated as medicines under the *Therapeutics Goods Act 1989* (the Act). TGA states that traditional claims for herbal remedies be allowed, providing general advertising requirements are complied with and providing such claims are justified by literature references.

China

The State Pharmaceutical Administration of China, the Division of Drug Administration in the Ministry of Health, and the Division of Traditional Chinese Medicine in the Traditional Chinese Medication Administration Bureau were merged into the State Drug Administration (STA) in 1999. The new organization revised major provisions of herbal drug regulation that had lagged behind the times and added new provisions and guidance's. These regulations covered the drug registration procedure, new drug protection and technology transfer, Good Clinical Practices (GCP), and Good Laboratory Practices.

European Union

European Union, after giving due consideration to increasing popularity of herbal products have recently released a comprehensive directive which allows simplified registration of Traditional Herbal Medicinal Products (THMP). However in order to be eligible for simplified registration these traditional herbal remedies should be in use for more than15 years in any of the EU member countries in addition to more than 30 years in country of origin.

Germany

An independent division of the German Federal Health Agency; Commission E established in 1978 evaluates the safety and efficacy of herbal medicines (phytotherapy and herbal substances). The Commission E has 24 members, which comprise of: physicians, pharmacists, pharmacologists, toxicologists, industry representatives and laypersons. Commission E has published about 300 herbal monographs: 200 positives and 100 negatives. The commission evaluates the herbal medicines on the basis of following methods and criteria 1) traditional use; 2) chemical data; 3) experimental, pharmacological and toxicological studies; 4) clinical studies; 5) field and epidemiological studies; 6) patient case records submitted from physician's files, and 7) additional studies, including unpublished proprietary data submitted by manufacturers. It separates two kinds of monographs: mono preparations and fixed combinations and three kind of herbal drugs categories for marketing: 1) temporary marking authorization for old herbal drugs until they are evaluated for safety and efficacy; 2) monographs of standardized marketing authorization, and 3) individual marketing authorization. Evaluations are published in the form of monographs that approve or disapprove the herbal drugs for over-the-counter use. Herbal medicines are sold in pharmacies, drugstores and health food stores. Some herbal medicines are controlled by a physician's prescription.

India

Central Drugs Standard Control Organization (CDSCO) and Department of AYUSH (ayurveda, unani, siddha, homoeopathic medicines, naturopathy and yoga) Ministry of Health and Family Welfare, Government of India are the drug regulatory bodies for approval and control of ayurvedic, unani and siddha medicines. The Chapter IVA section 33C of The Drugs and Cosmetics Act, 1940 and The Drugs and Cosmetics Act and rules, 1945 has laid down the provisions relating to ayurvedic siddha and unani drugs.

United States of America

Herbal medicines have been regulated under the Dietary Supplement Health and Education Act (DSHEA) of 1994. On the basis of this law, herbal medicines are not evaluated by the FDA and most important, these products are not intended to diagnose, treat, cure, or prevent diseases, However, herbalist may also apply under existing guidelines for approval of new herbal drugs, but this will be a huge financial burden similar to the total cost of bringing a new pharmaceutical drug.

The US government has established the Office of Alternative Medicine at the National Institutes of Health (NIH) with the following aims: 1) to explore the potential role of dietary supplements in the improvement of health; 2) to promote the scientific study of supplements for maintaining health and preventing chronic diseases; 3) to compile a database of scientific research related to supplements; 4) to coordinate NIH funding for dietary supplements related to the treatment of chronic disease. The regulatory lockout of natural remedies has crippled natural products research in US universities and hospitals. There is no dedicated level of support by the Federal Government for herbal medicine research.

Recently USFDA have released the guidance on herbal drugs and it contains the guiding principles for application of herbal products as drugs.

UK

The MHRA (Medicines and Healthcare Products Regulatory Authority) is the executive arm of the UK's Drug Licensing Authority and is responsible for all aspects of the regulation of medicines in the UK. In January 2002, the European Commission adopted formal proposals for a Directive on Traditional Herbal Medicinal products. The MHRA held a full public consultation during the summer of 2002 which was extended following a request from Ministers for a greater degree of dialogue between the herbal sector and the Agency. Informal consultation continued through 2003 with representatives of the herbal sector attending meetings to discuss many aspects of the Directive, as proposed at that time. The MHRA and the herbal sector agreed that key priorities in the negotiations were greater flexibility in relation to acceptance of evidence of traditional use from outside the European Union, and the possibility for companies to include vitamins and minerals with traditional herbal remedies. These objectives were achieved in European negotiations.

Preclinical or Safety Aspects

The approval for marketing of traditional herbal medicine in several countries (for example, ayurvedic medicine in India) does not need the preclinical/ clinical trial data. This, however, should not be surprising in view of their long-term usage and relatively low toxicity, if at all, exhibited and reported with traditional/ herbal medicines.

With regard to safety evaluation a guiding principle should be that if the product has been traditionally used without demonstrated harm, no specific restrictive regulatory action should be undertaken unless new evidence demands a revised risk-benefit assessment. A review of the relevant literature should be provided with original articles or references to the original articles. If official monograph/review results exist, reference can be made to them. However, although long-term use without any evidence of risks may indicate that a medicine is harmless, it is not always certain how far one can rely solely on long-term usage to provide assurance of innocuity in the light of concern expressed in recent years over long-term hazards of some herbal medicines. Reported side effects should be documented according to normal pharmacovigilance practices. Toxicological studies, if available, should be part of the assessment. Literature should be indicated as above.

As a basic rule, documentation of a long period of use should be taken into consideration when assessing safety. This means that, when there are no detailed toxicological studies, documented experiences of long-term use without evidence of safety problems should form the basis of the risk assessment. However, even in cases of drugs used over a long period, chronic toxicological risks may have occurred but may not have been recognized. The period of use, the health disorders treated, the number of users, and the countries with experience should be specified. If a toxicological risk is known, toxicity data must be submitted. The assessment of risk, whether independent of dose or related to dose, should be documented. In the latter case, the dosage specification must be an important part of the risk assessment. An explanation of the risks should be given, if possible. Potential for misuse, abuse, or dependence must be documented. If long-term traditional use cannot be documented or there are doubts on safety, toxicity data should be submitted.

Ayurvedic recipes range from food products to therapeutic foods to OTC and dispensed or prescribed ayurvedic medicines. Since ayurvedic product development was based upon wide ranging experiments and experiences, need to validate the safety of these products was never felt. However, in the current times, quality of drugs have been affected due to several factors, Improper manufacturing process; Contaminants; Irrational use of ayurvedic medicine; use of metal based ayurvedic products; quality of ayurvedic medicine and abuse/ adulteration, etc. These factors have led to the need for evidence of safety of ayurvedic products. ICMR (2000), guidelines provide a guiding principle for conducting toxicity studies, if required.

REGULATORY ASPECTS ON CONDUCTING THE CLINICAL TRIALS

Considering long term usage of traditional/herbal medicines in several countries including India and China, clinical trials have not been made mandatory by the regulatory authorities as a prerequisite to market authorization. Recent resurgence of herbal/traditional medicines has generated interest among the scientific community and they have started demanding the evidence of efficacy through the clinical trials. Most of the clinical trials currently are conducted to generate the data to validate the claim. In the absence of any harmonized guideline on clinical trials on traditional/herbal medicines, *sui generis* systems are being followed by the enthusiasts.

Few organizations have developed broad directional guidelines, which are summarized below.

Indian Council of Medical Research (ICMR) Guidelines

ICMR guidelines (2000) have classified herbal drugs in the three categories and have suggested to follow different approaches of their clinical evaluation.

The herbal products can belong to either of the three categories given below:

- A lot is known about the use of a plant or its extract in the ancient ayurveda, siddha or unani literature or the plant may actually be regularly used by physicians of the traditional systems of medicine for a number of years. The substance is being clinically evaluated for same indication for which it is being used or as has been described in the texts.
- When an extract of a plant or a compound isolated from the plant has to be clinically evaluated for a therapeutic effect not originally described in the texts of traditional systems or, the method of preparation is different, it has to be treated as a new substance or new chemical entity (NCE) and the same type of acute, sub acute and chronic toxicity data will have to be generated as required by the regulatory authority before it is cleared for clinical evaluation.

  An extract or a compound isolated from a plant, which has never been in use before and has not ever been mentioned in ancient literature, should be treated as a new drug, and therefore, should undergo all regulatory requirements before being evaluated clinically.

It is important that plants and herbal remedies currently in use or mentioned in literature of recognized traditional system of medicine is prepared strictly in the same way as described in the literature while incorporating GMP norms for standardization. It may not be necessary to undertake phase I studies. However, it needs to be emphasized that since the substance to be tested is already in use in Indian systems of medicine or has been described in their texts, the need for testing its toxicity in animals has been considerably reduced. Neither would any toxicity study be needed for phase II trial unless there are reports suggesting toxicity or when the herbal preparation is to be used for more than 3 months. It should be necessary to undertake 4 - 6 weeks toxicity study in 2 species of animals in the circumstances pointed out in the preceding sentence or when a larger multicentric phase III trial is subsequently planned based on results of phase II study.

Clinical trials with herbal preparations should be carried out only after these have been standardized and markers identified to ensure that the substances being evaluated are always the same. The recommendations made earlier regarding informed consent, inducements for participation, information to be provided to the subject, withdrawal from study and research involving children or persons with diminished autonomy, all apply to trials on plant drugs also. These trials have also got to be approved by the appropriate scientific and ethical committees of the concerned Institutes. However, it is essential that such clinical trials be carried out only when a competent ayurvedic, siddha or unani physician is a co-investigator in such a clinical trial. It would neither ethically acceptable nor morally justifiable, if an allopathic physician, based on references in ancient literature of above-mentioned traditional systems of medicine, carries out clinical evaluation of the plant without any concept or training in these systems of medicine. Hence, it is necessary to associate a specialist from these systems and the clinical evaluation should be carried out jointly.

When a folklore medicine/ethnomedicine is ready for commercialization after it has been scientifically found to be effective, then the legitimate rights/share of the tribe or community from whom the knowledge was gathered should be taken care of appropriately while applying for the intellectual property rights and / patents for the product.

World Health Organization (WHO) Guidelines

The WHO has published guidelines in order to define basic criteria for evaluating the quality, safety, and efficacy of herbal medicines aimed at assisting national regulatory authorities, scientific organizations and manufacturers in this particular area (WHO, 2000). Furthermore, the WHO has prepared pharmacopeia monographs on herbal medicines and the basis of guidelines for the assessment of herbal drugs (WHO, 1999; 2001). Originally, WHO guidelines for GCP are adapted from ICH guidelines. These guidelines specify the requirements for clinical trial protocol and protocol amendment(s); background information about the name and description of the investigational product(s); trial objectives and purpose and trial design selection and withdrawal of subjects; treatment of subjects; assessment of efficacy and safety; statistics; direct access to source data/documents; quality control and quality assurance; description of ethical considerations relating to the trial; data handling and record keeping financing and insurance if not addressed in a separate agreement; publication policy; if not addressed in a separate agreement; pharmaceutical assessment of preparations; stability and safety aspect.

Good Clinical Practices (GCP) Guidelines

GCP is an international ethical and scientific quality standard for designing, conducting, recording and reporting trials that involve the participation of human subjects.

Compliance with this standard provides public assurance that the rights, safety and well being of trial subjects are protected; consistent with the principles that have their origin in the Declaration of Helsinki, and that the clinical trial data are credible. Objective of ICH GCP Guideline is to provide a unified standard for the European Union (EU), Japan and the United States to facilitate the mutual acceptance of clinical data by the regulatory authorities in these jurisdictions. The ICH guideline was developed with consideration of the current good clinical practices of the European Union, Japan, and the United States, as well as those of Australia, Canada, the Nordic countries and the World Health Organization.

Ethical Issues

Ethical and economical issues are important in the management aspects of herbal medicines research. The main players in the exploitation of herbal medicines include the traditional medicine practitioner, the research scientists, pharmaceutical industry that will bring forth the medicines and medicinal products of research to the public and the larger society that will ultimately benefit in health and disease. National governments are also involved as they have responsibility of ensuring the welfare and safety of citizens. All the parties mentioned are interested in developing herbal medicines for public use. However, in the clinical development of herbal traditional medicines, the tripartite relationship between the researcher, the traditional practitioner and the research participant is most paramount.

Treating physicians have the obligation of judging the material risks of their medical treatments, and this may include the risks associated with complementary medicine. Most patients and many healthcare professionals view traditional medicine as virtually risk free, a notion that is often misguided. Complementary medicine is likely to become relevant to the informed consent obligation of GPs (Ernst E, 2004).

Informed Consent

Informed consent (IC) is an ethical, legal, and regulatory instrument of communication between researchers and their clients. It is an integral part of research by which we create understanding on the research projects. Informed consent is a 'process of weighing up the any possible risks and benefit to be derived'. IC has become the cornerstone of research ethics because it affords the research participants the ability to exercise their rights to beneficence and autonomy. Nevertheless, informed consent as contained in the international guidelines focuses mainly relationship between the researcher and the research participant. As the popularity of complementary medicine grows, and as informed consent becomes more and more comprehensive, its relevance for clinical trial practice is important. At present, however, GPs' ethical obligations still exceed the legal ones.

Traditional medicine may be less risky than most conventional therapies but it is not totally devoid of adverse effects. Treating physicians have the obligation of informing about the adverse events. Many modern practitioners believe that all forms of traditional medicine lack evidence of efficacy. This is clearly not the case. If Cochrane reviews are anything to go by, several herbal remedies are of proven efficacy. For instance, St John's wort is an effective symptomatic treatment for mild to moderate depression (Kessler et al, 1995), so is horse chestnut seed extract for primary venous insufficiency (Creamer et al, 2001), and so is ginkgo for dementia (Stein et al, 2000)

Researchers should also remember that herbal medical care is a long time cultural duty of the traditional medicine practitioner within the community. He or she holds this responsibility on trust for the community but it is also his/her source of livelihood. These are important considerations in the consent process. Therefore, the need for understanding IC before research commences is strongly advocated. The concerns and benefits of all the stakeholders who share in the burden of herbal medicines research should be defined and determined. This measure should be considered as part and parcel of submissions to regulatory and ethical review committees (Karniyus and Carel, 2004). They should be clear terms on outcome of research regarding benefit and royalties. This should be included in the IRB/EC review process of herbal traditional medicines.

REVIEW OF CLINICAL TRIAL DESIGNS ON TRADITIONAL/HERBAL MEDICINES

Katiyar CK (2006) reviewed the representative clinical trials conducted in India, through National Center of Complementary and Alternative Medicines (NCCAM), USA and other international studies with a view to analyze the clinical trial designs followed. The search was conducted using internet search engines Pubmed and Google, studies compiled by Central Council for Research in Ayurveda and Siddha (CCRAS), New Delhi, Indian research journals published by CCRAS, Indian Council of Medical Research (ICMR), New Delhi, Indian Journal of Clinical Practice and other Indian Journals. Phytomedicine, International Journal of Complimentary and Alternative Medicine, Journal of American Medical Association, New England Journal of Medicine and other relevant journals were also screened for the purpose besides the NCCAM web site.

The review of clinical trials collated using above mentioned resources (without modifying the words used to describe the designs followed) revealed that several researchers have conducted clinical trials on ayurvedic/herbal medicines in India. These researchers belong to both modern medicine as well as traditional medicine streams. It was observed that there was no harmonization in the trial designs of 68 Indian clinical trials reviewed and shown in Table 19.2.

Among the 68 trials reviewed from India, 28 (approx 41%) were randomized open trials, followed by 13 (approx 19%) open comparative trials. Only 7 (approx 10%) were double-blind placebo controlled trials. These trials were conducted on single herbal ayurvedic medicines (viz *Pluchea lanceolata, Pterocarpus marsupium,*

Table 19.2 Designs followed in Indian clinical trials on ayurvedic/ herbal medicines		
Number of trials reviewed (India) : 68		
S. No.	*Trial design*	*No. of trials*
1	Double blind placebo-controlled	7
2	Double blind comparative	3
3	Open comparative placebo-controlled	3
4	Single blind placebo-controlled	5
5	Open non-comparative	1
6	Randomized open	28
7	Open add-on	1
8	Flexi-dose open	1
9	Double blind cross-over	1
10	Open add-on comparative	1
11	Open comparative	13
12	Single blind reference controlled	4

Glycyrrhiza glabra, Emblica officinalis, Withania somnifera, Crataeva nurvala, Clerodendrum serratum, Boswellia serrata, Picrorhiza kurroa, Bacopa monniera, Saraca asoka, Swertia chirayata, Terminalia arjuna, Commiphora wightii, Inula racemosa, Smilax china, Streblus asper, Tecoma undulata, Acorus calamus, Centella asiatica, Terminalia belerica, Hedychium spicatum, Gymnema sylvestre, Tribulus terrestris, Bergenia lingulata and Zingiber officinale), poly herbal and herbo-mineral formulations (viz Ayush-64, Rhumayog, Rhumayog Gold, K-4, Brihat Vata Chintamani Rasa, Shweta Parpati and Kshaar sutra).

Clinical trials conducted through NCCAM, USA were also reviewed to find out the designs followed for these studies. Table 19.3 provides the analysis of the same.

It was observed that, 23 (46%) were randomized double-blind placebo controlled parallel trials and 9 (18%) were randomized open and other trials were conducted using different designs. The trials have been conducted on Black Cohosh (9), Red Clover (6), Borage Oil (4), Gingko (3), Garlic (3), Mistletoe (1), Chamomile (1), Cranberry (2), Echinacea (3), Dehydro-epiandrosterone (1), Flax seed (1), Ginger (1), St. John's Wort (6), Milk Thistle (1), Soya Isoflavones (4), Pycnogenol (1), Saw Palmetto (1), Valerian (1) and Broccoli (1).

In the 179 clinical trials conducted internationally on herbs and herbal products, the methodologies, which have been adopted, are listed in Table 19.4. The herbs or products on which these trials have been conducted are *Cimicifuga racemosa* (10), *Serenoa repens* (18), *Hypericum perforatum* (35), *Zingiber officinale* (20), *Ginkgo biloba* (45), *Piper methysticum* (15), *Valeriana wallichii* (10) and *Echinacea purpurea* (26).

Out of these 179 clinical trials, 111 (62%) were found to be randomized double-blind placebo controlled studies, 33 (approx 19%) were double blind comparative and 17 (approx 10%) were single blind placebo controlled studies.

Table 19.5 depicts the comparative percentage of randomized double blind placebo-controlled (RDBPC), single blind placebo-controlled (SBPC) and double blind

Table 19.3: Analysis of reviewed clinical trials conducted through NCCAM

Number of trials reviewd (NCCAM): 50

S. No.	*Trial Design*	*No. of trials*
1	Randomized double-blind placebo controlled, parallel	23
2	Non-randomized open uncontrolled	3
3	Randomized open	9
4	Open label	3
5	Non-randomized open active control crossover	1
6	Randomized double blind placebo controlled crossover	2
7	Randomized double blind placebo controlled paralled dose-escalation	2
8	Randomized double blind active control parallel	1
9	Non-randomized open active control	1
10	Randomized double blind active control crossover	1
11	Non-randomized single blind placebo controlled	1
12	Randomized single blind placebo controlled	2
13	Randomized double blind	1

comparative (DBC) clinical trials conducted in India, through NCCAM, USA and other studies conducted internationally.

Single herbal drugs subjected to clinical trials using any one of the above designs have recently been reported to be ineffective in few papers published in international journals. Some of them are Echinacea for cold (Taylor et al, 2003), Guggulu for high cholesterol (Szapary et al, 2003) and more recently Saw Palmetto for benign prostrate hypertrophy (Stephen Bent et al, 2006). This is in contrast to the several other studies on the same products proving their efficacy in earlier conducted clinical trials using almost similar designs. Moreover review of the trial methodologies and results obtained provided the debatable conclusion that none of the above methods followed for conducting clinical trials are fool proof with respect to traditional medicines, which includes ayurvedic/ herbal medicines as well. Numerous trials on same product even using conventional design for clinical trial give inconsistency in results. Therefore, the conventional approach of conducting clinical trials on single drug as a component of treatment may not be appropriate for traditional/herbal medicines.

Table 19.4: Analysis of reviewed clinical trials (international)

Number of trials reviewed (International) : 179

S. No.	Trial design	No. of trials
1	Randomized double blind placebo controlled	111
2	Double blind comparative	33
3	Cross-over double blind	4
4	Single blind placebo-controlled	17
5	Placebo controlled single blind comparative	2
6	Parallel group comparative	12

Table 19.5: Trial design wise comparative percentages

Trial Methodology	India	NCCAM	International
RDBPC	10%	41%	62%
SBPC	7%	4%	10%
DBC	5%	-	19%

LIMITATION WITH HERBAL/TRADITIONAL MEDICINE WITH REFERENCE TO CLINICAL TRIALS

Several factors make the task of conducting clinical trials on traditional/herbal medicines daunting. Few important ones are discussed below.

i. Limitation of blinding.
ii. Limitation of placebo.
iii. Limitation of therapy.
iv. Limitation of clinical equipoise.
v. Limitation of conventional clinical trials methods.
vi. Limitation of standardization or quality of products

Limitation of Blinding

Blind assessment is a critical component of conventional evaluation of therapeutic interventions. Though treatment blinding in the evaluation of herbal medicines should adopt the approach of conventional medicines, e.g. using active and control formulations with similar color, taste, aroma, etc. However, in the evaluation of efficacy of traditional therapies, it can be difficult, impractical or impossible for the practitioner to be kept ignorant of what treatment the patients are receiving. It is important, however, to reduce any bias introduced by non-blinded treatment by carrying out a blinded assessment of the primary outcomes of the study. If the herbal medicine cannot be administered in a predetermined standardized formulation, it will be impossible to keep the treatment blinded.

Limitation of Placebo

Use of a placebo may not always be possible as they may involve ethical issues as well as technical problems. For example, it may be not possible to have a placebo control if the herbal medicine has a strong or prominent smell or taste, as is the case for products containing certain essential oils. In addition, patients who have been treated previously with the herbal medicine under investigation that has a characteristic organoleptic property cannot be randomized into control groups. In the case of herbal medicines with a strong flavour, placebo substances with the same flavour may have a similar function. This problem may become more compounded in case of semi solid formulations like Chyawanprash. In such cases, it may be advisable to use a low dosage of the same herbal medicine as a control. Alternatively, a positive control, such as well-established treatment, can be used.

Limitation of Clinical Equipoise

Ayurveda or herbal medicine does not have another herbal clinical equivalent, rather clinical trial with herbal equipoise are discouraged. Herbal traditional medicine research, comparing the activities of the herbal remedies to standard care is paramount in order to achieve clinical *equipoise*. Without *equipoise*, the research will not be scientifically valid as some of the participants may receive inferior treatment and the effort will not contribute to increasing knowledge about best treatment. The draw back in this approach is that some of the intangible holistic values of the herbal remedies are masked by the western approach and are not put into consideration. Therefore, the control group in herbal medicines research should be placed on the standard clinical care of allopathic medicines where it is available. Furthermore, we suggest that the issue of continued care after completion of the study should be raised in such studies before commencement.

Limitation of Therapy

Ayurveda or other traditional systems of medicine seldom use mono herb based therapy. In most of the cases traditional medicine physicians follow the approach of multiple therapies coupled with dietary and behavioral modalities to achieve therapeutic effectiveness. Rheumatoid arthritis is a typical example in which case oral drugs (mostly poly herbal), topical application of medicated oils along with strict dietary restrictions are common features.

Limitation of Standardization or Quality Control

Plants are polypharmacy themselves containing hundreds of constituents and some of them are present at very low concentrations. Standardization of herbal products is a burning issue being discussed and debated from academic to regulatory fora. Quality of the finished product depends upon the quality and authenticity of the crude raw material, geographical location of collection, time of collection, method of harvesting, storage, processing, microbial load, heavy metal contamination, etc. Most critical point to achieve standardization is identification, isolation and characterization of the marker compounds. It is followed by developing appropriate analytical methods to test the qualitative and quantitative presence of the compounds not only in the crude plant material, but also in the intermediates like extracts and their finished formulations.

Intense efforts are ongoing globally to evolve and develop the pharmacopeial standards of the medicinal plants used in the traditional medicines.

WHO have laid down certain specific requirement for assessment of quality; pharmaceutical assessment for Crude plant material; Plant preparations; finished product and all procedures should be in accordance with Good Manufacturing Practices; Stability studies; Assessment of safety; Toxicological studies and Documentation of safety based on experience (WHO, 2000).

CLINICAL TRIAL DESIGNS, APPROACHES AND METHODOLOGIES

According to WHO guidelines (WHO, 2000) the starting point in the design of a research protocol is a complete literature review, including the traditional use of the proposed practice and existing scientific research in the field. Where little or no literature exists, the oral tradition and the source of this tradition need to be clearly stated.

A review of the literature should identify the current level of evidence of efficacy and safety for the proposed intervention. Evaluation of the literature should follow well-established and accepted guidelines. However, meta-analysis in traditional medicine may be difficult, mainly due to the lack of large clinical trials of good quality. In addition, the efficacy of a particular treatment may also vary according to the skill and experience of the practitioner. These issues must be considered and kept in mind.

Complementary and alternative medicine presents special challenges in the design and execution of studies, with respect to both internal validity and generalizability. These problem relates to the tension between specifying the intervention sufficiently that others can apply it and desire to study traditional medicine as it is applied in traditional medicine practices; they also concern the difficulties in controlling expectation bias (the systematic effect on the results of the participants belief that a certain therapy will help them). Most traditional medicine interventions are investigated only after they are so widespread that they can no longer be ignored, and by that time, the traditional medicine practices are highly diversified in practices, personal experiences, biases, and expectations. A single research strategy will not fit all circumstances and all traditional medicine interventions; hence, there is need for flexibility in designing of trials likes randomized trial, single case, black box, ethnographic, etc. The study design may be chosen from a whole spectrum of clinical research designs, which are suitable for assessing traditional medicine (WHO, 2000).

Randomized Controlled Trials

Clinical trial is an artificial event; however, it is fair to say that with in mainstream medicine large numbers of patients do routinely receive the same treatment, this is never the case in herbal medicine. The most powerful method for testing the effect of a conventional medical intervention is Randomized clinical trial is not suitable for many traditional medicines. Standard randomized controlled trials (RCTs) consist of two or three study arms, large numbers of patients in each study arm, one specific, standard treatment or dose of treatment per study arm, and 1 or 2 years of follow-up may be ill-suited to answer questions about the long-term effects of complementary and alternative medicine. For many other traditional medicine therapies, however, the conceptual basis for the therapy requires an interaction between the practitioners and patient that modifies the therapy to the individual. Indian traditional medicines especially an Ayurvedic medicine require individualization of treatment based on an examination and understanding of the patient's condition using concepts that do not have an analogue in western allopathic medicine. Consequently, traditional medicine/ CAM advocates have criticized randomized clinical trials that reported no effect for not having allowed the necessary tailoring of the intervention.

A survey of published results over 10 years revealed that approximately one in six studies were randomized controlled trials and 50 percent of them were observational descriptive studies, of those that were actual experiments, one third lacks the control and another one third utilized non randomized controls. Thus, the use of non classical randomized control trial is not widespread as might be thought. This is because its limitations are well recognized and not all treatments can be subjected to such analysis. For these reason, "pragmatic" or observational trials are frequently advocated for studying traditional medicines.

Single-case Design

WHO General Guidelines for Methodologies on Research and Evaluation of Traditional Medicine (WHO, 2000), describes advantage of single case design being adaptable to the clinical needs of the patient and the therapeutic approach of the practitioner, but have limitations due to their lack of generalization to other patients. Guidelines say single case designs are appropriate for the development of research hypotheses, testing those hypotheses in daily clinical practice and refining clinical techniques. Guidelines advocates single-case designs using a common protocol—if the protocol can be systematically followed for collaborative research among practitioners from different backgrounds. For example, single-case designs can evaluate the effectiveness of various specialized acupuncture methods in patients with a variety of individual differences. In a single-case design, the patient is his or her own control. Treatment can be randomized for a patient, rather than the patient being randomized for a treatment.

Black-box Design

The study of traditional medicine can also be undertaken in a "black-box" manner (WHO, 2000). This means that the treatment and all of its components are delivered, as they would be in the usual clinical situation. In this type of study, no component of the treatment "package" is isolated and studied independently. This allows the effectiveness of traditional medicine to be determined either within its own theoretical framework or within that of conventional medicine. However, 'Black box designs' are much less convincing and will increase the data requirements regarding robustness and persuasiveness of study results. The credibility of study results is low as a clear dose-response relationship or a clear chain of events cannot be identified (for example, drug exposure to target occupancy, to dynamic measures, to clinical outcome).

Ethnographic Design

Ethnographic studies that document the social and cultural context in which a traditional practice emanates may be appropriate in situations where there is no available scientific literature or other documentation (WHO, 2000). These and other qualitative studies can provide baseline information from which hypotheses may be generated, and can lead to further research.

Observational Trial

Observational studies collect findings on a therapeutic or prophylactic treatment under routine conditions. The special feature of these studies is that they seek, as far as possible, not to influence the individual doctor-patient relationship with respect to indications, and the selection of and carrying out the treatment. These studies may be conducted with or without a control group. The specific details of the study (e.g. the time and extent of examination for each individual patient, the number of patients involved) and the envisaged methods (e.g. data recording and evaluation) must be adapted to the question investigated in the study (e.g. safety or appropriate posology). Observational studies have specific advantages in studying aspects of clinical safety. The use of such studies to prove efficacy is limited because bias in patient selection may occur. Nevertheless, the level of evidence on efficacy of traditional medicine can be significantly increased by well-designed observational studies (WHO, 2000).

An observational trial is different from a clinical or treatment trial in a number of ways. In an observational trial, no specific treatment is being studied. Subjects are not randomized into different groups and are not given either an experimental treatment or placebo. Instead, subjects are enrolled and observed over a period of time. Different types of data are collected from the participants and analyzed to look for trends and correlations that may inform us better about the disease and how to conduct a clinical trial involving experimental treatments. For example, data collected may include biological (e.g., blood or tissue analyzed for genetic factors or other biological substances), imaging (e.g., magnetic resonance imaging (MRI) or computed tomography (CT), family history, medical history (e.g., what treatments are being or have been used), clinical, behavioral, etc. Observational studies can be very powerful in terms of defining the natural history of a disease and gathering, in a systematic way, information about patients experiences with different forms of treatment. However, because observations studies are not controlled as in a treatment trial, they cannot make conclusions about cause and effect of particular treatments.

For example, a study might consider a group of 100 elderly women, 50 of whom have taken herbal therapy, and 50 of whom have never taken herbal medicine. If the incidence of Alzheimer's disease is lower among the 50 women taking herbal therapy than among the 50 women who are not taking herbal therapy, then the researchers might conclude that herbal therapy helps prevent Alzheimer's disease. Observational trials are most useful for suggesting a previously unsuspected link between a medication or lifestyle pattern and a disease (or prevention of a disease). For these reasons, once an apparent relationship has been detected in observational trials, the next step is for researchers to conduct clinical trials. Continuing the example above, the clinical trial might consider 100 randomly selected women, give half HRT and half an inactive placebo pill, and then see whether the women on HRT really are less likely to develop Alzheimer's disease.

A classical example of observational research using an integrated ayurvedic approach was recently published in first annual report on Integrated Approach for the Treatment of Migraine (Balendu Prakash, 2006). This report is unique, wherein the disease definition and categorization was in accordance to the international conventional system of medicine, while treatment was based on ayurvedic approach. An ayurvedic physician based on his own experience, developed protocol for ayurvedic treatment of migraine. This treatment protocol was shared with 5-6 ayurvedic practitioners all over India and details of the patients, observations, and treatment outcomes were recorded on similar case report forms basis actual practice. The data was analyzed at the central place. Post card system is being used for follow up of these patients. The data generated on actual documented practice on about 250 patients so far was published in VCPC first annual report and demonstrated fair to good efficacy in 67 percent patients (Balendu Prakash, 2006). This project of simultaneous documentation of actual clinical practice is a unique experiment of observational research in India and will probably lead by example.

Pragmatic Trials

In a pragmatic trial, patients are assigned to a traditional practitioner rather than a tightly specified traditional therapy (Hugh MacPherson, 2004). The traditional practitioners can provide their treatments in their usual fashion, individualizing the therapy for each particular patient (Paul et al, 2005). While this strategy allows the conventional practice to occur in its traditional fashion, it makes blinding or otherwise controlling expectation bias very difficult.

Furthermore, while in one way individualizing the therapy increases generalizability, it also increases the sensitivity of the results to the skill of the practitioners. Since the intervention relies on practitioner expertise in understanding the patient and delivering the therapy, the study results are more difficult to apply to other practitioners. Thus, pragmatic trials should discuss the training and experience of the traditional practitioner. Large pragmatic trials that include many practitioners and that compare a traditional therapy with a credible control or alternative therapy would be particularly useful in assessing traditional medicine (Paul et al, 2005).

Pragmatic trials, of course, do not compare traditional therapies with sham treatment. However, a patient's expectation of how likely it is that a therapy will be beneficial for their condition can substantially influence the results. In a study comparing massage, acupuncture, and usual care for patients with chronic low back pain, patients were asked their expectation before treatment. When patients were randomly assigned to treatments they thought more likely to be effective, they in fact reported greater efficacy (Kalauokalani et al, 2001). While blinding of patients or providers is clearly not possible in a pragmatic trial, it is possible to use outcome assessors who are blind to treatment. If feasible, such use should be considered a methodological strength. In sum, this variability in sham therapies across studies presents a challenge. If sham groups do vary in important ways, they cannot all be equated and treated as generic control groups. The investigator must examine each sham treatment thoroughly, just as active-treatment groups are assessed. Categories of sham therapies may need to be constructed and each study classified. This categorization may result in a loss of sample size, since fewer studies will be comparable. Investigators should consider choosing the active treatment of interest, and then constructing effect sizes for alternative therapies versus this reference (Assendelft et al, 2003).

Preference Trial

A common problem in randomized controlled trials arises when patients (or their clinicians) have such strong treatment preferences that they refuse randomization. The absence of these patients from trials may restrict generalization of the results, as participants may not be representative. A further potential source of bias exists when patients with strong treatment preferences are recruited and randomized. When it is not possible to blind patients to their treatment allocation for their preferred treatment they may poorly comply (Bradley C, 1993). On the other hand, patients receiving their preferred treatment may comply better than average. There may, therefore, be a treatment effect, which results from patient preferences and not from therapeutic efficacy.

Patients may be placed in one of three groups according to preference and willingness to be randomized: (*a*) patients who have no strong preferences and therefore consent to randomization; (*b*) patients with a preference who still consent to randomization; and (*c*) patients who refuse randomization and opt for their treatment of choice.

To cope with patient preferences the use of a comprehensive cohort design (Olschewski and Scheurlen, 1985) or the patient preference trial has been suggested (Brewin and Bradley, 1989) Patients with treatment preferences are allowed their desired treatment; those who do not have strong views are randomized conventionally. Hence, in a trial of two interventions, A and B, we end up with four groups: randomized to A; prefer A; randomized to B; prefer B. The analysis of such a trial is uncertain. Any comparison using the non-randomized groups is unreliable because of the presence of unknown and uncontrolled confounders (Silverman and Altman, 1996). At least one analysis should, therefore, be a comparison between the two randomized arms alone. Analyses, which include the unrandomised groups, should be treated as observational studies with known confounding factors adjusted for in the analysis. Olschewski and Scheurlen (1985) have suggested that an analysis using randomization status, as a covariate might be helpful. A further limitation of the patient preference approach is that it may increase the size and cost of trials.

Patient preference designs complement, but do not replace randomized trials. However, measuring patient preferences within a fully randomized design deserves further use as this conserves all the advantages of a fully randomized design with the additional benefit of allowing for the interaction between preference and outcome to be assessed.

Non-inferiority Trial (NIT) and the Equivalence Trial (ET)

Non-inferiority trials (NITs) are designed to answer that one therapy is not worse than other, while ETs are aimed to finding out whether one treatment is neither better nor worse than another. At first glance, NITs and ETs look very much like conventional studies. They have a comparison group; can be randomized and even double blind. Yet there is one crucial difference: while conventional studies aim to test whether there is a difference between the experimental and the control treatment, NITs and ETs aim to test whether both interventions yield the same (equivalent) result (Jadad AR, 1998). Like many other areas of medicine, in herbal or alternative medicine it is also relevant to ask, is therapy A as good (i.e. efficacious) as therapy B (i.e. another treatment used for the same condition).

Despite the fact that such studies seem ideally suited to answer many research questions in herbal medicine, they are associated with several major drawbacks.

First, the sample size of a typical NIT or ET has to be substantially larger than that of a typical conventional trial. For a conventional superiority trial, one needs to define what is clinically different (e.g. a difference of 5 points on a scale to arrive at an estimated sample size). For a NIT or an ET, one has to define what is clinically non-superior or equivalent and this must be less (e.g. plus or minus 2 points on the scale), thus the sample size of a typical NIT/ET needs to be larger. Analysis is different too: NITs and ETs require confidence intervals. One also needs to be quite clear whether one is doing a strict ET, i.e. no better and no worse, or a NIT, i.e. no worse. The implications can be considerable, where recruitments/ availability or ethics approval for number of patients are low. For example, while a conventional (placebo-controlled) study with, say, 200 patients is (at least sometimes) approvable, one with 400 patients is rarely (Edzard Ernst, 2005).

Equivalence or non-superiority, however are undertaken with the comparator treatment of proven efficacy and one must make sure that, in the trial, one gives the comparator treatment its best chance of success. This usually means using it under the same conditions as those in which it was originally shown to be effective, and on a similar population. In other words, doses, inclusion and exclusion criteria, etc. must be the same as in the original trials. This can be a problem for traditional medicine where one often wants to treat mild to moderate symptoms, whereas in a typical superiority trial one might opt to exclude mild to moderate symptoms (Edzard Ernst, 2005).

Important implications arise here for complementary or alternative medicine: situations where a therapeutic option of proven efficacy exists are few and far between. If the comparator treatment is not of proven efficacy, establishing equivalence or non-inferiority between the experimental and the two treatments can be interpreted in at least two different ways: treatment A is equally effective as B, or it is equally ineffective as B. In the latter case, the result would obviously be less than informative (Yueh et al, 2003). The usual herbal scenario is a setting where several herbal therapies are used but none are of proven efficacy. Some would even insist that lack of proof of efficacy is a hallmark of alternative medicine (Eisenberg et al, 1993), in which case NITs or ETs of one form of alternative medicine versus another hardly seem to be a good idea. NITs and ETs of one form of complementary or alternative medicine versus an orthodox therapy, on the other hand, may encounter some of the above-listed problems typical of placebo-controlled studies, e.g. reservations of participating patients

In conclusion, NITs and ETs seem to be an attractive alternative to conventional, placebo-controlled, superiority trials of alternative medicine. Hence, there is need to undertake more and more of such investigations. However, it is crucial to ensure that they are properly designed and that their conclusions are correct. Studies incorrectly posing as NITs or ETs can be seriously misleading.

THE CONTROL ARM AND USE OF PLACEBO

A well-conducted and controlled clinical trial could provide sufficient evidence to establish a relationship between the use of an herbal medicine or traditional procedure-based therapy and the prevention, diagnosis, improvement or treatment of an illness, provided there is a supporting body of evidence from observational or mechanistic studies.

Randomized controlled trials require one or more control groups for purposes of comparison. The selection of control groups depends on the objectives of the study. In the evaluation of traditional medicine, a concurrent control group should be used. The control groups may involve one or more controls such as a well-established treatment or non-treatment or different doses of the same treatment or sham or placebo treatment or full-scale treatment or minimal treatment or alternative treatment.

Different controls can be used in clinical trials to answer different questions. The use of a placebo, when possible, is desirable, because it generates evidence of better quality. Placebo-controlled trials are intended to establish whether treatment is valuable over and above what might be achieved by a control treatment, and not whether treatment is valuable at all. Thus, it allows researchers to distinguish specific from non-specific effects of treatment in order to determine whether the additional cost, risk and effort of a specific treatment are worthwhile. It is also important for understanding the mechanism of a treatment. This is true for the evaluation of all drugs. It is not only of academic interest, but is also of practical value, especially for developing new treatments from traditional ones. However, in some cases, placebo-controlled trials may not be possible (WHO 2000). The traditional way to manage expectation bias in drug trials to use a matched placebo has been disputed for several reasons (Heusser et al, 1999). Many clinicians feel that giving placebo to suffering patient is unethical. The declaration of Helsinki advocates placebo controlled trial only for conditions for which no therapy of proven efficacy exists. The magnitude of a potential "placebo response," or even its existence at all, is controversial. However, there is agreement that the placebo response is particularly important in studies that use subjective patient measures of outcome, especially pain. Because chronic painful conditions account for a large proportion of the reasons patients seek traditional therapies, the use of placebo controls is especially important.

It is preferable to compare traditional/herbal medicine with both a well-established treatment and another control group (from the list of control groups) to determine whether the herbal medicine is useful in the context of current best practice. One specific problem in clinical research of traditional medicine is the simultaneous conventional treatment of patients (e.g. cancer patients) in a study. It may not be ethically possible to withdraw the conventional treatment. Therefore, in such cases, the focus of research may be on the additional or supportive effects of traditional medicine. Research on combinations of traditional and conventional medicine should always consider potential therapeutic interactions and side effects.

Two herbal medicines cannot be tested against each other because it will be difficult to know whether either is better than nothing, or indeed which one will be better than the standard care. Even if one is found to be better than the other, it may still be difficult to ascertain the extent of benefit conferred since the interventions may differ markedly in other ways e.g. cost or toxicity (Karniyus and Carel, 2004). Therefore, in herbal traditional medicine research, comparing the activities of the herbal remedies to standard care is paramount in order to achieve clinical *equipoise*. Without *equipoise*, the research will not be scientifically valid as some of the participants may receive inferior treatment and the effort will not contribute to increasing knowledge about best treatment. The draw back in this approach is that some of the intangible holistic values of the herbal remedies are masked by the western approach and are not put into consideration. Therefore, the control group in herbal medicines research should be placed on the standard clinical care of allopathic medicines where it is available (Karniyus and Carel, 2004).

For alternative medicine double blind placebo controlled trial design poses a much greater challenge especially in conditions where single drug is almost never prescribed. We, however, suggest a novel method of double blind placebo controlled drug trials in this situation also. For example a typical prescription of Sandhigata Vata (Osteo-Arthritis) comprises (1) Brihat Vata Chintamani Rasa – Mercurial preparation, (2) Maha Yogaraj Guggulu – Herbo-mineral preparation, (3) Rasna Saptak Kwatha – Herbal preparation, (4) Maha Narayan Taila (Local application)- Oil and (5) Diet restrictions: Curd, Spices, Lady-finger, Brinjal, etc; so if we are assessing the clinical efficacy of Maha Yograj Guggulu the regimen for the control group should comprise the same treatment regime except this Yograj Guggulu should be replaced by placebo in the trial group. Table 19.6 depicts this model more clearly.

Since the effectiveness of ayurvedic treatment in osteoarthritis is due to sum effect of total treatment regime rather than single drug, obviously the treatment outcome when compared would not show significant difference in the two groups leading to erroneous conclusion that 'Maha Yogaraj Guggulu' is ineffective in sandhigata vata (osteoarthritis).

Blinding of Trial

Treatment blinding in the evaluation of herbal medicines should adopt the approach of conventional medicines, e.g. using active and control formulations with similar color, taste and weight. However, if the herbal medicine cannot be administered in a predetermined standardized formulation, it will be impossible to keep the treatment blinded. Treatment blinding is also difficult to implement in most types of traditional procedure-based therapies. It is important, however, to reduce any bias introduced by non-blinded treatment by carrying out a blinded assessment of the primary outcomes of the study (WHO, 2000).

One mechanism for assessing the success of the "blinding" ability of a sham therapy is to survey patients after receipt of the therapy and ask them to guess whether they

Table 19.6: Suggested new methodology for conducting placebo controlled clinical trials on ayurvedic/ herbal medicines

Drug group	*Placebo group*
Brihat Vata Chintamani Rasa	Brihat Vata Chintamani Rasa
Maha Yogaraj Guggulu	Placebo
Rasna Saptak Kwatha	Rasna Saptak Kwatha
Maha Narayan Taila (Local application)	*Maha Narayan Taila (Local application)*
Diet restrictions: curd, spices, lady finger, brinjal, etc.	Diet restrictions: curd, spices, lady finger, brinjal, etc.

received active or sham therapy. Similar responses in patients receiving active and sham therapy are good evidence that the sham was successful in controlling expectation bias. Successful sham therapies have been reported for acupuncture and spinal manipulation (Triano et al, 1995; Sherman et al, 2002; Shen et al, 2000).

Randomization

Ideally, we wish to obtain an unbiased estimate of the effect of the treatment being investigated compared to placebo or to another active compound and, for this reason, every effort should be made to randomize patients from the beginning of the therapeutic testing phase. The goal of obtaining an unbiased estimate of the size of effect is true in studies in small populations as well as large trials for common diseases. Thus, in developing any treatment, a comparative trial will usually be preferable but may not always be possible. In serious and life-threatening diseases where no alternative treatments exist, there can be a tendency to grasp at any treatment seemingly offering some hope to patients. Anecdotal reports of patients responding then make it practically very difficult to persuade patients to take part in subsequent controlled trials.

Study Outcome Measures

It is essential that the outcome measures chosen be appropriate to the research question. Appropriate outcomes may include quantitative and qualitative outcomes; primary and/or secondary outcomes; and generic and/or highly specific outcomes. Traditional medicines are usually used in chronic conditions and there is a reasonable perception that these drugs do improve quality of life. In clinical trials on traditional/ herbal medicines, therefore, QOL parameters assume strong significance.

Selection of Patients

WHO (2000), have given general guidelines for selection of patients for a clinical trial. It is essential that the sample represent the target population of patients to which the results would be generalized. Publication of the study requires a clear description of the patients using both traditional and conventional terms. The reliability of the categorization/diagnostic criteria used in the study should be considered and stated. The source of the patients under study should be comprehensively described along with details of the recruitment process. The inclusion and exclusion criteria should be completely described and rationalized. Any potential bias in patient selection, recruitment and enrolment should be excluded. Investigators should be aware of any potential errors that may occur when studying traditional medicine out of context and without reference to its traditional theories and concepts. For example, most of the patients who are not responding to conventional therapies look for the alternative therapies and recruitment of such patients are more likely in alternative or traditional medicine trials, hence, thereby increases the chances to negative outcomes. In a recently published study (Stephen et al, 2006) Saw Palmetto was shown to be ineffective in benign prostate hypertrophy, a condition in which it is commonly used and efficacy has been backed by several other clinical trials. Detailed analysis revealed that the patients included in the trial were having advanced disease while the product was reported to be effective in stage 1 or 2 of the disease.

When the research involves techniques that depend on skills that may differ between practitioners, more than one practitioner should conduct such research in order to increase the generalization of the results.

Sample Size

The number of patients in a study needs to be adequate, in order to be able to determine any clinically important differences between the study groups. With respect to the study design, the statistical methods used should be appropriate to the proposed analysis of the study's outcome.

Adverse Events or ADR

Although most traditional therapies are presumed to be safe, there is still the problem of how to assess and quantify the possibility of very rare, but potentially devastating, adverse events. Serious event is enough to tip the scales against use of the alternative medicine therapy. If the benefit for any alternative medicine therapy is modest or unproven, then the presence of even a very small increased risk for a serious event is enough to tip the scales against use of the alternative medicine therapy.

RCT data will almost never be sufficient to prove or disprove a causal relationship between a alternative medicine therapy and a rare adverse event. Indeed, for a future randomized trial to have sufficient power to assess adverse events occurring at a rate of 1 per million, it was calculated that such a study would need to enroll about 3 million treated patients (Paul et al, 2005). Clearly, this threshold will not be crossed for any interventions for that matter. With RCT data insufficient to draw conclusions, the next place to look for evidence is hypothesis testing observational studies. The case– control study is the traditional epidemiologic tool for evaluating possible relationships between exposure and rare events (Paul et al, 2005).

IMPORTANT CONSIDERATION IN CLINICAL TRIALS ON HERBAL/ TRADITIONAL MEDICINES

Differentiating features of herbal drugs have been discussed elsewhere in this chapter. Given below are some important points, which should be kept in view while conducting or planning to conduct a clinical trial on traditional/herbal medicines.

- It is suggested that the consent process in herbal medicine development be extended to the traditional practitioners through the IRB and the medicines being investigated.
- In order to achieve clinical *equipoise*, the standard care (where available) should be used in the control arm of the clinical trial of herbal traditional medicines and not placebo.
- The pre-clinical data requirements for ethical review of studies on herbal medicines should only target specific questions about specific products, which are needed to fill the gap of necessary information on safety that cannot be assumed from the traditional application.
- Phase I clinical trial in the study of herbal traditional medicines that are already in use should be reviewed because the study in normal volunteers will not maximize benefit and minimize risks as much as the study on patient volunteers from the same community would. The pharmacokinetic profile of herbal formulation is usually not feasible, as it comprises several unknown active or non-active constituents; however in some cases the known constituents may be profiled.
- It is suggested that only phases II and III clinical trials should be considered to be valid and ethical. Overall, the need for review of the ethical guidelines for studies involving herbal traditional medicines is suggested.
- Clinical trial to be undertaken in the communities where it has been traditionally used. There is often a very high social desirability in herbal research within the local communities whereby participants are often eager to enroll not merely for economic reasons, but sometimes based on the desire to see their own medicines accepted, developed and used. This places additional responsibility on the researcher to ensure true understanding on the risks and benefits of the entire study through the informed consent process.

NEED FOR ALTERNATIVE METHODS OF CLINICAL TRIAL FOR AYURVEDIC MEDICINES

There is a quest for appropriate method for assessment of ayurvedic or herbal products. ayurveda does not consider body as separate from mind and soul and treat these three components together for complete healing of individuals.

An integrated/holistic approach is essential while undertaking the clinical trial with ayurveda drug and the following factors need to be considered as variables individually and should be accommodated while designing the clinical trial protocols for ayurvedic/ herbal medicine.

Essential elements of an ayurvedic therapeutic regimen are DEEDS, DIET and DRUGS in addition to the following:

i. Complex (individualistic) treatment approach — Psychosomatic constitution (*prakriti*), etc.
ii. Multifactorial *Rogi* (patient) and *Rog*a (disease) *pariksh*a (examination)
iii. Interventions at different stages of disease (*kriyakal*a)
iv. Close relationship of food (Pathya Apathya), medicine, *anupana* (vehicle), time of drug administration, etc.
v. Quality of drug to be tested (batch-to-batch consistency)
vi. Doctor-patient relationship
vii. Use of treatment regimen rather than single drug.

Complex (Individualistic) Treatment Approach — Psychosomatic Constitution (*Prakriti*)

Prakriti of an individual is determined at the time of conception and can be defined as a 'psychosomatic constitution' of individual. Total population can be divided in 7 psychosomatic types. Prakriti pariksha is based on physical and mental traits and influenced by Tridosha (Vata, Pitta and Kapha). Ayurvedic system of medicine believes in individualistic treatment. This is the reason while different patients with same disease are prescribed different drugs depending upon several factors including their psychosomatic constitution. This may also partly explain why most of the ayurvedic medicines are polyherbal in composition.

Multifactorial Patient (*Rogi*) and Disease Examination (*Pariksha*)

Integrated/holistic approach of ayurveda does not differentiate the disease from the patient. Rather both are considered simultaneously. This approach puts insurmountable challenges in deciding the inclusion and exclusion criteria in clinical trial of ayurvedic medicines following ayurvedic principles.

Interventions at Different Stages of Disease (*Kriyakala*)

Ayurveda proposes different interventions at different stages of disease (Kriyakala) in the same patient providing another variable in a clinical trial.

Pathya-apathya (diet)

Diet component may also affect the treatment outcome in clinical trial. Administration of Maha Yogaraj Guggulu (a formulation having anti-inflammatory effect) with restriction of rice, curd, brinjal, etc. will give positive outcomes, however, in similar kind of patients without restriction of rice, curd, brinjal, etc. will give negative outcomes of therapy.

Anupana (Vehicle for drug administration)

Component of ayurveda is also accountable for therapeutic efficacy of ayurvedic medicines. Most of the time the drug is recommended to be administered with a specific vehicle like honey, sugar, jaggery, buttermilk, curd, *ghee*, warm water, expressed juice of a herb, etc. An 'Anupana' is a half-medicine in itself. An interesting example is of Mrityunjaya Rasa used for fever in ayurveda, is given with different anupana (vehicle) in different kind of fevers. For example in vataja jwara with buttermilk, in sannipata jwara with ardraka swarasa (Ginger juice), in ajirna jwara with nimbu swarasa (Lemon juice), in vishama jwara with krishna jeeraka and jaggery.

WAY FORWARD

Last few decades have witnessed tremendous resurgence of interest in herbal medicines globally. This trend has attracted the attention of scientists of various disciplines as well. People with scientific temper started demanding the evidence of efficacy of herbal medicines, taking safety for granted basis their traditional use. Institutions involved in traditional medicines initiated some research using their own methodologies, however, the technological advancements in related put their endeavors far behind. Continued interest in herbal medicines gave way to interdisciplinary research and soon it was observed that apart from the physicians, pharmacologists, biochemists, biotechnologists, agriculturists etc jumped into the fray. As a result today we know that gugulipid work by FXR inhibition (Urizar et al, 2002), and Boswellic acids exhibit their anti inflammatory activity through are Cox 2 inhibition. It can be said that most of the convincing researches on herbal drugs have been conducted in the past few decades only and it has been possibly only due to convergence of various streams of scientists as a team.

Concept of evidence based medicine necessitated clinical evaluation of traditional medicines preferably following the gold standard randomized placebo controlled clinical trials. After few attempts it was realized that gold standard of evaluating the efficacy of conventional drug does not do justice with traditional medicines. Soon the realization dawned upon the clinical researchers that there is a need of identifying newer techniques to evaluate the clinical efficacy of traditional/ herbal medicines.

Normally, clinical research of all types of conventional medicine considers both efficacy and safety, and is conducted according to WHO's guidelines for good clinical practice and the Declaration of Helsinki. Safety evaluation, however, may not be the main focus of clinical research in traditional medicine, because of the long history of traditional medicine. Herbal traditional medicines evolved from traditional knowledge rather than laboratory experimentation. Their development process works backwards from actual use to scientific/laboratory evidence or correlation, often referred to as reverse pharmacology. As drug development process in western medicine is prospective in nature, from preclinical and clinical research, it is reverse in case of knowledge based traditional/herbal medicine (Nicholas AC, 1992). Since the two approaches are fundamentally different, their strategies for development should also differ. Based on their extensive use in humans, herbal traditional medicines may have sufficient information to support limited pilot clinical study with little pre-clinical testing especially when the herbal remedies are prepared in the same way, used in the original form as the traditional practitioner and if the trial is to be carried out in the same community that use them. However, new compounds, isolates or new formulations of the herbs may bear different characteristics and scientific behavior from the original products. These should therefore undergo full-scale pre-clinical and clinical evaluation to establish their traditional validity using current standards.

The conventional methods of controlled and randomized clinical trial is considered gold standard, however, while applying it on evaluation of traditional or alternative medicine especially ayurvedic medicines, its limitations came to fore. Hence, there is need for a paradigm shift in the clinical research on herbal medicines. Different methodologies should be adopted while evaluating the safety and efficacy of traditional medicine through clinical trials.

Keeping above observations in view, some of the methodological approaches specific to the assessment of traditional medicines through clinical research are given below.

- Evaluate traditional medicine in its own theoretical framework-this approach is related to clinical evaluation of holistic multipronged therapeutic approach basis of the traditional system of medicine practices. For example in case of Ama Vata (Rheumatoid arthritis) ayurvedic holistic therapeutic approach should be evaluated in totality rather than reducing it to drug trial.
- Evaluate traditional medicine in the theoretical framework of conventional medicine- this approach refers to certain cases of Ayurvedic drugs where single herbs are used as stand alone medicine in traditional medicine e.g. Guggulu for hyperlipidemia.
- Compare the efficacy of different traditional practices within a system of traditional medicine- this approach refers to clinical evaluations of non-therapeutic or semi therapeutic practices e.g. panchakarma that involve use of medicated oil or yogic practices which do not involve any medicine.
- Evaluate the efficacy of pure active phytochemicals under the rigorous current scientific procedures or conventional methods for clinical trials e.g. artemisinin, paclitaxel, etc.

The most appropriate method to generate efficacy data on classical ayurvedic therapeutic regimen appears to be observational research as it involves:

- Efficacy of whole treatment regimen
- It is conducted in real life situation
- Data generated by this method can be used by other physicians as well.
- Change in mind set is required among traditional medicine physicians to start proper documentation of their practice to generate the data, though.
- It will be acceptable to both WHO as well as to drug regulatory agencies as documented evidence of traditional use.

The pragmatic approach (Paul et al, 2005) of conducting the clinical trial is also suitable for traditional medicines. However, these trials need to be conducted in such a way as to take into account the international guidelines that define such studies. Standardized mixtures can also be tested in the same way as pure drug compounds provided they are used as stand alone drugs in actual clinical practice traditionally. Increasing popularity also invites cynicism followed by criticism. This some times leads to innovative solutions to the vexed problems. Identification and validation of one universally acceptable method of conducting clinical trials on traditional/ herbal drugs would remain a dream if top brains do not converge to look at this issue after understanding the basic philosophies behind the traditional systems of medicines. Till that happens let us accept that "one size fits all" is not true for knowledge based traditional medicines. Let us hope that current chaos in clinical trial methodologies on herbal drugs would ultimately lead to more disciplined approaches which would be universally acceptable to the scientific community and regulatory authorities alike.

ACKNOWLEDGEMENTS

The authors are thankful to Dr Navin Sharma, Sr Research Scientist for providing invaluable inputs.

SUGGESTED READING

1. Angell M, Kassirer JP. Alternative medicine—The risks of untested and unregulated remedies. N Engl J Med 1998;339(12):839-41.
2. Assendelft WJ, Morton SC, Yu EI, Suttorp MJ, Shekelle PG. Spinal manipulative therapy for low back pain. A meta-analysis of effectiveness relative to other therapies. Ann Intern Med 2003; 138(11):871-81.
3. Balendu Prakash. Integrated approach in the treatment of Migraine, First Annual report, VCPC Research Foundation (SIROs), Dehradun, 2006.
4. Bensky D, Gamble A. Chinese Herbal Medicine: Materia Medica (revised edition), Eastland Press Inc., Seattle 1993.
5. Bradley C. Designing medical and educational intervention studies. Diabetes Care 1993;16: 509-18.
6. Brewin CR, Bradley C. Patient preferences and randomised clinical trials. BI Med J 1989;299: 313-35.
7. Brody JE. Alternaive medicine makes inroads, but watchout for curves. New Yorrk Times. 1998; Apri 28: F7.
8. Charak Samhita, edited and Translated by PV Sharma, Chaukhamba Orientalia, Varanasi, 2005.
9. Creamer M, Burgess P, McFarlane AC. PTSD: findings from the Australian National Survey of Mental Health and Well-Being. Psychol Med 2001; 31: 1237-47.
10. Edzard Ernst. Equivalence and Non-inferiority Trials of CAM. Evid Based Complement Alternat Med. 2004; 1(1): 9-10.
11. Eisenberg DM, Kessler RC, Foster C, Norlock FE, Calkins DR, Delbanco TL. Unconventional medicine in the United States. N Engl J Med 1993; 328: 246-52.
12. Ernst E. Complementary medicine: implications for informed consent in general practice British Journal of General Practice 2004, 54, (499): 82-3.

13. Farnsworth NR, Morris RW. Higher plants: the sleeping giant of drug development. Am J Pharm 1976; 3/4:46.
14. Farnsworth NR, O'Akerele AS, Bingel DD, Soejarta, Eno Z. Medicinal plants in therapy. WHO Bull 1985;63(6):965-81.
15. Hugh MacPherson. Pragmatic clinical trials. Complementary Therapies in Medicine 2004; 12: 136-40.
16. ICMR. Ethical Guidelines for Biomedical Research on Human Subjects. Indian Council of Medical Research New Delhi, 2000.
17. Jadad AR. Randomised controlled trials. A use guide. London UK: Br Med J Books 1998.
18. Kalauokalani D, Cherkin DC, Sherman KJ, Koepsell TD, Deyo RA. Lessons from a trial of acupuncture and massage for low back pain: patient expectations and treatment effects. Spine 2001; 26(13):1418-24.
19. Karniyus SG, Carel IJ. Ethical challenges posed by herbal traditional medicines research. Global Forum for Health Research Forum 8, Mexico City, November 2004.
20. Katiyar CK. Clinical Trials on Herbal Drugs: Limitation and Way Forward: In Ray A and Gulati K- Text Book on Recent Trends in Pharmacology. IK International Press. Delhi 2006; In Press.
21. Katiyar CK. Safety Aspects of Ayurveda: In Ayurveda and its Scientific aspects: opportunities for globalization: Dept of Ayurveda , Yoga and Naturopathy, Unani, Siddha and Homeopathy, Ministry of Health and Family welfare and CSIR Government of India, New Delhi, 2006:110-22.
22. Kessler RC, Sonega A, Bromet E, et al. Post-traumatic stress disorder in the National Comorbidity Survey. Arch Gen Psychiatry 1995; 52: 1048-60.
23. Maurie Markman. Safety Issues in Using Complementary and Alternative Medicine. Journal of Clinical Oncology 2002, 20, 18S: 39s-41s.
24. Nicholas AC. Ethics are local: Engaging cross cultural variations in the ethics for clinical research. Soc Sci Med 1992; 35(9):1079-91.
25. Olschewski M, Scheurlen H. Comprehensive cohort study: An alternative to randomised consent design in a breast preservation trial. Meth Inform Med 1985; 24:131-34.
26. Paul GS, Sally CM, Marika JS, Nina B, Carol F. Challenges in Systematic Reviews of Complementary and Alternative Medicine Topics. Annals of Internal Medicine 2005; 142 (12): 1042-47.
27. Silverman WA, Altman DG. Patient preferences and randomised trials. Lancet 1996; 347:171-74.
28. Solecki RS. Shanidar IV, a Neanderthal flower burial of northern Iraq. Science 1975; 190: 880.
29. Stein MB, McQuaid JR, Pedrelli P, et al. PTSD in the primary care medical setting. Gen Hosp Psychiatry 2000; 22: 261-69.
30. Stephen B, Christopher K, Katsuto S, John N, Esther SH. Saw Palmetto for Benign Prostatic Hyperplasia. N Eng J Med 2006;354(6):557.
31 Szapary PO, Wolfe ML, Bloedon LT, Cucchiara AJ, DerMarderosian AH, Cirigliano MD, Rader DJ. Guggulipid for the treatment of hypercholesterolemia: a randomized controlled trial. Journal of the American Medical Association 2003; 290; 6: 765-72.
32. Taylor JA, Weber W, Standish L, Quinn H, Goeslsing J, McGann M, Calabrese C.. Efficacy and Safety of Echinacea in treating upper respiratory tract infections in children. Journal of the American Medical Association 2003; 290 (21); 2824-30.
33. TGA (Therapeutic Goods Administration).The regulation of complementary medicines in Australia: An overview; April 2006.
34. TGA (Therapeutic Goods Administration). Therapeutics Goods Act 1989 (the Act).
35. Urizar NL, Liverman AB, Dodds DT, Silva FV, Ordentlich P, Yan Y, Gonzalez FJ, Heyman RA, Mangelsdorf DJ, Moore DD. A natural product that lowers cholesterol as an antagonist ligand for FXR. Science 2002; 296(5573):1703-06.
36. WHA31.33 Medicinal plants. Thirty-first world health assembly Geneva, 8-24 MAY 1978 Hbk Res., Vol. II (2nd ed.), 1.10.1.

37. WHA42.43 Traditional medicine and modern health care. Forty-Second World Health Assembly-Thirteenth plenary meeting, Committee A, fourth report) Geneva, 8-19 MAY 1989 Hbk Res., Vol. II (1989), 1.15.4.
38. WHO. WHO Expert Committee on Specifications for Pharmaceutical Preparations. WHO Technical Report Series No. 863, thirty-fourth report. Geneva, World Health Organization, 1996: 178-84.
39. WHO. General Guidelines for Methodologies on Research and Evaluation of Traditional Medicine. WHO/EDM/TRM/2000.1
40. WHO. World Health Organization Guidelines for the Assessment of Herbal Medicines. Programme on Traditional Medicines, Geneva, 1991.
41. WHO. Monographs on selected medicinal plants; Volume 1, World Health Organization, Geneva, 1999.
42. WHO. Monographs on selected medicinal plants; Volume 2, World Health Organization, Geneva, 2001.
43. WHO. Report of a WHO global survey on National policy on traditional Medicine and regulation of herbal medicines. WHO Press, 2002 Avenue Appia, 1211 Geneva 27, Switzerland
44. Yueh B. On equivalence trials and alternative medicine. Arch Otolaryngol Head Neck Surg. 2003; 129:403-4.

20 Investigational New Drug Applications

Kala Suhas Kulkarni, Ravindra Ghooi

INTRODUCTION

Regulations of drugs were originally concerned with their quality. The quality of a drug is primarily determined by its identity and purity. Current regulations are however, an integral part of every aspect of discovery, development, manufacturing, presentation, marketing, distribution and use of drugs, and are country specific. The present chapter deals more with the regulations in the US, on which model the regulations of other countries are based.

Since regulations regarding the introduction of new drugs are country specific, organizations developing new drugs are put to often unnecessary efforts and expenses when they attempted to register their products in different countries. This leads to an overall increase drug prices, since the innovators had to recoup the expenses incurred. Recognizing this problem extensive efforts were made to achieve global harmonization in terms of policies, standards, monograph specifications, analytical methods and acceptance criteria.

These activities spearheaded by USA, Europe and Japan led to the establishment of Good Clinical Practices, which specified requirements for testing of drugs. Though originally meant to insure mutual recognition of new drugs among the member countries, these guidelines have gained acceptance world wide because of their clarity. Additionally economic compulsions make these guidelines acceptable all over the world since all countries would like to market their products in these member countries, which constitute the world's largest pharmaceutical markets.

The safety and efficacy of new drugs have to be demonstrated and confirmed before they can be introduced into clinical practice. In Europe, the principal document guiding the clinical development plan is ICH Harmonized Tripartite Guideline for Good Clinical Practice (GCP). GCP incorporates a series of requirements imposed by the USFDA during 1970s, and those introduced in Europe and Japan. This common standard has allowed globalization of the Pharmaceutical Industry to progress significantly over the past two decades.

In the US, the FDA, and elsewhere other regulatory agencies ensure that foods, cosmetics, drugs, medical devices and radiation emitting products are safe and effective. These agencies oversee regulations of drugs and medical devices, with respect to both clinical development and marketing of such products. The regulations also ensure that clinical studies on these products are conducted in such a way that subject's welfare is guarded. Innovators are required to complete preclinical studies and incorporate them in the investigational new drug application (IND) that is required to be approved before clinical trials can be initiated.

In the US the Federal law requires that a drug be the subject of an approved marketing application before it is transported or distributed across state lines. Because a sponsor will probably want to ship the investigational drug to clinical investigators in many states, it must seek an exemption from that legal requirement. The IND is the means through which the sponsor technically obtains this exemption from the FDA.

Investigational New Drug applications are of many types and can be submitted by different stakeholders. The different types of INDs include the following:

Investigator IND

Is submitted by a physician who both initiates and conducts an investigation and under whose immediate direction the investigational drug is administered or dispensed. A physician might submit a research IND to propose studying an unapproved drug, or an approved product for a new indication or in a new patient population.

Emergency Use IND

This allows the FDA to authorize use of an experimental drug in an emergency situation that does not allow time for submission of IND. It is also used for patients who do not meet the criteria of an existing study protocol.

Treatment IND

This is submitted for experimental drugs showing promise in clinical testing for serious or immediately life-threatening conditions while the final clinical work is conducted and reviewed by the FDA.

INDs can also be classified as a Commercial and non-Commercial. A commercial IND permits the sponsor to collect the data on the clinical safety and effectiveness needed for application for marketing in the form of a New Drug Application (NDA). A non-commercial IND permits the sponsor to use the drug in research or early clinical investigations to obtain the advanced scientific knowledge of the new drug, and there is no plan to market the product.

The most important component of an IND is Clinical Development. Plan for particular pharmaceutical new chemical entity (NCE) or other types of therapeutic agent. The clinical development plan may include all trial phases and some trials for specific subject populations like those with renal and hepatic impairment.

The IND application must contain information in the following broad areas:

- Pharmaceutical information on the dosage form, its composition, stability, methods of analysis etc.
- Animal Pharmacology and Toxicology Studies - Preclinical data to permit an assessment as to whether the product is reasonably safe for initial testing in humans.
- Manufacturing Information - Information pertaining to the composition, stability, and controls used for manufacturing the drug substance and the drug product. Regulatory authorities assess this information to ensure that the manufacturer can produce and supply the drug of adequate quality and in adequate quantity.
- Clinical Protocols and Investigator Information – Detailed protocols for proposed clinical studies to assess whether the initial-phase trials will expose subjects to unnecessary risks. Information on the qualifications of clinical investigators-professionals who oversee the administration of the experimental compound to assess whether they are qualified to conduct the clinical trials. Finally, commitments to obtain informed consent from the research subjects, to obtain review of the study by an institutional review board (IRB), and to adhere to the investigational new drug regulations.

The IND application must contain information in three broad areas:

- Animal Pharmacology and Toxicology Studies - Preclinical data to permit an assessment as to whether the product is reasonably safe for initial testing in humans. Also included are any previous experiences with the drug in humans (often foreign use).
- Manufacturing Information - Information pertaining to the composition, manufacturer, stability, and controls used for manufacturing the drug substance and the drug product. This information is assessed to ensure that the company can adequately produce and supply consistent batches of the drug.
- Clinical Protocols and Investigator Information - Detailed protocols for proposed clinical studies to assess whether the initial-phase trials will expose subjects to unnecessary risks. Also, information on the qualifications of clinical investigators-professionals (generally physicians) who oversee the administration of the experimental compound-to assess whether they are qualified to fulfill their clinical trial duties. Finally, commitments to obtain informed consent from the research subjects, to obtain review of the study by an institutional review board (IRB), and to adhere to the investigational new drug regulations.

RESOURCES FOR IND APPLICATIONS

A number of resources have been made available by the authorities for preparing INDs these include guidelines, review principles, policies and procedures.

Pre-IND Consultation Program

CDER offers a Pre-Investigational New Drug Application (IND) Consultation Program to foster early communications between sponsors and new drug review divisions in order to provide guidance on the data necessary to warrant IND submission. The review divisions are organized generally along therapeutic class and should be contacted before the preparation of IND begins.

GUIDANCE DOCUMENTS FOR INDs

Guidance documents represent the Agency's current thinking on a particular subject. These documents are prepared for FDA review staff and applicants/sponsors to provide guidelines to the processing, content, and evaluation/approval of applications and also to the design, production, manufacturing, and testing of regulated products. They also establish policies intended to achieve consistency in the Agency's regulatory approach and establish inspection and enforcement procedures. Because guidance is not a regulation or a law, it is not enforceable, either through administrative actions or through the courts. An alternative approach may be used if such approach satisfies the requirements of the applicable statute, regulations, or both. For information on a specific guidance document, please contact the originating office.

Guidance documents to help prepare INDs include:

- Guidance for Industry: INDs – Approaches to Complying with CGMP's for Phase 1 Drugs (Draft)
- Guidance for Industry: Exploratory IND Studies
- Content and Format of Investigational New Drug Applications (INDs) for Phase 1 Studies of Drugs Including Well-Characterized, Therapeutic, Biotechnology-Derived Products.
- Q and A - Content and Format of INDs for Phase 1 Studies of Drugs, Including Well-Characterized, Therapeutic, Biotechnology-Derived Products.
- Bioavailability and Bioequivalence Studies for Orally Administered Drug Products - General Considerations.
- IND Exemptions for Studies of Lawfully Marketed Drug or Biological Products for the Treatment of Cancer.
- Drug Master Files.
- Required Specifications for FDA's IND, NDA, and ANDA Drug Master File Binders.
- Immunotoxicology Evaluation of Investigational New Drugs

LAWS, REGULATIONS, POLICIES AND PROCEDURES

Laws enacted by the US. Congress are enforced by the Food and Drug Administration, their principal aim is to protect the consumer's health, safety, and pocket. *The Federal Food, Drug and Cosmetic Act* is the basic food and drug law of the US. With numerous amendments it is the most extensive law of its kind in the world. The law is intended to assure consumers that foods are pure and wholesome, safe to eat, and produced under sanitary conditions; that drugs and devices are safe and effective for their intended uses; that cosmetics are safe and made from appropriate ingredients; and that all labeling and packaging is truthful, informative, and not deceptive.

The FDA is itself made up of a number of offices each of which regulates a particular aspect of drug regulations. The various components of FDA are:

FDA Components

- Center for Food Safety and Applied Nutrition
- Center for Drug Evaluation and Research
- Center for Devices and Radiological Health
- Center for Biologics Evaluation and Research
- Center for Veterinary Medicine
- Office of Regulatory Affairs
- National Center for Toxicological Research.

The above centers between them regulate the following:

Food

(Including foodborne illness, nutrition, dietary supplements, etc.)

Drugs

(Including prescription, over-the-counter, generics, etc.)

Medical Devices

(Including pacemakers, contact lenses, hearing aids, etc.)

Biologics

(Including vaccines, blood products, etc.)

Animal Feed and Drugs

(Including livestock, pets, exotic animals, etc.)

Cosmetics

(Including manufacture, safety, labeling, etc.)

Radiation-Emitting Products

(Including cell phones, lasers, microwaves, etc.)

Combination Products

CODE OF FEDERAL REGULATIONS (CFR)

The Code of Federal Regulations is a compilation of the proposed rules, final rules, meeting notices, etc. published daily in the Federal Regulations. The *CFR* is divided into 50 titles that represent broad areas subject to Federal regulations. The FDA's portion of the *CFR* interprets the *Federal Food, Drug and Cosmetic Act* and related statutes. Section 21 of the *CFR* contains most regulations pertaining to food and drugs. The regulations document all actions of all drug sponsors that are required under Federal law.

The following regulations apply to the IND application process:

21CFR Part 312	Investigational New Drug Application
21CFR Part 314	INDA and NDA Applications for FDA Approval to Market a New Drug (New Drug Approval)
21CFR Part 316	Orphan Drugs
21CFR Part 58	Good Lab Practice for Nonclinical Laboratory [Animal] Studies
21CFR Part 50	Protection of Human Subjects
21CFR Part 56	Institutional Review Boards
21CFR Part 201	Drug Labeling
21CFR Part 54	Financial Disclosure by Clinical Investigators

MANUAL OF POLICIES AND PROCEDURES (MAPPs)

In turn the CDER's publishes a Manual of Policies and Procedures (MaPPs). MaPPS are approved instructions for internal practices and procedures followed by CDER staff to help standardize the new drug review process and other activities. MaPPs define external activities as well. All MaPPs are available for the public to review to get a better understanding of office policies, definitions, staff responsibilities and procedures. MaPPs of particular interest to IND sponsors include:

- 5240.4 Submission of an IND Application to the Office of Generic Drugs (OGD). OGD policy and procedures regarding submissions on INDs for bioequivalence studies. These INDs are called Bio-INDs to distinguish them from clinical INDs submitted to CDER's new drug reviewing divisions.
- 6030.1 IND Process and Review Procedures (Including Clinical Holds). Includes general IND review principles, policies and procedures for issuing clinical holds of INDs, and processing and responding to sponsors' complete responses to clinical holds.

- 6030.2 INDs: Review of Informed Consent Documents
- 6030.4 INDs: Screening INDs. This MaPP describes procedures for the review of multiple active moieties or formulations under the single investigative new drug application (IND) called a screening IND.
- 6030.8 INDs: Exception from Informed Consent Requirements for Emergency Research.

IND FORMS AND INSTRUCTIONS

An Investigational New Drug Application (IND) is a request for Food and Drug Administration (FDA) authorization to administer an investigational drug to humans. Such authorization must be secured prior to interstate shipment and administration of any new drug that is not the subject of an approved new drug application. The important Forms for use in submitting INDs include:

- FDA 1571 Investigational New Drug Application (see Appendix I)
- FDA 1572 Statement of Investigator (See Appendix II)

These forms come with Instructions for completing FDA forms 1571 and 1572.

The instructions for filling the FDA 1571 is both exhaustive and self explanatory, it helps sponsors file the relevant data for consideration by the CDER for permission to conduct human studies. FDA 1572 helps the regulators to assess the investigators, their facilities and the IRB, with a view to ascertain the safety of the trial subjects.

TARGETED PRODUCT INFORMATION (TPI) PROJECT

After a 12-month collaborative effort between FDA and the Pharmaceutical Research Manufacturers Association (PhRMA), FDA's Office of Drug Evaluation IV (ODE IV) started a pilot test of a tool that may improve the drug development process. This tool is the Targeted Product Information (TPI) Document. The sponsor writes the TPI to guide the design, conduct, and analysis of clinical trials so that at the end of the development program, the sponsor will have gathered the necessary data to support the sponsor's desired outcome – the approval and appropriate labeling, or package insert, of the drug under development.

GENERAL PRINCIPLES OF THE IND SUBMISSION

FDA's primary objectives in reviewing an IND are, in all phases of the investigation, to assure the safety and rights of subjects, and, in Phase 2 and 3, to help assure that the quality of the scientific evaluation of drugs is adequate to permit an evaluation of the drug's effectiveness and safety. Therefore, although FDA's review of Phase 1 submissions will focus on assessing the safety of Phase 1 investigations, FDA's review of Phases 2 and 3 submissions will also include an assessment of the scientific quality of the clinical investigations and the likelihood that the investigations will yield data capable of meeting statutory standards for marketing approval.

The amount of information on a particular drug that must be submitted in an IND to assure the accomplishment of the objectives described above depends upon such factors as the novelty of the drug, the extent to which it has been studied previously, the known or suspected risks, and the developmental phase of the drug.

The central focus of the initial IND submission should be on the general investigational plan and the protocols for specific human studies. Subsequent amendments to the IND that contain new or revised protocols should build logically on previous submissions and should be supported by additional information, including the results of animal toxicology studies or other human studies as appropriate. Annual reports to the IND should serve as the focus for reporting the status of studies being conducted under the IND and should update the general investigational plan for the coming year.

The IND format set forth in FDA 1571 should be followed routinely by sponsors in the interest of fostering an efficient review of applications. Sponsors are expected to exercise considerable discretion, however, regarding the content of information submitted in each section, depending upon the kind of drug being studied and the nature of the available information.

A sponsor-investigator who uses, as a research tool, an investigational new drug that is already subject to a manufacturer's IND or marketing application should follow the same general format, but ordinarily may, if authorized by the manufacturer, refer to the manufacturer's IND or marketing application in providing the technical information supporting the proposed clinical investigation.

A sponsor-investigator who uses an investigational drug not subject to a manufacturer's IND or marketing application is ordinarily required to submit all technical information supporting the IND, unless such information may be referenced from the scientific literature.

IND CONTENT AND FORMAT

A sponsor who intends to conduct a clinical investigation subject to this part should submit an "Investigational New Drug Application" (IND) including, in the following order:

A. Cover Sheet (Form FDA–1571).

A cover sheet for the application containing the following:

1. The name, address, and telephone number of the sponsor, the date of the application, and the name of the investigational new drug.
2. Identification of the phase or phases of the clinical investigation to be conducted.
3. A commitment not to begin clinical investigations until an IND covering the investigations is in effect.
4. A commitment that an Institutional Review Board (IRB) that complies with the requirements set forth in part 56 will be responsible for the initial and continuing

review and approval of each of the studies in the proposed clinical investigation and that the investigator will report to the IRB proposed changes in the research activity in accordance with the requirements of part 56.

5. A commitment to conduct the investigation in accordance with all other applicable regulatory requirements.
6. The name and title of the person responsible for monitoring the conduct and progress of the clinical investigations.
7. The name(s) and title(s) of the person(s) responsible under for review and evaluation of information relevant to the safety of the drug.
8. If a sponsor has transferred any obligations for the conduct of any clinical study to a contract research organization, a statement containing the name and address of the contract research organization, identification of the clinical study, and a listing of the obligations transferred. If all obligations governing the conduct of the study have been transferred, a general statement of this transfer—in lieu of a listing of the specific obligations transferred—may be submitted.
9. The signature of the sponsor or the sponsor's authorized representative. If the person signing the application does not reside or have a place of business within the United States, the IND is required to contain the name and address of, and be countersigned by, an attorney, agent, or other authorized official who resides or maintains a place of business within the United States.

B. Table of Contents

C. Introductory Statement and General Investigational Plan

1. A brief introductory statement giving the name of the drug and all active ingredients, the drug's pharmacological class, the structural formula of the drug (if known), the formulation of the dosage form(s) to be used, the route of administration, and the broad objectives and planned duration of the proposed clinical investigation(s).
2. A brief summary of previous human experience with the drug, with reference to other IND's if pertinent, and to investigational or marketing experience in other countries that may be relevant to the safety of the proposed clinical investigation(s).
3. If the drug has been withdrawn from investigation or marketing in any country for any reason related to safety or effectiveness, identification of the country(ies) where the drug was withdrawn and the reasons for the withdrawal.
4. A brief description of the overall plan for investigating the drug product for the following year. The plan should include the following:
   a. The rationale for the drug or the research study;
   b. The phase and the type of study to be conducted with details about the comparator drugs.
   c. Brief method of eliminating bias and randomization of patients
   d. Number of centers and expected number of patients to be enrolled at each center.

e. Methods for evaluating efficacy and safety of the investigation product.
f. Methods of data analysis.

D. Investigator's Brochure

Investigational New Drugs are new and information on them is not in the public domain. Investigators are therefore not likely to have detailed information about them. In order to ensure the safety of their patients they need to be provided with as much information as necessary to ensure the safety of their patients.

E. Study Protocol

The study protocol is an exhaustive document that details each aspect of the clinical trial. The contents of the protocol for submission have been described elsewhere, and templates are also available for reference. One such template from the University of Minnesota is currently on the internet and can be accessed for study (http://ahc.umn.edu/img/assets/11663/ 2006_02_10_GCP_protocol_Template_Final.doc).

F. Investigator, Facilities and IRB Data

The FDA requires details on the investigator, the facilities and the IRB. This data is filled in FDA 1572 (see Appendix II). Additionally a series of commitments by the investigator are also required in the aforesaid form.

G. Chemistry, Manufacturing and Control Data

The IND must be accompanied by detailed information on the chemistry of the investigational drug, the specifications and the method of analysis of the same. The method of preparation and testing of the formulation to be investigated is also required. The FDA also requires a statement on the possible impact of the manufacturing process on the environment.

H. Pharmacology and Toxicology Data

The pharmacology and toxicology data forms by far the most important part of the IND. The regulators review the detailed pharmacological data to assess whether the compound, proposed to be investigated, indeed possesses the pharmacological potential. They look both for the novelty of the action as well as that of the mechanism of action. Review of the toxicological data helps them assess the safety of the drug, and is the most important part to be studied before the grant of "First in Human Study" permission.

Before the human studies can begin, an IND must be submitted to the Agency containing, among other things, information on any risks anticipated based on the results of pharmacologic and toxicological data collected during studies of the drug in animals. These basic safety tests are most often performed in rats and dogs. The studies are designed to permit the selection of a safe starting dose for humans, to gain an understanding of which organs may be the targets of toxicity, to estimate the margin of safety between a clinical and a toxic dose, and to predict pharmacokinetic and pharmacodynamic parameters. These early tests are usually resource intensive, requiring significant investment in product synthesis, animal use, laboratory analyses, and time.

Many resources are invested in, and thus wasted on, candidate products that subsequently are found to have unacceptable profiles when evaluated in humans — less than 10 percent of INDs for new molecular entities (NME) progress beyond the investigational stage to submission of a marketing application (NDA). In addition, animal testing does not always predict performance in humans, and potentially effective candidates may not be developed because of resource constraints.

Existing regulations allow a great deal of flexibility in terms of the amount of data that need to be submitted with any IND application, depending on the goals of the proposed investigation, the specific human testing proposed, and the expected risks. The FDA believes that sponsors have not taken full advantage of that flexibility. As a result, limited, early phase 1 studies, such as those described in this guidance, are often supported by a more extensive preclinical database than is required by the regulations. It may therefore be a good practice to consult the FDA prior to making a detailed study of the investigational drug.

The FDA also puts out regular guidance documents for the industry and reviewers. Many of the documents are drug class specific and give details of the studies that the FDA considers adequate to support an IND. A generic guidance document is also available that deals with the subject in general, entitled "Guidance for Industry, Investigators Reviewers – Exploratory IND Studies (http://www.fda.gov/CDER/guidance/7086fnl.htm)

I. Previous Human Experience

In a large number of INDs, the drug has been exposed to humans, either in another country or for another indication. Very often this data is of extreme importance in seeing an IND through. However in a large number of cases where the application is for a phase I study no such data would be available.

Recent changes in FDA rules allow early Phase I studies where microdose studies are conducted. Potentially useful study designs include both single- and multiple-dose studies. In single-dose studies, a sub-pharmacologic or pharmacologic dose is administered to a limited number of subjects. For example, microdose studies usually involve the single administration of a small dose with the goal of collecting pharmacokinetic information or performing imaging studies, or both.

REVIEW OF IND

The review of an IND is a multidisciplinary one and involves a number of experts. The general flow chart of the review process is shown in appendix III. At the CDER the Medical, Chemical, Pharmacological/Toxicological and Statistical data are reviewed prior to a safety review. It is only after this a Clinical Hold decision may be taken. In such cases the sponsor is asked to provide additional data for review. Only after satisfaction of the concerned experts permission for Phase I trial is granted.

CONCLUSIONS

The process of filing an IND is a complicated process and the data required differs for different drugs. The FDA has a large number of guidelines that have been issued for the use of the sponsors. As stated earlier, in the light of economy and saving time, it may be useful to go in for a pre IND consultation, to understand exactly what the agency expects from the sponsor. The general guidance of the agency on the Investigational New Drug Process is an important document that can guide the preparation of the IND. Reference to this document (http://www.fda.gov/cder/regulatory/applications/ind_page_1.htm) cannot be overemphasized.

SUGGESTED READING

1. Guidance for Industry, Investigators Reviewers – Exploratory IND Studies (http://www.fda.gov/CDER/guidance/7086fnl.htm)
2. http://ahc.umn.edu/img/assets/11663/2006_02_10_GCP_protocol_Template_Final.doc
3. http://www.fda.gov/cder/regulatory/applications/ind_page_1.htm
4. ICH Harmonized Tripartite Guideline for Good Clinical Practice.

Appendix-I

DEPARTMENT OF HEALTH AND HUMAN SERVICES FOOD AND DRUG ADMINISTRATION **STATEMENT OF INVESTIGATOR** *(TITLE 21, CODE OF FEDERAL REGULATIONS (CFR) PART 312)* (See instructions on reverse side.)	Form Approved: OMB No. 0910-0014. Expiration Date: May 31, 2009. *See OMB Statement on Reverse.* **NOTE:** No investigator may participate in an investigation until he/she provides the sponsor with a completed, signed Statement of Investigator, Form FDA 1572 (21 CFR 312.53(c)).

1. NAME AND ADDRESS OF INVESTIGATOR

2. EDUCATION, TRAINING, AND EXPERIENCE THAT QUALIFIES THE INVESTIGATOR AS AN EXPERT IN THE CLINICAL INVESTIGATION OF THE DRUG FOR THE USE UNDER INVESTIGATION. ONE OF THE FOLLOWING IS ATTACHED.

☑ CURRICULUM VITAE ☐ OTHER STATEMENT OF QUALIFICATIONS

3. NAME AND ADDRESS OF ANY MEDICAL SCHOOL, HOSPITAL OR OTHER RESEARCH FACILITY WHERE THE CLINICAL INVESTIGATION(S) WILL BE CONDUCTED.

4. NAME AND ADDRESS OF ANY CLINICAL LABORATORY FACILITIES TO BE USED IN THE STUDY.

5. NAME AND ADDRESS OF THE INSTITUTIONAL REVIEW BOARD (IRB) THAT IS RESPONSIBLE FOR REVIEW AND APPROVAL OF THE STUDY(IES).

6. NAMES OF THE SUBINVESTIGATORS *(e.g., research fellows, residents, associates)* WHO WILL BE ASSISTING THE INVESTIGATOR IN THE CONDUCT OF THE INVESTIGATION(S).

7. NAME AND CODE NUMBER, IF ANY, OF THE PROTOCOL(S) IN THE IND FOR THE STUDY(IES) TO BE CONDUCTED BY THE INVESTIGATOR.

FORM FDA 1572 (5/06) PREVIOUS EDITION IS OBSOLETE. **PAGE 1 OF 2**

PSC Graphics (301) 443-1090 EF

8. ATTACH THE FOLLOWING CLINICAL PROTOCOL INFORMATION:

☐ FOR PHASE 1 INVESTIGATIONS, A GENERAL OUTLINE OF THE PLANNED INVESTIGATION INCLUDING THE ESTIMATED DURATION OF THE STUDY AND THE MAXIMUM NUMBER OF SUBJECTS THAT WILL BE INVOLVED.

☐ FOR PHASE 2 OR 3 INVESTIGATIONS, AN OUTLINE OF THE STUDY PROTOCOL INCLUDING AN APPROXIMATION OF THE NUMBER OF SUBJECTS TO BE TREATED WITH THE DRUG AND THE NUMBER TO BE EMPLOYED AS CONTROLS, IF ANY; THE CLINICAL USES TO BE INVESTIGATED; CHARACTERISTICS OF SUBJECTS BY AGE, SEX, AND CONDITION; THE KIND OF CLINICAL OBSERVATIONS AND LABORATORY TESTS TO BE CONDUCTED; THE ESTIMATED DURATION OF THE STUDY; AND COPIES OR A DESCRIPTION OF CASE REPORT FORMS TO BE USED.

9. COMMITMENTS:

I agree to conduct the study(ies) in accordance with the relevant, current protocol(s) and will only make changes in a protocol after notifying the sponsor, except when necessary to protect the safety, rights, or welfare of subjects.

I agree to personally conduct or supervise the described investigation(s).

I agree to inform any patients, or any persons used as controls, that the drugs are being used for investigational purposes and I will ensure that the requirements relating to obtaining informed consent in 21 CFR Part 50 and institutional review board (IRB) review and approval in 21 CFR Part 56 are met.

I agree to report to the sponsor adverse experiences that occur in the course of the investigation(s) in accordance with 21 CFR 312.64.

I have read and understand the information in the investigator's brochure, including the potential risks and side effects of the drug.

I agree to ensure that all associates, colleagues, and employees assisting in the conduct of the study(ies) are informed about their obligations in meeting the above commitments.

I agree to maintain adequate and accurate records in accordance with 21 CFR 312.62 and to make those records available for inspection in accordance with 21 CFR 312.68.

I will ensure that an IRB that complies with the requirements of 21 CFR Part 56 will be responsible for the initial and continuing review and approval of the clinical investigation. I also agree to promptly report to the IRB all changes in the research activity and all unanticipated problems involving risks to human subjects or others. Additionally, I will not make any changes in the research without IRB approval, except where necessary to eliminate apparent immediate hazards to human subjects.

I agree to comply with all other requirements regarding the obligations of clinical investigators and all other pertinent requirements in 21 CFR Part 312.

INSTRUCTIONS FOR COMPLETING FORM FDA 1572
STATEMENT OF INVESTIGATOR:

1. Complete all sections. Attach a separate page if additional space is needed.
2. Attach curriculum vitae or other statement of qualifications as described in Section 2.
3. Attach protocol outline as described in Section 8.
4. Sign and date below.
5. FORWARD THE COMPLETED FORM AND ATTACHMENTS TO THE SPONSOR. The sponsor will incorporate this information along with other technical data into an Investigational New Drug Application (IND).

10. SIGNATURE OF INVESTIGATOR	11. DATE

(**WARNING:** A willfully false statement is a criminal offense. U.S.C. Title 18, Sec. 1001.)

Public reporting burden for this collection of information is estimated to average 100 hours per response, including the time for reviewing instructions, searching existing data sources, gathering and maintaining the data needed, and completing reviewing the collection of information. Send comments regarding this burden estimate or any other aspect of this collection of information, including suggestions for reducing this burden to:

Department of Health and Human Services
Food and Drug Administration
Center for Drug Evaluation and Research (HFD-143)
Central Document Room
5901-B Ammendale Road
Beltsville, MD 207052-1266

Department of Health and Human Services
Food and Drug Administration
Center for Biologics Evaluation and Research (HFM-99)
1401 Rockville Pike
Rockville, MD 20852-1448

"An agency may not conduct or sponsor, and a person is not required to respond to, a collection of information unless it displays a currently valid OMB control number."

Please DO NOT RETURN this application to this address.

FORM FDA 1572 (5/06) **PAGE 2 OF 2**

Appendix-II

DEPARTMENT OF HEALTH AND HUMAN SERVICES FOOD AND DRUG ADMINISTRATION **STATEMENT OF INVESTIGATOR** *(TITLE 21, CODE OF FEDERAL REGULATIONS (CFR) PART 312)* (See instructions on reverse side.)	Form Approved: OMB No. 0910-0014. Expiration Date: May 31, 2009. *See OMB Statement on Reverse.* **NOTE:** No investigator may participate in an investigation until he/she provides the sponsor with a completed, signed Statement of Investigator, Form FDA 1572 (21 CFR 312.53(c)).

1. NAME AND ADDRESS OF INVESTIGATOR

2. EDUCATION, TRAINING, AND EXPERIENCE THAT QUALIFIES THE INVESTIGATOR AS AN EXPERT IN THE CLINICAL INVESTIGATION OF THE DRUG FOR THE USE UNDER INVESTIGATION. ONE OF THE FOLLOWING IS ATTACHED.

☐ CURRICULUM VITAE ☐ OTHER STATEMENT OF QUALIFICATIONS

3. NAME AND ADDRESS OF ANY MEDICAL SCHOOL, HOSPITAL OR OTHER RESEARCH FACILITY WHERE THE CLINICAL INVESTIGATION(S) WILL BE CONDUCTED.

4. NAME AND ADDRESS OF ANY CLINICAL LABORATORY FACILITIES TO BE USED IN THE STUDY.

5. NAME AND ADDRESS OF THE INSTITUTIONAL REVIEW BOARD (IRB) THAT IS RESPONSIBLE FOR REVIEW AND APPROVAL OF THE STUDY(IES).

6. NAMES OF THE SUBINVESTIGATORS *(e.g., research fellows, residents, associates)* WHO WILL BE ASSISTING THE INVESTIGATOR IN THE CONDUCT OF THE INVESTIGATION(S).

7. NAME AND CODE NUMBER, IF ANY, OF THE PROTOCOL(S) IN THE IND FOR THE STUDY(IES) TO BE CONDUCTED BY THE INVESTIGATOR.

FORM FDA 1572 (5/06) PREVIOUS EDITION IS OBSOLETE. **PAGE 1 OF 2**

PSC Graphics (301) 443-1090 EF

8. ATTACH THE FOLLOWING CLINICAL PROTOCOL INFORMATION:

☐ FOR PHASE 1 INVESTIGATIONS, A GENERAL OUTLINE OF THE PLANNED INVESTIGATION INCLUDING THE ESTIMATED DURATION OF THE STUDY AND THE MAXIMUM NUMBER OF SUBJECTS THAT WILL BE INVOLVED.

☐ FOR PHASE 2 OR 3 INVESTIGATIONS, AN OUTLINE OF THE STUDY PROTOCOL INCLUDING AN APPROXIMATION OF THE NUMBER OF SUBJECTS TO BE TREATED WITH THE DRUG AND THE NUMBER TO BE EMPLOYED AS CONTROLS, IF ANY; THE CLINICAL USES TO BE INVESTIGATED; CHARACTERISTICS OF SUBJECTS BY AGE, SEX, AND CONDITION; THE KIND OF CLINICAL OBSERVATIONS AND LABORATORY TESTS TO BE CONDUCTED; THE ESTIMATED DURATION OF THE STUDY; AND COPIES OR A DESCRIPTION OF CASE REPORT FORMS TO BE USED.

9. COMMITMENTS:

I agree to conduct the study(ies) in accordance with the relevant, current protocol(s) and will only make changes in a protocol after notifying the sponsor, except when necessary to protect the safety, rights, or welfare of subjects.

I agree to personally conduct or supervise the described investigation(s).

I agree to inform any patients, or any persons used as controls, that the drugs are being used for investigational purposes and I will ensure that the requirements relating to obtaining informed consent in 21 CFR Part 50 and institutional review board (IRB) review and approval in 21 CFR Part 56 are met.

I agree to report to the sponsor adverse experiences that occur in the course of the investigation(s) in accordance with 21 CFR 312.64.

I have read and understand the information in the investigator's brochure, including the potential risks and side effects of the drug.

I agree to ensure that all associates, colleagues, and employees assisting in the conduct of the study(ies) are informed about their obligations in meeting the above commitments.

I agree to maintain adequate and accurate records in accordance with 21 CFR 312.62 and to make those records available for inspection in accordance with 21 CFR 312.68.

I will ensure that an IRB that complies with the requirements of 21 CFR Part 56 will be responsible for the initial and continuing review and approval of the clinical investigation. I also agree to promptly report to the IRB all changes in the research activity and all unanticipated problems involving risks to human subjects or others. Additionally, I will not make any changes in the research without IRB approval, except where necessary to eliminate apparent immediate hazards to human subjects.

I agree to comply with all other requirements regarding the obligations of clinical investigators and all other pertinent requirements in 21 CFR Part 312.

INSTRUCTIONS FOR COMPLETING FORM FDA 1572
STATEMENT OF INVESTIGATOR:

1. Complete all sections. Attach a separate page if additional space is needed.
2. Attach curriculum vitae or other statement of qualifications as described in Section 2.
3. Attach protocol outline as described in Section 8.
4. Sign and date below.
5. FORWARD THE COMPLETED FORM AND ATTACHMENTS TO THE SPONSOR. The sponsor will incorporate this information along with other technical data into an Investigational New Drug Application (IND).

10. SIGNATURE OF INVESTIGATOR	11. DATE

(**WARNING:** A willfully false statement is a criminal offense. U.S.C. Title 18, Sec. 1001.)

Public reporting burden for this collection of information is estimated to average 100 hours per response, including the time for reviewing instructions, searching existing data sources, gathering and maintaining the data needed, and completing reviewing the collection of information. Send comments regarding this burden estimate or any other aspect of this collection of information, including suggestions for reducing this burden to:

Department of Health and Human Services
Food and Drug Administration
Center for Drug Evaluation and Research (HFD-143)
Central Document Room
5901-B Ammendale Road
Beltsville, MD 207052-1266

Department of Health and Human Services
Food and Drug Administration
Center for Biologics Evaluation and Research (HFM-99)
1401 Rockville Pike
Rockville, MD 20852-1448

"An agency may not conduct or sponsor, and a person is not required to respond to, a collection of information unless it displays a currently valid OMB control number."

Please DO NOT RETURN this application to this address.

FORM FDA 1572 (5/06) **PAGE 2 OF 2**

Appendix-III

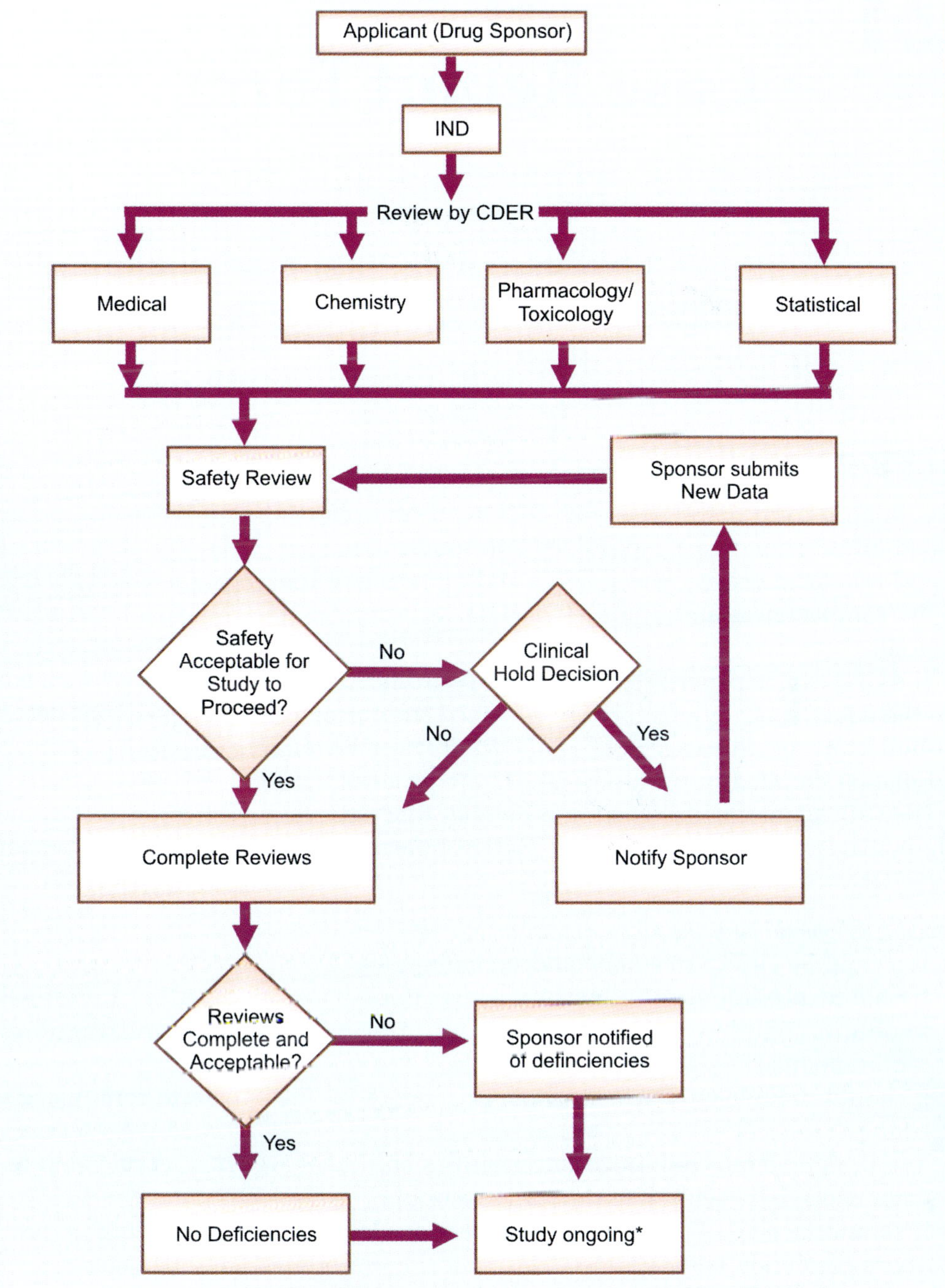

*While sponsor answers any deficiencies

21 Case Report Form

Anoop K Agarwal, Pratibha Nadig, Praveena Koteshwar, Raveena Nath

INTRODUCTION

Case Report Form (CRF) is a trial document for collecting and recording patient-related information in a standardized and uniform manner. This is important for the clinical trial team because the analysis and reporting of trial outcome is largely based on the completeness and accuracy of data recorded from each patient recruited in the trial.

The CRF can be paper-based or in the electronic format allowing direct data entry into the database. CRF must be distinguished from protocol which provides detailed methodology of all aspects of trials whereas, CRF enables to collect subject's information enrolled in the study as per the protocol.

The CRF should be designed in a manner that aids the investigator, monitor and data manager to record and review patient information, which is vital for outcome of a trial.

A good CRF should have the following characteristics:

i. It should be clear, systematic and unambiguous.

ii. It should provide comprehensive instructions to be followed by investigator to obtain complete information as per approved protocol and regulatory requirements.

iii. It should provide guidance on eligibility criteria for the patient to continue in the trial.

iv. The design should minimize uncertainties and facilitate entry verification (e.g., cross-check between related data) by monitor.

v. It should facilitate in designing and creating clean database requiring minimum query resolution between the investigator, monitor and data manager.

Ideally, the CRF should be critically reviewed by designer, quality assurance department, monitor, investigator, data manager and statistician meeting the objectives of a trial.

REGULATORY GUIDELINES FOR CRF

All CRF must comply with ICH-GCP guidelines and fulfill regulatory requirements, which get reviewed along with clinical study report by regulatory authorities.

It has often been observed that the protocols are approved without CRF resulting in discrepancies as both are addressed independently during the study. The Section 8.2.2 of ICH-GCP clearly describes that CRF should be a part of protocol when finalized and submitted for approval. The practice also helps in streamlining the processes and procedures described in the protocol. The protocol and CRF should compliment each other once approved and adopted.

The steps and guidelines for CRF designing are generally described in Standard Operating Procedures (SOPs) and other in-house documents. However, its use and completion should be in according to ICH-GCP requirements, since the quality and integrity of data collected decides the fate of the trial. Moreover, in some cases CRF may be regarded as a source data. The success is ensured when instructions to investigators' inspire them to instructions comply with regulatory requirements.

CRF DESIGN AND DEVELOPMENT

A good CRF design invites significant contribution and repeated reviewing by expert team member to meet the objectives. The team consists of:

i. CRF designer
ii. Medical advisor
iii. Clinical monitor
iv. Data entry leader
v. Data manager
vi. Statistician.

The CRF designer prepares a frame work based on protocol. The initial version shows the visits and various assessments on each visit, which are reviewed in the backdrop of the latest copy of protocol (ideally final approved version). Any change in protocol must be informed immediately for necessary amendments in the CRF.

The designer should in accordance with GCP standards and SOP requirements follow standard format to maintain uniformity. The protocol requirements have to be translated into simple and clear questions with appropriate space for recording patient responses using design pointers. At the same time, 'instructions' are generated to guide and remind the investigator regarding various assessments and actions required at each visit.

As a part of quality control process, the first CRF version thus prepared is checked against the protocol and for internal consistency by an independent reviewer. The first version is subsequently circulated to all team members for review and suggestion invited for appropriate amendments circulating same copy avoids duplication of suggested changes. Thereafter, all team members meet to discuss the implications of the suggested changes and guide the designer to incorporate the essential changes in the CRF.

The CRF designer will subsequently generate the second version which is again reviewed by the team for fine tuning. No meeting is required unless the protocol has changed demanding major amendments in CRF.

In the meantime, the designer will select and brief the printers regarding design characteristics, type and size of paper and card required, font size, number of CRFs required and deadlines for distribution.

The comments on second version are considered for final version which for quality assurance review and later sent to project manager for approval. Once approved, the printer should provide a finished proof copy of the CRF. The Project manager finally reviews the finished proof copy of the CRF (material, blinding, format, etc) and orders for printing multiple copies.

As per GCP guidelines, copies of each version, annotations, review meeting decisions, quality control/quality assurance checks and all approval documents must be retained and archived as they represent raw data for the trial.

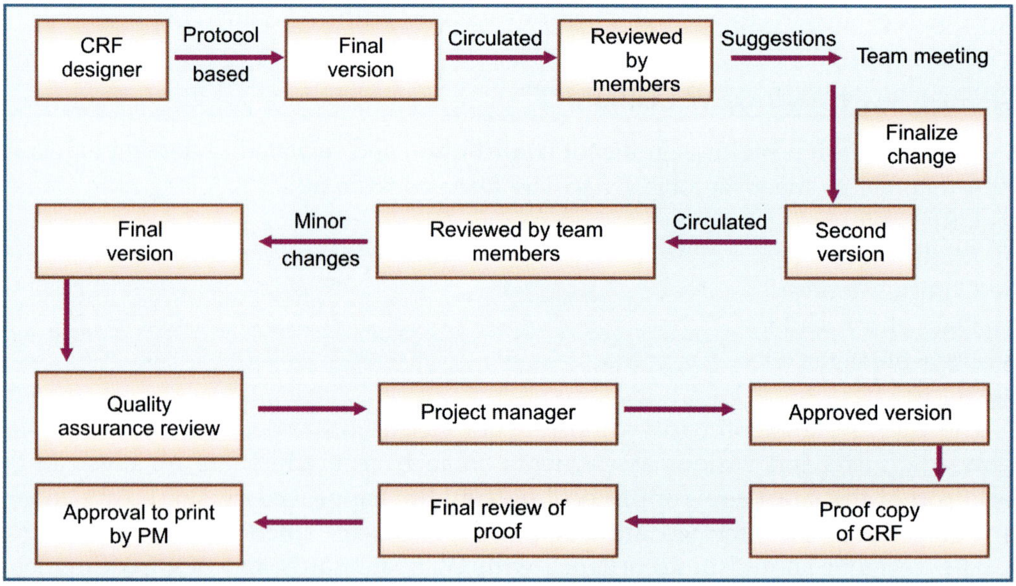

PURPOSE OF INFORMATION TO BE COLLECTED

The data collected through CRF should address two main issues:

1. Study hypothesis.
2. Drug safety.

The CRF should provide the accurate data to achieve the objectives proposed in the study protocol. The honest and complete recording of information in a GCP compliant pattern avoids discrepancy and speeds up drug approval process.

Recording additional information on the CRF beyond the protocol requirement, out of academic interest shall make the CRF lengthy and complicated. Moreover, the data need to be cleaned of unwanted information which delays data processing and analysis.

Thus, a good CRF should have following characteristics to be accepted and owned by all members involved in the trial:

1. Simple and quick to complete with no ambiguity.
2. Collects precise information as required by the protocol.
3. Presents clear information in a logical sequence maintaining uniformity.
4. Facilitates interpretation by data entry staff.
5. Provides clear instructions to review the subject's eligibility for continuing in the trial.
6. Display questions and assessment parameters in sequence to minimize queries.

CRF LAYOUT

Identification of CRF

CRF builds a link between the sponsor, investigator, patient and data manger and should, therefore, be attractive and good in appearance and quality. The language should be simple, clear and easy to read and understand.

The identification code of every CRF and of each page within CRF should be unique for that particular trial, study centre and the subject. The subjects are identified by a code system to maintain confidentiality. This code generally consists of subject's initial and trial identification number.

Each CRF page should be complete in following respects:

i. Name of sponsoring company.
ii. Patient identification number/bar code label.
iii. Trial identification code or protocol number.
iv. Centre code.
v. Visit number for each assessment.
vi. Study day reference including date.
vii. Page number (Page 'n of nn')
viii. Identification of CRF copies when printed on no-carbon required (NCR) paper.

These items help in two ways:

i. Detached CRF pages can be correctly located and allocated to the study.
ii. All CRFs can be easily verified for missing pages by the data manager.

Formatting CRF

The assessment parameters should be presented in a logical sequence, which ensures careful and accurate completion of CRF is important for quick data processing.

A complicated CRF is an invitation to error and misinterpretation at all steps particularly in the hands of a busy investigator. Thus, a good quality CRF ensures complete, credible and reliable data generation.

1. Ideally, multiple assessments done on each patient should appear in the CRF in the same format and sequence as performed, for all visits. This not only helps the investigator to complete all assessments but also assists in database building and quick data entry.
2. The various assessments should be separated by white space not to be utilized for writing notes/remarks by the investigator. However, a separate global comments page should be provided with the CRF for his remarks.
3. An easily readable font style should be selected which encourages detailed review of the CRF and its filling. (e.g. Helvetica or Arial)
4. All text should preferably be 12 point size, which is neither too small not too large. Moreover the text should be well-spaced with proper page breakup for easy reading.
5. The margins should be identical in all CRF pages.
6. If text needs to be turned 90 degrees e.g., column holders, the text should be turned as complete words and not printed as individual letter, stacked on top of each other.

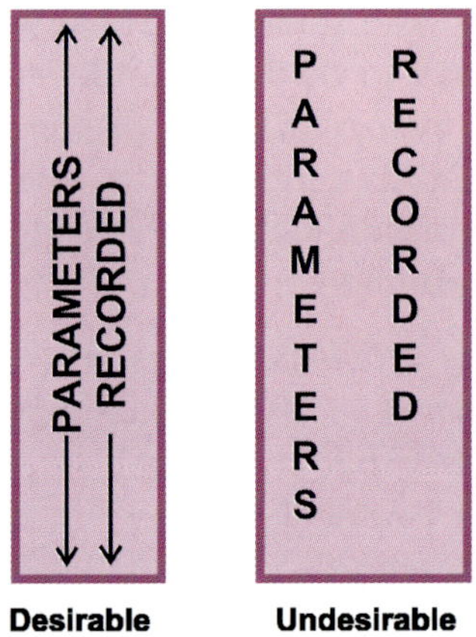

7. Avoid using hyphenation in the CRF text. It may convey a different meaning if used liberally e.g., therapist may read as the-rapist.

Uniformity

The layout for all CRFs used in different trials of a particular drug should be uniform. It helps to collect information in a similar fashion when used in different trials.

It helps in three ways:
1. The designer maintains a standard CRF format saving time and energy.
2. The investigator gets used to a particular design and directions, committing minimum errors.
3. The data manager can economize on database design favoring faster data entry and query management.

AVOIDING TRANSCRIPTION PROBLEMS

All information in the CRF has to be ultimately entered into the database. Thus, a good CRF design and nicely framed questions are very helpful in avoiding misunderstandings, incorrect entries, and incomplete information which minimize data cleaning and queries before locking the database. As a consequence, the report generation is also accelerated.

Many transcription problems can be overcome simply by numbering the lines where similar information is appearing repeatedly e.g., on adverse events or concomitant medication pages. Moreover, the database should also be sequentially numbered to match the CRF pages encouraging easy transcription of CRF data.

ENTERING DATA INTO DATABASE

1. The CRF should be formatted such that repeated observations taken on same day (e.g., temperature, blood pressure, pulse etc) can be recorded in separate lines rather than single line running horizontally. For example,

Format A

Date	Time 1	Temperature	Time 2	Temperature	Time 3	Temperature
17.7.06	7 AM	99.0° C	1 PM	99.1° C	8 PM	98.7° C

Format B

Date	Time	Temperature
17.7.06	7 AM	99.0° C
	1 PM	99.1° C
	8 PM	98.7° C

Desirable format

Format B is simple and easier to complete. Moreover, it helps the entry personal to read and transcribe the same on to the database.

2. The units of all measurements should be specified in the CRF to maintain uniformity, and appropriate boxes should be provided to avoid confusion.

For example, weight of the patient.

0	8	4	kg

Or

Weight (gm)

0	8	4	0	0	0

3. The CRF entries should be neatly written preferably in block letters to avoid errors. Appropriate space should be provided in each column to avoid overriding, abbreviations or cryptic comments overflowing the allotted space.

The data management personnel may have tough time to figure out the medical terms, medication, microbial species, laboratory tests, etc., if the text is illegible. This becomes more pronounced in multinational studies since different nations have different fonts.

4. Attempts should be made to minimize graphical data e.g., visual Analogue Scale. The linear scale may be intercepted in different ways causing inconsistency. If graphics are unavoidable, the CRF designer should first decide on data coding for the database in consultation with the data manager and then design the graphic to reflect that code.

TYPES OF CLINICAL TRIAL DATA

Generally, four types of data are collected in clinical trials.

1. Baseline data	:	Demographics Inclusion and exclusion criteria Clinical signs and symptoms Physical examination Laboratory investigations Previous medications.
2. Efficacy data	:	Assessments specific to the objectives of the study.
3. Safety data	:	Ongoing record of vital signs Physical examination Laboratory values Adverse events.
4. Compliance data	:	Accounting of test medication Concurrent medication Withdrawal/end-of-study records.

Many of the above observations such as baseline data, concurrent, medication, ADR etc., are common to all trials and thus can become a standard CRF module that would require minimum modification for different trials and different products.

INSTRUCTIONS FOR CRF COMPLETION

The investigator should be provided clear instructions for CRF completion with respect to subject eligibility, assessments on every visit, subject's compliance, concomitant medication, adverse event recording reporting etc. The instructions can be presented in the form of instruction manual or instruction page that accompanies CRF. This includes the general instructions for collecting the data, completion of CRF and dealing with correction of entries made in error. Date and time format should also be explained at this point. Moreover, the page should also guide to account for missing or unknown data.

Graphics are helpful in conveying instructions when English is not the first language of the investigator, especially in global trials. The designer must consider this fact while designing CRF for a multinational study. It may be good to include a list of assessments (or flow chart) to be carried out at the beginning of each visit, which will remind the investigator to ask the relevant questions and take appropriate actions. Moreover, reminders should appear at appropriate places in the CRF e.g., enquiring adverse events, ensuring laboratory reports, ECG etc., for recording and completing the CRF. Method to record dosages and frequency should be indicated. Similarly, list of prohibited medicines can be put against the concomitant page. Instructions for deviations from CRF items should also be highlighted. There may be a separate instruction for certain assessments where numeric codes are being used to indicate route of administration for concomitant medication or approach following an adverse event.

Finally, prompts placed along-side of inter-related entries will reduce inconsistently between inter-related information filled on different pages of the CRF, which will minimize data management queries e.g., for adverse event treated by medication, a corresponding entry should appear on the concomitant medication page.

FRAMING THE QUESTIONS FOR CRF

As we have seen in the earlier sections, a good CRF should be clean, precise and easy for the study co-ordinator or the investigator to enter the data with no ambiguity. Therefore, it is essential that the questions be framed in a manner that elicits a suitable answer. The question and response formats in a CRF are grouped as follows:

a. Alphanumeric and free text.
b. Multiple choice including binary options.
c. Matrix arrays.
d. Analogue scales.

A CRF designer uses a combination of these sets.

Alphanumeric and Free Text

This method is used to indicate certain data such as the patient identification adverse event and treatment responses. The responses utilize words and/or numbers. To enter these data, either a free space or constrained space with character separators is provided. Free space gives psychological freedom to the investigator/CRC but, increases the chances of wrong entries, cancellations and re-entries. Character separators ensure that the first entry is the right entry. However, wrong entries may be overwritten by the CRC resulting in an undecipherable data. Therefore, the most preferred approach is to use a free space with restricted length, e.g. an inch space can be used for eight characters of a standard handwriting.

For example: Patients name : __________

The data for information such as Date of Birth, however, needs to use character separators but indicating the day, month and year as shown below:

Y	Y	Y	Y		M	M		D	D

The responses that indicate measurements can be made more specific by mentioning the units after the spaces. This will ensure uniformity in the CRF at all centers.
For example:

Blood Pressure (1) sitting	[ ][ ][ ] [ ][ ][ ] mmHg Systolic Diastolic
Heart rate (1) sitting:	[ ][ ][ ] Beats/minute

Multiple Choice Questions

In certain instances like collection of demographic data, it is easier for a CRC/ investigator to tick an answer from the options given rather than writing a self-generated answer. Multiple choice questions are, therefore, the most preferred format of questionnaire that saves time and also reduces the ambiguity. The number of options could range from two to six depending on the type of data to be collected. The most common multiple choice question is a binary type where the CRC has to choose between the two options e.g., YES and NO. Using this format in as many number of places as possible is encouraged not only in the interest of the CRC but also for the data manager who can create a specific database with less difficulty.

Designing these questions must be done skillfully. Although the answers appear simple, the questions must be specific and the expected answer should not have any other options than the mentioned ones. Furthermore, the lay out of questions must also be considered. For instance, while framing questions on eligibility criteria, it is always advisable that the answer is YES as the desired option for all inclusion criteria and NO for all the exclusion criteria for the patient to be included in the study as shown in the following example:

Inclusion criteria

Age: 18-30 yrs [√] YES [ ] NO
Type II diabetes [√] [ ] YES
NO
Non-smoker [√] YES [ ] NO
Not an insulin [√] YES [ ] NO

Exclusion criteria

Received additional medication within 30 days	☐ YES	☑ NO
Hypertensive	☐ YES	☑ NO
Suffering from any concurrent illness	☐ YES	☐ NO

The advantage is that a quick glance on the responses gives comprehensive information. If there is more than one choice, clear instructions must be given whether the investigator can choose more than one answer. This is especially true with reference to the data on adverse events where more than one expected adverse events may be enlisted.

For example: Adverse events after the first dose

☑ Nausea	☑ Vomiting
☐ Diarrhea	☐ Belching

Matrix Arrays

These are utilized to obtain specific information on different categories collectively. The questions are usually arranged in rows and each question has an option from the choices arranged in columns. The options for each question can be ticked.

This format provides comprehensive information during analysis.

Concurrent illness	*None*	*Confirmed but not under treatment*	*Confirmed and under treatment*
Tuberculosis			
Leprosy			
HIV			

Analogue Scales

In a clinical trial, it is necessary to asses the progress of the disease or the response to the treatment by comparing the base line observations with the ones observed in the follow-up visits. Analogue scales are often used for some of the assessments. These scales are valuable in transforming the subjective information into a quantifiable data. The visual analogue scale used for assessment of an analgesic response is one such example represented as a scale represented as a 10 cm graduated line graded from 0 to 10. It is instructed to the subject that zero indicates no improvement and 10 indicates maximum response to treatment (no pain). The CRC puts a slash mark or a cross on the horizontal line after interacting with the subject to indicate the severity of the desired response at every visit. This data can be subsequently coded for the computer input by converting the reading into a quantifiable data.

FORMATTING A QUESTIONNAIRE

Sections of CRF may involve a questionnaire to be filled by the patients valuable especially in cases of evaluations of quality of life. The questionnaires need to be designed keeping in mind that they are to be filled by patients speaking different languages of different backgrounds, age group, etc.

General guidelines

a. Use simple and non-technical language.
b. Use examples wherever necessary.
c. Minimize free text entry.
d. The duration of recording in daily card should preferably not exceed 2-4 weeks. Fresh cards are to be provided after two weeks.
e. Font size should be more than 10 to enable comfortable reading by the aged.

PRINTING REQUIREMENTS

The efforts of designing and formatting the CRF can be translated into use only if good printing is ensured. Printing plays an important role in adding values to the quality of CRF. It is desirable to coordinate between the project manager and the printer resolving queries.

The printer needs to be well-informed about various requirements of a CRF such as:

a. The dimensions of the paper to be used.
b. The weight and the colour of the paper.
c. The margin to be allocated so that binding does not go through the printed text.
d. Font sizes for header, footer and the text.
e. Color of ink to be used.
f. Logo formats.

If the material is supplied to the printer as an electronic file, the printer must have an access to the same program and templates that have been used in the design.

PACKAGING AND ORGANIZING THE CRF BOOK

Once the final version is ready for printing, it has to undergo a proofreading by at least two members of the team, after which it is approved for final printing. The next step is to decide the number of copies required per page. Ideally three copies should be printed per page considering one for the investigative site, second for the sponsor and third to be used as a worksheet for corrections. It is advisable to use a different color for each of these copies to be identified by the recipient. To ease the data entry by the investigator/CRC, the usage of No Carbon Required (NCR) paper is recommended.

The enormous data collected in the case report form necessitates that the forms be bound in copies the form of a booklet. This ensures the ease of usage and integrity of the data. The CRFs can be prepared by doting different types of binding such as:

- Stapled
- Stitched and glued
- Spiral bound
- Wire bound
- Three ring binder.

Three ring binders are most commonly used. This type of binding has an advantage that any form (page) can be detached for data entry and refiled after usage. Secondly, it has a provision for storing the source documents and notes until the data is transcribed into the database. The disadvantage is that the CRF becomes expensive and bulky. Moreover, the forms may be lost or misplaced once detached.

Once the binding is determined, the organization of forms needs to be considered. The forms can be organized based on their type or visits. The convenient method is arranging the papers according to visit so that the entire information required during a particular visit can be incorporated without referring to the protocol. To demarcate the visits, thick sheets can be inserted at appropriate place indicating the visit number, a formatted planner for scheduling the list of all the forms required for that particular visit and next visit.

ROLE OF CRA IN DESIGNING AND DEVELOPMENT OF CRF

The Clinical Research Associate (CRA) is a key person in the performance of a clinical trial. CRA's involvement in the development of CRF varies with nature of project. A sponsor may designate people or departments within his company or may outsource the job to companies that have specialized in CRF designing.

CRF design is the basic factor, which determines the quality of the data generation. A poorly designed CRF poses a major problem to the CRA while reviewing the form at the investigative site. A CRF that is ambiguous in terms of questions and format will have more number of errors committed by the co-coordinator. For example, it has been observed by the CRA's that more number of errors in the CRF occurs in the data entered in the lower one-third of the forms. This input was considered and the CRF was improvised including the critical data in the upper third of the forms.

MONITORING OF THE CRF

Monitoring is the responsibility of the CRA and the critical review of the CRF is a challenging job. The prime duty of the CRA is to review the case report form and source documents. The CRA should ensure that the data entered in the CRF is consistent and derived from the source document in accordance with the protocol. The discrepancies, if any, should be explained.

Source document is the one in which the observations are first recorded. The source data includes all the information of clinical findings, observations or other activities in original records in a clinical trial necessary for the reconstruction and evaluation of the trial.

Examples of source documents are:

a. Hospital records
b. Clinical and office charts
c. Lab reports (central and local)
d. Subjects evaluation checklist (case sheet)
e. Pharmacy dispensing records
f. X-ray
g. ECG tracings etc.

All discrepancies with respect to the source document and the CRF have to be corrected by the persons authorized to make entries and/or corrections in CRF (either the CRC or the investigator.).

A CRA must review the CRFs in a systematic manner, starting with the new subjects enrolled after his last monitoring visit. A CRF review can be successfully accomplished by finishing one subject at a time. The CRFs of all each new subject should be collected and reviewed for completeness and consistency with the source documents.

ROLE OF CRC IN CRF DOCUMENTATION

CRC is the one who deals with the CRF at the site. He may be involved in the filling, handling and archiving the CRFs. The CRC is the first person to look into the completeness and quality of the CRF with the help of following checklist:

CRC Checklist

1. The data entered in the forms should be accurate, complete, and legible.
2. Check that each section has been completed and no space is left unattended.
3. Check the header and the footer, information on each page for integrity.
4. Check whether the values are in normal range.
5. Check if the form is signed by the investigator.
6. During the visits.
   a. Check for the date of visit, and confirm that it falls within the allowed window period. Every visit date should be scheduled with reference to the first visit (and not from the last).
   b. Enters data in order of sequence specified.

c. Enters the concomitant medication and the adverse events in appropriate section during each visit.
d. Check the consistency of the data across the visit.

Last but not the least, is the identification of the subject during visits with their ID number, initials and other identification features mentioned.

Errors in CRF Entry

Inspite of the instructions and guidelines provided for CRF completion several errors have been identified during monitoring visits and at data entry level. Incomplete and missing information leads to poor quality of data which may affect the study outcome. All the errors identified need to be rectified before data entry and analysis. The common errors encountered in the filled CRF are as follows:

1. Inconsistencies between the source document and CRF
2. Missing data
3. Inconsistencies across the visits
4. Illegible data
5. Spelling errors
6. Blank 'mandatory comment fields'
7. Unacceptable terminology
8. Missing investigators signature.

Errors identified in the CRF have to be dealt with the help of an query form that is specific to the CRF of the particular study provided by the sponsor.

Procedure for Making Correction in the CRF

Query can be generated by the CRA or data entry operator. The identified errors must be discussed by the CRA with the investigator and CRC to obtain the explanation. The CRC must make the necessary corrections by striking a line through the incorrect entry, entering the correct data with date and initials. The reason for the change has to be explained. The original entry should not to be whiteout or erased from the CRF as one must be able to see the original incorrect value, i.e. no corrections should obscure the original entry.

For example, hemoglobin = 10g%

The investigator should also retain records of the changes and corrections made in the CRF.

ELECTRONIC CASE RECORD FORM (eCRF)

Among the various challenges in the drug developmental process, one of the key challenges faced by the sponsor, investigators and CROs is how to manage the large volume of clinical data generated in an efficient, secure and cost effective manner.

Electronic version of Case Report Form is getting importance due to the ease of application as compared to the paper based CRF. Due to the advancement of information technology and the need for better data management, the present focus has been shifted to electronic version CRF.

Electronic CRF initially started as scanned copy of filled paper CRF. This partially solved the problems associated with data analysis, but data was still recorded on paper. With the advent of electronic data transfer and electronic signature, the security of data was well assured and it made the remote data entry possible. This minimized the data entry errors and reduced the time required to lock the database at the end of the study. This has to be in compliance with international standards as described in 21 CFR Part 11.

The use of electronic device/software that enables the investigator to enter the patient data directly into eCRF electronically is called electronic data capture (EDC) process. Among the different types of data, laboratory results get entered directly into eCRF. The results generated from analytical instruments and from automated machines get transferred electronically into electronic database. Though vital parameters can be recorded digitally, usually they are first recorded in paper CRF and later gets transcribed to eCRF. Various methods of electronic data capture such as Interactive Voice Response System (IVRS), Interactive Web Response System (IWRS), etc. are employed to collect data and the same is electronically represented in eCRF.

Electronic data capture (EDC) has been an effective tool to speed up the process of data entry and enhancing the quality of data obtained during a trial. With the advent of Internet Based Clinical Trials (IBCT) and Clinical Data Interchange Standards Consortium (CDISC), many pharmaceutical companies have initiated enforcing *e*CRF based *e*Trials.

It is a fundamental GCP requirement for investigator to "maintain" a copy of eCRF as per 21 CFR 312 62.b section. These are the investigator's records, which must be prevented from being modified without their knowledge.

Types of eCRF

eCRF exists in two formats

1. Tagged Image File Format (TIFF)
2. Portable Document Format (PDF)

TIFF based eCRF is the most commonly used variety as it accurately depicts the image of scanned paper CRF. This is an electronic document which is programmed to accept only the valid data in the relevant fields, thus reducing queries generated during data entry.

PDF based eCRF is the latest format applied. It has ADOBE controlled specifications designed for sharing document information. It is a PDF document with in built edit checks but no facility to recognize data errors. It represents single viewing interface.

The issues concerning the PDF format are the big file size and problems associated with printing of PDF files.

Designing of eCRF

Designing of a CRF is an important process since it is essential to collect all the data specified in the protocol. The process of designing an eCRF involves various steps. Designer should draft the first version of CRF based on the protocol requirements and sponsor's specifications. Once the basic design of CRF is drafted, the programmer can begin to generate the data entry screens of eCRF. This will be reviewed by the original designer for accuracy and errors detected in the design will be rectified. During this review period, online edit checks too will be programmed into eCRF by providing sites with immediate feedback to correct the errors or missing data, thereby ensuring clean data which helps in locking the database. It will be further subjected to scrutiny for overall navigation layout (the visits and forms associated with each visit), form content and edit checks for both accuracy and completeness of eCRF, after which the final version will be approved and released.

While designing eCRF, the attributability of the data should be the utmost consideration, thereby fulfilling the key component of the ALCOA provisions (attributable, legible, contemporaneous, original, accurate) — highlighted in the Guidance on Computerized Systems Used in Clinical Trials.

Data Entry in eCRF

It follows three different patterns:

1. Copying from completed paper CRF into eCRF.
2. Direct entry into eCRF at the site via internet explorer to the central data base as a complete web based system.
3. Data entry into CRF loaded in a dedicated laptop at the site, a partial web based system.

Sites have the ability to begin entering data within a few weeks from the start of the design process. And if an eCRF needs to be modified, it is possible to deploy a new eCRF quickly without delaying the study. This is important for sponsor and CRO as they are ultimately responsible for driving the study and hitting timelines.

Differences between eCRF versus Paper CRF

Though there are intrinsic differences between electronic and paper CRF, visual impressions of both should remain the same.

1. Paper CRF can be viewed as a booklet, whereas, in eCRF only a single page is displayed on the screen.
2. In a paper-based CRF, cleaning and reviewing data is a difficult and time consuming process which has been simplified with eCRF.

3. High cost and delay associated with printing, binding, shipping, tracking of paper CRF can be avoided with eCRF. It also minimizes the generation of wastes arising from unused printed CRF records.
4. Unlike paper CRF, eCRF avoids double key data entry, spelling errors and issues regarding legibility while entering the data.
5. Recording of surplus information in paper CRF may lead to overcrowding which can be avoided in eCRF, just by clicking on the icon "add another."
6. The problems associated with archival of paper CRF *viz.*, space, storage conditions, retrieval of data, etc. is not encountered with eCRF.
7. The confidentiality of data is high in eCRF in comparison with paper CRF due to security provided through password protection.
8. The quality of data can be checked by remote review without any personal visit to the site and timelines of data entry can be controlled in eCRF which is not possible with paper CRF.

However, eCRF has its own limitations too.

1. Setting up the infrastructure for designing and implementing eCRF involves high cost and time.
2. Adopting eCRF requires the training and motivation of clinical research professionals.
3. Technical problems arising with eCRF demands immediate attention and support from help desk.
4. Failure of internet and communication systems may interfere with the continuity of the trial.

CHANGING ROLE OF CRA

In the present scenario of eTrials, CRA should develop electronic data management skills, in addition to the traditional monitoring. CRA can be a part of eCRF designing team too. CRA has the highest responsibility to motivate and train the site personnel to use the EDC facilities, to enter the data directly into eCRF and to use the help desk if required. DEO at site should be educated about the password, timelines and expiry of unused password.

With direct access to the data at the sites, CRA can review the same from home-office for quality purposes before each monitoring visit and queries can be generated and ideally resolved by site personnel beforehand. When the CRA arrives on site, he or she can perform source data verification (SDV) on clean data. Timely implementation of query resolution will significantly improve data quality, minimizes the errors and reduces the number of monitoring visits; subsequently resulting in less travel time.

Adopting EDC, CRA is relieved of retrieving the pages of CRFs, data clarification requests, separating out originals and copies, searching for missing pages of CRF, completing tracking logs and dispatch originals to data managers. Visit follow-up activities, such as sending reminders to the site and generating reports, will be simplified because basic information is available on the system and does not need to be duplicated.

SUGGESTED READING

1. Code of Federal Regulations, Title 21, Part 11 (US Government Printing Office, Washington, DC); also available at www.access.gpo.gov/nara/cfr/.
2. Food and Drug Administration, Guidance for Industry: Computerized Systems Used in Clinical Trials (FDA, Rockville, MD, April 1999); also available at www.fda.gov/cder/ guidance.

22 Clinical Trial Logs

Ravindra Ghooi, Sachin Manocha

INTRODUCTION

Managing clinical trials and studies is no different from managing materials, machines and people. Successful trial site borrow heavily from management methods used in large industrial projects. Careful record keeping serves as an important back up source of information if questions arise about study related dates or events.

Logs and lists are important tools in meticulous execution of complex activities, such as clinical trials. The likelihood of forgetting a particular item of activity increases in proportion to the number of items that need to be done. Using lists and logs ensures that every item, however, minor is not overlooked, but given equal importance. Most regulatory authorities recognize the importance of logs and demand that they be maintained and produced during audits as evidence of good clinical practice.

TYPES OF LOGS AND LISTS

Various logs and lists are recommended for use during clinical trials, each log covering one aspect of the trial. Commonly used logs and lists include but are not limited to the following:

- System master list
- Master check list
- Communication log
- Adverse event log
- Patient screening log
- Monitoring checklist
- Subject identification log
- Study appointment log
- Patient sign in log

- Laboratory specimen log
- Drug accountability log
- Device exposure log
- Device accountability log

Some organizations split up the logs and lists into a smaller ones breaking up the activities and grouping them under related heads. In such cases a systems master list detailing all lists and logs used in the study are listed.

To enable a thorough understanding about the role of logs and lists, a brief description of individual logs or lists follows:

Systems Masterlist

The systems master list provides a check for all lists used in the study. Copies of this list are filled periodically, say monthly to ensure that all logs and lists have been duly filled during the month. When filed chronologically these lists give an overview of the health of the system.

Master Checklist

The master checklist is a comprehensive list, which details all the activities to be undertaken during the trial. Ideally this list can be filled in at the specific time points in the trial, such as beginning of recruitment, or end of recruitment or end of trial. This list running in numerous pages provides an overview of all the activities to be undertaken during the period to which the list pertains.

Communication Log

The role of written letters is a gradually eroding, and letters are being replaced with telephone calls and e-mails. However, it is easy to forget a particular e-mail or a conversation unless it is recorded on paper. Most organizations insist on the maintenance of logs to record the highlights or every conversation between the trial managers and sponsors or site personnel. Communications logs can be maintained on paper or directly in a computer. A web based communications log known as Commlog, containing a study directory and communications database has been developed.

CommLog is based on multitiered component based architecture, with security systems to prevent access by unauthorized persons. Developed by teams of experts from the Purdue and Vanderbilt Universities, it has been validated in a number of phase III trials

Adverse Events Log

Adverse events are one of the most important findings in a clinical trial. In fact the frequency and severity of adverse events decide the fate of the investigational product.

Adverse events are required to be documented and reported to both the sponsors and regulatory authorities. A record of adverse events in the form of a log provides a backup for the adverse event reporting system.

Patient Screening Log

This list provides details of all the patients who were contacted for the trial. Some patients appearing in this list may not consent to the trial or may not be eligible to enter the trial. If reasons for non-participation were also listed, then a study of the same would provide an answer about recruitment rates.

Monitoring Checklist

Monitoring is one of the most important activities in a trial; the outcome of any trial depends upon the competence and thoroughness of monitoring. Additionally monitoring is an activity carried out on the site, and often by a single individual, in such a situation a monitoring checklist provides support to the monitor in carrying out the activity with thorough competence. This checklist contains all activities to be conducted before during and after the monitoring visit, and it may be split-up into the three parts.

The monitor may, after preparing the checklist, get it checked by superiors so that inadvertently no action is missed. This list additionally monitors the monitor, ensuring that all monitoring activities are carried out as planned.

Delegation of Duties Log

According to GCP regulations the responsibility of each function has to be assigned to a member of the investigator's team, and that person will be held accountable for the proper conduct of the function. At the beginning of the trial it is necessary that the principal investigator prepares a log for the delegation of duties. Each function has to be identified and the person responsible named, along with the signature of the person indicating that he/she accepts the responsibility.

The investigator may name more than one person as responsible for each function, but then it is preferable that the investigator defines the hierarchy of responsibility, so that accountability can be individualized.

Subject Identification Log

Requirements of confidentiality dictate that identifiable information of the subjects should not be made available to one and all involved in the trial. Hence most documents carry only a subject number or initials of the patient. It is therefore necessary to have a document that connects the coded identity of the subject with identifiable information of the subject. In the absence of such a log, the trial staff would themselves be unable to identify the subject correctly and CRF entries could be erroneous.

While transferring data to the sponsor, care has also to be taken to ensure that identifiable information is not sent, unless necessary. When trials involve devices or agents which have long term effects, the sponsor may need to know the identity of the subjects, should there be need to contact the subjects even after the end of the trial.

Study Appointment Log

This log maintains a record of every appointment, the date, time and purpose, during the trial. The log also reveals whether the subjects keep every appointment or not. This serves as an important tool for assessing patient compliance.

Patient Sign-in Log

The patient sign-in log is a simple notebook in which the subject signs during each of his/her visit. This log is an important back-up for the study appointment log.

Laboratory Specimen Log

Most trials involve a number of laboratory tests, at different intervals. A log detailing the number of tests ordered and the reports received and entered in the source documents. In studies involving a large number of laboratory tests this log is a useful tool to ensure the timely receipts of laboratory reports. If this log is reviewed daily, it serves as a control for ensuring prompt order of tests, dispatch of laboratory samples and receipt of laboratory reports.

Drug Accountability Log

Many drugs used in clinical trial are INDs, which have not yet been approved for widespread medical use. Under these circumstances it is essential to maintain a very accurate account of every single tablet or capsule of the investigational product. The sponsor would like to ensure that not even a single unit of investigational drug is misplaced and so would the regulator. It is therefore imperative that the investigator has a complete account of the investigational drug. The drug accountability log is an important tool to ensure that drug is not misplaced and every unit is accounted for.

This log contains details of total number of units received, their batch number and date of receipt. If any units or packages were found to be damaged, then this is also mentioned. Every time units are dispensed they should be entered in the log, so that at the end of the trial one is able to account for every unit of the drug. During the close out visit this log can be handed over to the CRA, and even used during audits and inspections to demonstrate control over use of investigational products.

Device Exposure Log

Devices are classified on the basis of duration of exposure of the subject to the device. This log records the device identity and exposure time, while also noting defective or devices with problems of sterility etc. This log is an important back-up of trial documentation, and helps in reconciliation of devices at the end of the trial.

Device Accountability Log

The use, disposition and return of devices used in trials is very important for both sponsors and regulators. This is to ensure that devices are not removed from the trial and used in other patients under treatment at the study site.

In addition to the above, organizations can prepare additional logs and lists, which they find useful for good clinical practice. With use in each trial, these tools undergo refinement, which improves their vale to the conduct of the trial. Nonetheless, it should be remembered, these tools do not ensure compliance with GCP, but when used judiciously, help in complying with GCP.

I. SYSTEMS MASTER LIST

Study code:
Study protocol title:
Centre no.:
Investigator and site: Date:

		Completion			
S No	*Log or list*	*YES*	*NO*	*NA*	*Comments*
1	Master checklist	☐	☐	☐	
2	Communication log	☐	☐	☐	
3	Delegation of responsibilities log				
4	Adverse event log	☐	☐	☐	
5	Patient screening log	☐	☐	☐	
6	Monitoring checklist	☐	☐	☐	
7	Subject identification log	☐	☐	☐	
8	Study appointment log	☐	☐	☐	
9	Patient sign in log	☐	☐	☐	
10	Laboratory specimen log	☐	☐	☐	
11	Device exposure log	☐	☐	☐	
12	Device accountability log	☐	☐	☐	

Comments:____

Name:______________________________

Signature:______________________________

Date:______________________

II. MASTER CHECKLIST

Study code:
Study protocol title:
Centre no.: Date of visit:
Investigator and site:

A. Checklist of SMF

S. No.		YES	NO	NA	Comments
1.	DCGI approval letter	☐	☐	☐	
2.	Ethics Committee/IRB approval letter of the all version(s) of the protocol /ICD	☐	☐	☐	
3.	EC letter contains date, place and protocol, ICD, IB version no approved	☐	☐	☐	
	• Is the chairman of EC, a member of the institution	☐	☐	☐	
	• Is the investigator a member of the EC	☐	☐	☐	
	• If yes , did the investigator vote	☐	☐	☐	
4.	Was there a quorum maintained at the time of the EC approval (Please note that investigator should not vote)	☐	☐	☐	
5.	Were the following documents reviewed by The EC				
	• Latest protocol version	☐	☐	☐	
	• Latest IB	☐	☐	☐	
	• CRF	••			
	• ICD along with translations	☐	☐	☐	
	• Advertisement if any	☐	☐	☐	
	• Any protocol amendment	☐	☐	☐	
6.	Letter informing the ethics committee about the amendment	☐	☐	☐	
7.	Letter of approval of amendment from EC/ IRB, if any	☐	☐	☐	
8.	All version (s) of the IB	☐	☐	☐	
9.	All version (s) of the Protocol	☐	☐	☐	
10.	All version(s) of the CRF	☐	☐	☐	
11.	All version(s) of the ICD with translations	☐	☐	☐	
12.	Delegation document (signed and dated)	☐	☐	☐	
13.	Any change in delegation document (signed and dated)	☐	☐	☐	
14.	Laboratory selection report	☐	☐	☐	
15.	Laboratory reference range	☐	☐	☐	
16.	Any change in laboratory reference range	☐	☐	☐	
17.	Lab investigations cost sheet	☐	☐	☐	
18.	Subject screening log is signed and dated	☐	☐	☐	
19.	Patient identification code list	☐	☐	☐	
20.	Drug accountability form reviewed	☐	☐	☐	
21.	Emergency code break envelops (sealed)	☐	☐	☐	
22.	Any seal broken	☐	☐	☐	
23.	Investigator agreement letter with the sponsor	☐	☐	☐	
24.	Protocol agreement (signed and dated)	☐	☐	☐	

Contd...

Contd...

S. No.	*YES*	*NO*	*NA*	*Comments*
25. Financial agreement with the sponsor	☐	☐	☐	
26. CT shipment supply record(s)	☐	☐	☐	
27. Payment receipt(s)	☐	☐	☐	
28. Shipment record(s)	☐	☐	☐	
29. Proposal letters	☐	☐	☐	
30. Investigator undertaking	☐	☐	☐	
31. CVs of investigators	☐	☐	☐	
32. CVs of delegated person(s)	☐	☐	☐	
33. Site visit log	☐	☐	☐	
34. CT research grant receipt form(s)	☐	☐	☐	

B. CRF review

S.No.	*YES*	*NO*	*NA*	*Comments*
35. Patient initials checked on each sheet	☐	☐	☐	
36. Patient number checked	☐	☐	☐	
37. Randomization number checked	☐	☐	☐	
38. Centre number checked	☐	☐	☐	
39. Have all the corrections in CRF been signed and dated by the investigator/delegated person	☐	☐	☐	
40. Has patient attended the visit within the prescribed visit date (including window period)	☐	☐	☐	
41. CRF checked against in patient case records/source data	☐	☐	☐	
42. CRFs are signed by investigator on every page	☐	☐	☐	
43. Are there any protocol deviations	☐	☐	☐	
44. If yes, has the investigator asked for any protocol waivers	☐	☐	☐	
45. Has the waiver request form been duly filled and returned	☐	☐	☐	

C. Laboratory data verification

S.No.	*YES*	*NO*	*NA*	*Comments*
46. Date of sample collection/report	☐	☐	☐	
47. Any missing data	☐	☐	☐	
48. If yes, is file to note generated	☐	☐	☐	
49. Have comments been put on values outside the normal reference range	☐	☐	☐	

D. Adverse event/ SAE reporting

S.No.	*YES*	*NO*	*NA*	*Comments*
50. Any new SAE since last visit	☐	☐	☐	
51. Has SAE been reported to Ranbaxy within 24 hours of investigator becoming aware of it	☐	☐	☐	
52. Has SAE been reported to EC within 7 days of its occurence	☐	☐	☐	
53. If yes, has SAE form been filled	☐	☐	☐	
54. Has SAE resolved and follow up form filled	☐	☐	☐	

E. Source documents verification (100%)

S.No.		YES	NO	NA	Comments
55.	Pain Diary Cards	☐	☐	☐	
	• Data transcribed from diary card correctly	☐	☐	☐	
	• Check for any errors/ correction	☐	☐	☐	
	• Any data obliteration with pen/white ink	☐	☐	☐	

S.No.		YES	NO	NA	Comments
56.	Medication Compliance Cards (MCC)				
	• Data transcribed from MCC correctly	☐	☐	☐	
	• Check for any errors/correction	☐	☐	☐	
	• Any data obliteration with pen/white ink	☐	☐	☐	
57.	Has the MCC and Pain diary card filled in the same language as that of the ICD	☐	☐	☐	

F. Drug supplies storage check

S.No.		YES	NO	NA	Comments
58.	Drug supplies adequate	☐	☐	☐	
59.	Drug storage appropriate	☐	☐	☐	
60.	Drug accountability verified	☐	☐	☐	
61.	Temperature log checked	☐	☐	☐	

G. Have the following being discussed?

S.No.		YES	NO	NA	Comments
62.	New information about study medication or any update on information brochure.	☐	☐	☐	
63.	Any SAE at any other investigator site information given	☐	☐	☐	
64.	Any new adverse event information given	☐	☐	☐	
65.	Any protocol amendment information given	☐	☐	☐	
66.	Any change in regulatory requirements	☐	☐	☐	
67.	Recruitment status discussed	☐	☐	☐	
68.	Is the recruitment status satisfactory	☐	☐	☐	
69.	If no, does the investigator and sponsor want to take up any actions	☐	☐	☐	

Comments ____

____

____

Name ______________________

Signature______________________

Date:______________________

23 Standard Operating Procedures

Ravindra Ghooi

INTRODUCTION

ICH defines SOPs as "Detailed, written instructions to achieve uniformity of the performance of a specific function". (ICH E6 1.55) Quite simply, a standard operating procedure specifies in writing what should be done, when, where and by whom.

The pharmaceutical industry, and by default the New Drug Discovery process, is highly regulated, probably only next to the aeronautical industry. To regulate the new drug development process the International Conference on Harmonization (ICH) introduced the Good Clinical Practice (E6) as an ethical and scientific standard for designing, conducting, recording and reporting data that is accurate, credible and acceptable to regulatory authorities. In order to achieve this, quality and consistency is required in all its component processes.

For controlling the quality of the end products organizations set up standards for both raw materials and processes. Standardized inputs and processes reduce cost by preventing product failures in the long run. These are generally defined as Raw Material Standards (RMS), Standard Test Procedures (STPs) and Standard Operating Procedures (SOPs). SOPs find application in areas even other than manufacturing and have become the gold standards even for service industries.

Similarly raw materials and processes in the pharmaceutical industry, including new drug development must be consistent so that the end product stands the stringent scrutiny of regulatory authorities. This is controlled by Good Manufacturing Practices (ICH Quality Guidelines, Schedule M, Drugs and Cosmetics Act 1940).

Prior to 1996, every country had its own guidelines for conducting new drug development process. Registration of the drug in another country usually meant repetition of parts or whole studies as per the requirements of the target country. ICH Guidelines were formed to avoid this duplication of research leading to saving of time, money and efforts. To meet the requirements of these guidelines, SOPs became a necessity, whether for a pharmaceutical company, a sponsor, a contract research organization, an investigator site, an ethics committee or any other involved party. Strict adherence to SOPs by each involved party ensures data reliability and integrity in addition to efficiency of the clinical research operations.

BENEFITS OF SOPs

1. SOPs help to assure consistency of the procedure.
2. SOPs help to ensure compliance with ethical and applicable regulatory requirements.
3. SOPs enable personnel to delegate and may free up time for other activities.
4. SOPs help to avoid confusion and ensure role clarification.
5. SOPs are useful tools for training new members of staff.
6. SOPs provide a contribution to the audit process.

Most regulatory authorities recognize the value of SOPs and have made it compulsory to have written-down SOPs. The Drugs Controller General (India) requires that clinical trials are guided by SOPs and the sponsor, the investigator have documented SOPs to ensure compliance with ethical and regulatory requirements.

Organizations have standard procedures for different operations carried out in various functional areas. These procedures are time tested and most suited for the organization's needs, and prepared on the basis of expertise developed in-house. The objective of Standard Operating Procedures (SOPs) is to institutionalize this expertise so that despite changes in personnel at the operational level, procedures remain unchanged. In order to fulfill the objective of SOPs, they need to be developed after due consultation, documented in detail. Additionally all personnel must be trained in SOPs, so that the procedures are clearly understood and strictly adhered to at all times. SOPs are however not immutable, and can be amended so that they are in tune with changing circumstances. Indeed they must be periodically reviewed and revisions made whenever needed.

In addition to providing guidance for performing functions, they also specify who is responsible for performing them, when and how. SOPs also lay down the duration and the method for storing records generated. Standard Operating Procedures recognize that despite all training there will be instances when there is a failure to follow them, specific methods are prescribed for detecting such instances and fixing responsibilities for these. Not stopping at this, they provide information on corrective measures to be adopted.

Any discussion on SOPs must therefore include all aspects for preparation, use, review and amendment of these procedures. These are preceded by a study and establishment of an environment in which all functions are SOP driven. These aspects are discussed in detail in the foregoing parts.

THE ENVIRONMENT

Successful deployment of SOPs demands an environment, which is both transparent and well defined. The organization structure becomes the starting point for the preparation of SOPs, since SOPs define roles and responsibilities of individuals that form the organization. An organogram needs to be first prepared before any attempt is made to lay down SOPs.

In addition to reporting structure, the organogram depicts the responsibilities of individuals, thus preventing cross-functional interference that can lead to confusion among the staff. A separate document that details the succession plan and specifies the individuals to whom the responsibilities pass in case of a person being absent, adds value to the SOP based system.

Different organizations have different structures, some highly hierarchical and some flat. There is no overall advantage of one type of structure over another, and different organizations should adopt one that suits those most. Titles, positions and responsibilities too vary, and no single recommendation can be made to suit all. Figure 23.1 gives an example of an organogram, this is by no means a recommended one, and each organization should build its own. Such organograms can be constructed using MS Excel or any other suitable software package.

Since SOPs are meant for personnel to follow, they should not be imposed, but should come from the personnel themselves. Personnel should be explained the advantages of the SOPs so that they develop a sense of ownership. It is for this reason that the persons using the SOPs are known as process owners. Greater the sense of ownership to SOPs greater the compliance to them.

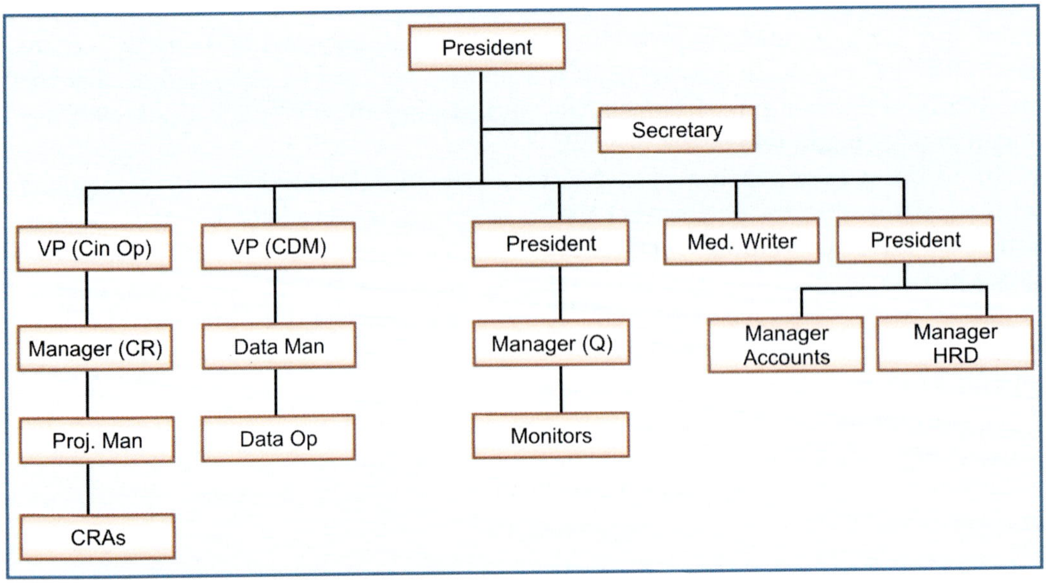

Fig. 23.1: A typical organogram

COMPLIANCE TO SOPs

Write down what you do, do what is written down

The European Clinical Trial Directive 2001/20/EC puts the magnifying glass onto the suitability of investigators, their supporting staff, and the quality of facilities when conducting clinical trials. With this, the directive also entailed the awareness and importance of the critical conditions in which clinical trials are conducted and managed at investigative sites. It is well known that there are big differences in standards of facilities, which vary in size, expertise, and organization.

The complex ICH-GCP guidelines are admittedly only meant for member states, yet countries around the world have recognized the primacy of the ICH member states in so far as the pharmaceutical market is concerned. If any country is to hope for its drugs to find acceptance in the ICH member states, ICH guidelines become regulations that must be followed. SOPs are therefore an important tool to ensure compliance to complex guidelines that GCP has propounded. The importance of SOPs rises in proportion to the complexity of the guidelines to be followed.

STEPS IN SOP PREPARATION

SOP generation in most organizations takes place as per the pattern given below:

- Process mapping
- SOP writing
- SOP authorization
- SOP distribution and archiving
- SOP training
- SOP review and revision.

Process Mapping

In any efficient industry processes follow a set pattern. Some begin simultaneously, while others are staggered or sequential. Mapping of processes helps in identifying the order in which processes should be taken up and completed. This also helps in identifying processes that need standardization, and has been applied to clinical research with good results.

An organization involved in clinical research would require SOPs for administrative and financial functions in addition to research functions. Such SOPs include but are not limited to the following:

- SOPs relating to human resources (e.g. recruitment and appointment of staff, working hours, leave, travel, allowances, monetary compensation, discipline, etc.)
- SOPs relating to purchase of materials and services (e.g. office equipment, consumables, courier services, communications, etc.)
- SOPs relating to finance (e.g. staff salaries, payments and receipts, budgets, and accounting, etc.)

If clinical trial data is to comply with ICH-GCP, it is essential that all people and sites involved in clinical studies have the appropriate SOPs in place in order to conduct clinical research and to assure compliance with the current regulations. The presence of these quality documents is essential when inspections take place since the most frequent reported deficiencies during inspections are the lack of written SOPs and/ or the failure to adhere to them. The risk of GCP non-compliance is high at organizations with a poor availability of clinical research specific SOPs.

When the ICH-GCP came into effect in July 1996, a lot of new SOPs had to be developed and reviewed by sponsors in order to comply with the guidelines. Some examples of new SOPs encompassed by the new clinical trials directive are:

- Procedures to be completed in the pretrial phase (e.g. site, investigator and laboratory selection, investigator and other agreements, collection of investigator's CVs, conflict of interest certificates, preparation of documents such as protocol, CRF, informed consent forms, translations and back-translations, etc)
- Procedures concerning the commencement of the clinical trial (e.g. Investigator's meetings, initiation meetings, obtaining regulatory clearance, applications to ethics committee, etc.)
- Procedures for the manufacturing and supply of the investigational products (IP), as well as their labeling, import and export procedures (e.g. maintenance of production equipment and facilities, production procedure, cleaning procedure, import and export of IP, storage and transport of IP, etc)
- Procedures concerning the conduct of clinical trials (e.g. translation of GCP requirements into SOP, storage/transport/dispensing and accounting of IP, informed consent procedure, contacts between sponsor — investigator — study site personnel - ethics committee - competent authorities, site management and site monitoring procedures etc, data management, laboratory analysis, etc)
- Procedures to assure the effective use of electronic records when using the clinical registration system and its safety reporting electronic counterpart, combined with the establishment of quality systems checking the accuracy, reliability, and completeness of the data entered into the database, etc
- Procedures concerning archiving and maintenance of study material and results (storage, privacy and security of study records, etc)
- Procedures concerning audits, inspections, etc

The total number of SOPs required in clinical research is large, and not limited to the above list. Each organization specializes in different areas of clinical research, often assuming different responsibilities in different studies; it is therefore not feasible to list out all the SOPs that it may require.

SOP Writing

Contrary to popular belief, writing SOPs is not exactly rocket science. The best advice to a beginner writing SOPs would be similar to one the Queen gave Alice,

"Start at the beginning and then go through till you come to the end." (Lewis Carol, Alice in Wonderland).

Once they realize that the SOP they write is merely for others to follow, most writers have no problem getting started. The most difficult thing for most authors is to stop. Writers feel the need to further explain everything that has already been stated quite clearly. This results in redundant sections that say the same thing already covered in an earlier section. This adds no extra value to the standard procedure and increases the chances of having conflicting information as time (and revisions) goes by.

While writing SOPs long complex sentences and paragraphs should be avoided; they make the standard procedure difficult to follow. Short, clear, and concise words and phrases convey clear and concise concepts in short paragraphs. Writing standard procedures is a form of technical writing. The writer should be cautioned that once a word or phrase is used to describe something, that same word or phrase should be used throughout the standard procedure. This will help keep the user focused and prevent confusion. If using jargon, abbreviations or initials, explanation and spelling in full, or citing the full title or name at the first use is recommended.

When a test method or process has been developed in-house, the individual who has designed the process and its controls, as described above, should write the procedure. The more knowledgeable the author, the more accurate the procedure will be. In addition, if the author is directly familiar with the work, the procedure will communicate effectively and the requirements of the work will be user-friendly.

Many procedures, however, are not designed or developed. Some of these are devised to meet some regulatory requirement, obviously SOP for such procedures are best written by some one who has wide experience in the procedure. Other procedures might be devised by consensus, as the most convenient way of performing a task. Again, the procedures should be written by an individual who performs the task routinely or someone who is directly responsible for the performance of the task.

There is no approved format by authorities such as ICH, for an SOP. Thus for an SOP to be valid, there is no need of a particular format. Nonetheless formats are commonly used, simply because they make the SOPs look standardized. An organization may choose any format for its SOPs, since the format is not the most important part of the SOP. A typical format is given in Figure 23.2, yet there are many other formats that could be used as per the choice of the organization. Whichever format is used it should provide facilities for recording each item required in the SOP.

Ideally the first SOP to be prepared should be one that specifies how SOPs are to be prepared. This SOP known as SOP of SOPs, is the master, and it lays down the procedures for making all the SOPs. The SOP begins by providing the layout and contents of all SOPs to be prepared and includes the following:

1. Title of the SOP
2. Pagination

Company Logo	Title of SOP	SOP Number
		Effective Date
		Version
		Next Revision

Prepared by		Date
Checked by		Date
Authorized by		Date

Confidential

Fig. 23.2: A typical format of SOP

3. Font type and size to be used for titles, sub-titles, headings and the text.
4. Version, effective date of the SOP and the date when the next revision is due
5. System for numbering the SOPs
6. Sections that should be included in the SOP
7. Signature section to identify personnel who prepare, check and authorize the SOP.
8. Appendix: logs, forms or templates
9. References.

Title of the SOP

The title should be descriptive, because a procedure describes how to do something, the title should use directive language to declare what is being done to what. An SOP titled "Import of Investigational Product" is not descriptive of the procedure's content; a more appropriate title would be, "Application for import of Investigational Product."

Pagination

Many of the SOPs run into a number of pages. In order to avoid confusion due to missing pages, each page should be numbered as page 1 of 5 or page 2 of 5, etc. This ensures the completeness of the SOP while enabling correct referencing.

Font

A very wide variety of fonts are available in MS-word. There is no specific font type or font size to be followed, but it is better to choose the most readable font. Once the font is chosen it should be stuck to, so that all documents are standardized. The final selected font type and size should be recorded in the SOP of SOPs, as follows (Table 23.1).

Table 23.1: Font types and size in SOP

S. no.	*Sections*	*Font types*	*Font size*
1.	Title of SOP	Times New Roman	16 Bold
2.	SOP number	Times New Roman	12 Bold
3.	Effective date	Times New Roman	12 Bold
4.	Version	Times New Roman	12 Bold
5	Next revision	Times New Roman	12 Bold
6.	Headings	Times New Roman	14 Bold
7.	SOP text	Times New Roman	12

Version and Dates

After the preparation of an SOP the personnel using the same may have to be trained. Only after this training can the SOP be implemented. For this reason the date of preparation of the SOP and the date of implementation (effective date) may differ, with the effective date being later than the preparation date.

An SOP is also not immutable. Changing conditions and continuous improvement of procedures may require changes in the SOP, in fact it is necessary to review the SOP periodically and revise it. If on review, no revision is called for then it should be renewed in its native form. To make this recognizable each revision should carry a version number and date. The date of the next due revision should also feature on the SOP so that it does not get used beyond its due date of revision.

SOP Numbering

Procedures must be uniquely identified. This identification supports accountability and traceability of the document throughout the facility and over time as it changes. The accountability and traceability of procedures are based on assigning them identification numbers or codes and control numbers or codes (e.g., revision or edition numbers).

Requirements for document identification and control, accountability and traceability, responsibilities, etc. must be included with every procedure. This can be accomplished by providing a consistent format and consistent document management requirements for every procedure.

Quick access to relevant SOPs is aided by systematic numbering and coding. Each SOP is coded on the basis of the department to which it pertains; giving clue to the activity it pertains. It is therefore customary to code SOPs as QA/AU/03 for an SOP pertaining to audits for the quality assurance department. There are many such codes, which an organization may choose from. Any code will do, so long as the code helps correct identification of the particular SOP.A master list of SOPs available with all personnel of the organization lists all SOPs in place helping them to search and retrieve the required SOP for reference.

Sections of the SOP

Several key sections should be included in the SOP. The common ones are given in Table 23.2.

Table 23.2: Key sections in SOP

S. no	*Sections*	*Particulars*
1	Purpose	Stating the general purpose of the SOP
2	Scope	Lists areas or parts of the procedure covered
3	Responsibility	Lists the person responsible for carrying out the activity in normal circumstances and to whom the responsibility may be transferred, under what circumstances
4	Procedure	Lists the procedure in simple words, including the steps to be taken in case of default of the procedures.
5	Records	Details site and duration of storage of the SOP.

Each section should be numbered so that sections and subsections become clear to the reader. An outline numbering system (1.1, 1.2, 1.3 and so on) has been found to be most suitable by some organizations.

In addition to those mentioned above the organization may add other sections depending upon its requirements.

Signatures

An SOP should clearly indicate the names of the persons who prepared it, who checked it and who authorized the document. Such signatures add to the responsibility and accountability of the procedures.

Appendix : Logs, Forms or Templates

During clinical trials activities are often tracked with the help of logs, these may pertain to visits by patients, dispensing of trial medication, clinical investigations etc. These logs form a part of the system and may be required by particular SOPs. Forms and templates are often included in SOPs for collection or transmission of information in a predefined format.

References

The use of references in standard procedures is a common practice. Putting the reference section (listing all the references in one place) in the standard procedure alerts the user that there might be other documents needed to correctly follow the standard procedure. Getting into the procedure and finding that another document, that is not at hand, is needed, can be frustrating. When making reference citations, use the phrase "current issue" instead of the actual date of any reference that is likely to change. This way the standard procedure will not be out of compliance if the reference document is changed before you can get your standard procedure revised. However, when a particular issue date of a reference is vital to your standard procedure, be sure to cite the necessary issue date. Citing other documents is easy and saves some writing; but overdoing the reference citations can produce a nightmare for the user.

SOP Authorization

An unauthorized SOP is not a valid document. After the preparation and review the SOP is finally released after authorization. This authorization is done by a person designated for this function.

SOP Distribution and Archiving

For every SOP developed, its distribution must be determined and noted in the master list. Restricting distribution of SOPs makes sense in more than one ways. It reduces chances of confusion among employees as well as leakage of sensitive organization owned procedures and methods.

An organization may have a few SOPs that are relevant to every employee; there could be others that are relevant to a particular department, while a few might be relevant to a select number of employees. Making every SOP available to every employee would most probably lead to an overload, with literally hundreds of SOPs, many of which are irrelevant.

A separate department or section (usually the Quality Assurance Department) should be responsible for the management of SOPs. This department is responsible for ensuring that all the SOPs in circulation are current versions and that all superseded SOPs are withdrawn. This ensures that obsolete procedures are not in use.

SOPs are classified and stamped as controlled and uncontrolled. Controlled SOPs have restricted distribution and are generally not meant for transmission outside the organization. Of late these are made available on company intranet and can neither be copied nor printed, thus ensuring that they are not leaked out.

Uncontrolled SOPs are more generic in nature and are made available to concerned employees. If required these SOPs may be supplied to sponsors or other parties on request.

The original signed SOP should be stored in a secure place under the supervision of a responsible person. The SOP archives should be protected from hazards like fire, flooding or pests. Older versions of SOPs are also required to be stored for reference, yet each organization can have its own policy about the number of versions to be archived. Normally the immediate prior version is stored as a rule, while other older versions are optional.

SOP Training

For the proper use of SOPs, personnel using the same should be trained to do so. A training session may be held by the quality assurance department in which the process owner takes the lead in training his or her colleagues. Maintenance of a training log indicates which of the employee has been trained and who has not been. It can be used to identify training requirements of the staff. Only after the training is complete for all the concerned employees should an SOP become effective.

SOP Review and Revision

Continuous improvement is one of the objectives of the quality system. Hence a constant effort in this direction would lead to revision of SOPs. Similar revisions may be required due to change in regulatory or organizational requirements. It is necessary to periodically review all SOPs, depending upon predefined timelines. In case the review suggests that no revision is called for, the SOP may be released as such, but version number may not change but the effective date is the date of the last review. Organizations could adopt any system which identifies the version as the current one.

LIMITATIONS OF SOPs

SOPs are a tool to maintain consistency of procedures. They help institutionalizing individual experience and knowledge, but have certain drawbacks. There has been unfounded criticism that they stifle creativity. Other objections to SOPs are:

1. Implementation of SOPs is time consuming.
2. They add to the costs of the organization.
3. Require a lot of effort in preparation and training.

However, a large number of organizations have implemented SOPs and found that in the long run they save time, effort and money for the organizations. The International Standards Organization, and their national counterparts have made detailed studies of the system and have demonstrated that SOPs are vital for an organization's growth and survival.

PROCEDURES THAT DO NOT NEED AN SOP

It is easy to define which procedure needs an SOP, but much more difficult to decide which does not. Organizations often go overboard and prepare SOPs for mundane activities. The enormous proliferation of SOPs makes employees wonder whether SOPs serve them or vice versa. The test to decide which procedure deserves an SOP and which does not a simple but very often ignored.

The main role of SOPs is to ensure consistent results, if the quality of the end product does not depend upon the procedure, then an SOP is clearly not required. For example, irrespective of how a photocopy machine is used, the quality of the copies is not significantly altered; hence the operation of the photocopy machine need not have an SOP. On the other hand a spectrophotometer is likely to produce inconsistent readings if not handled in a proper fashion, SOPs for this machine would therefore be useful.

Another point that troubles most people writing an SOP is the amount of detail to be entered. There is no rule or guideline for this. However, it would depend upon the level of training the end user of the SOP has had. If the procedure is to be followed by people who are not technically highly qualified, detailed instructions are called for, not, if they are well qualified.

AUDITS

An audit of the quality system is intended to determine to what extent the system achieves its objectives, conforms to requirements, complies with regulatory requirements, meets customer's contractual requirements, conforms to a recognized quality standards. Periodic internal audits ensure the health of the system, and prepare it for external audits. Employees trained in the technique of audits should periodically audit different departments and sections of the organization, to ensure that the system is operating well. Typically auditors should check for the following:

1. Whether the required SOPs are available at the point of use?
2. If the SOPs in use are the current ones?
3. If SOPs are regularly followed and if there are any deviations from the same?
4. In case of deviations, whether remedial actions are taken as prescribed?

Audits of the systems management department would be more rigorous and auditors would check every aspect of document management. At the end of the audit, auditors should prepare audit reports, which are reviewed by the top management. SOPs work best when meticulously followed and the management must lead by example to ensure that it succeeds.

A large number of SOPs prepared by bodies like the WHO are available on the internet. These may or may not be suitable for use as such, but could be used as a guideline for preparation of SOPs by newcomers in this field.

SUGGESTED READING

1. SOPs for investigators- http://www.who.int/tdr/publications/publications/pdf/sop.pdf
2. SOPs for ethics committees- http://www.who.int/tdr/publications/publications/pdf/ethics.pdf
3. SOPs for dams -http://www.who.int/tdr/publications/publications/pdf/operat_guidelines.pdf
4. SOPs for sponsors -http://www.crc.washington.edu/resources/GCPSOPsponsors. aspx (on payment).

24

Audits and Inspections in Clinical Trials

Kavita Singh

INTRODUCTION

Enormous importance has been directed in the International Conference of Harmonization (ICH) efficacy guidelines (E6) towards maintaining quality and reliability of the data generated from a clinical trial. The pertinent question remains "who is/are responsible for the same and who will ensure it?" The ICH- Good Clinical Practice (GCP) guidelines indicate that "the sponsor is responsible for implementing and maintaining Quality Assurance (QA) and Quality Control (QC) systems".

QC systems are the operational techniques and activities undertaken to verify the requirements for the quality of trial related activities. Without QC system in place, deficiencies in the trial procedures cannot be readily detected and rectified. QA is the planned and systematic action that ensures that the trial is performed and the data is generated, documented (recorded), analyzed and reported in compliance with GCP and the applicable regulatory requirements.

QC activities in a clinical trial are undertaken by the trial team members themselves; therefore carry an inherent potential for bias. Since the purpose is to have an unbiased appraisal of the quality and completeness of the trial, a person independent of the trial team should conduct it. Audit and inspection refer to such independent QA activities, which examine both 'the systems' and 'the specific study'. Hence, QA activities always form an integral part of a clinical trial. The best method to ensure quality at the end of a clinical trial is to build it right from its outset.

Audit refers to an independent examination of trial related activities and documents so as to determine whether or not the trial related activities are conducted in accordance with the study protocol, relevant SOPs, GCP and applicable regulatory requirements. The ultimate purpose is to ensure the quality, integrity and validity of investigational data. Inspection on the other hand is an official review of documents, facilities, records, and any other resources that are deemed by the authorities to be related to the clinical trial. It is a formal process that has legal implications. As per the "Medicines for Human Use (Clinical Trials) Regulations (2004)", inspections are mandatory for all commercial and non-commercial clinical trials.

AUDIT

An audit of a clinical trial provides the sponsor with independent appraisal of the quality and completeness of the trial. It identifies potential problems and helps in implementing solutions when corrective action is no longer an option. It is an informal, planned process and is usually conducted either by the sponsor or internally by the organization. Throughout the process of audit, general information is exchanged between the auditor and the person(s)/institution. This information is used to rectify the problems, train the staff and improve upon the quality of research conducted.

Different types of audits:
1. Sponsor audit of investigative site
2. IRB audit of investigative site
3. System audit of sponsor/CROs
4. Clinical laboratory audit
5. Clinical study report audit
6. Validation of computer system.

Sponsor Audit of Investigative Site

Section 5.19.1 of ICH (E6) mentions: "*The purpose of sponsor's audit, which is independent of and separate from routine monitoring or quality control functions, should be to evaluate trial conduct and compliance with the protocol, SOPs, GCP and the applicable regulatory requirements*". Also, the section 4.1.4. ICH-GCP states: "*The investigator/institution should permit monitoring and auditing by the sponsor, and inspection by the appropriate regulatory authority (ies).*" Thus, sponsor has the right to audit a site based both on the regulations as well as the contract signed between the investigator and the sponsor before the initiation of the trial. To fulfill these responsibilities, sponsor gets investigative sites audited either by sponsor's own quality assurance department or employs independent auditors. In addition to fulfilling the sponsor's responsibilities, site audit provides assurance to management and other staff that work is performed to the highest standards of GCP. The objectives of site audit are to assess whether: the subject's rights and safety have been maintained; company procedures for the conduct of clinical studies have been satisfactorily implemented during the course of the study and reliable, accurate and verifiable data has been obtained. It also points out the opportunities to improve the quality and SOPs for the future. In addition, it provides assurance to both the sponsor and the investigator that if a regulatory inspection subsequently occurs at the investigator site, no major problems have remained undetected and unresolved.

Types of Investigative Site Audit

Routine Audit

Routine audit may be done either when the study is in progress or after it has been completed. The ultimate aim is to ensure that the site is prepared for regulatory or IRB audit. Ideally such audits should not be a requirement if a monitor has been performing his role well.

For-cause Audit

Such audits are considered far more important and significant for both sponsor and investigator. These are commonly performed when non-compliance is suspected at the site, either with the protocol, regulations or with the SOPs. The sponsor is unlikely to inform the investigator the actual reason for audit.

Sponsors generally do not audit all investigators; the normal practice is to audit a sample of the centers. Few of the sampling criteria that may be considered include:

- Investigators recruiting large number of subjects
- Investigators performing more than one study
- Results of a previous audit for that investigator/monitor
- Investigators participating in a pivotal study.

The ICH-GCP guideline leaves it to the sponsor to determine audit frequency. As a thumb rule audits are usually scheduled when approximately one-third of study subjects have been recruited. However, a number of specific factors determine the sponsor's audit plan and procedures. Ideally the CRA (monitor), should accompany the auditor during the visit. This is because he/she is familiar with the site and at times may be able to answer a question more readily than the investigator. In fact, this is an excellent learning opportunity for both the monitor and the auditor with regard to each other's work.

Whenever an audit of investigator site is planned irrespective of the fact whether is a routine or for-cause audit, the steps in executing the "investigative site audit" are broadly divided as: before the audit, during the audit and after the audit.

i. *Before the Audit*

The audit process begins with the notification to the site. The auditor contacts the site to arrange for a mutually acceptable date. A detailed agenda mentioning the timings and the documents to be checked during the visit is informed. Just prior to the audit, the auditor reviews the protocol, Case Report Form (CRF), local regulations and guidelines, project specific guidelines, relevant SOPs, and in-house documentation. Before the audit the auditor also contacts the monitor to ask a few questions about the centre, e.g. are there any issues of which he (the auditor) should be aware of, ensure availabilility of documents etc. The auditor may also review, if available, a sample of completed CRFs, data queries and diary cards. The auditor will also select a sample, which covers a range of subject outcomes, e.g. serious adverse events, withdrawals in order to determine how different situations have been handled and documented.

ii. *During the Audit*

a. *Opening meeting:* An introductory meeting is held between the auditor and the site team. This provides an opportunity to meet the team members and establish communication. During this meeting the auditor briefs the site about the scope and proposed procedure of the audit. The opening meeting is also an opportunity for the investigator to ask any questions about the audit.

b. *Reviewing documents and collating information:* The auditor looks at both the study conduct and the available data. They can also conduct interviews with appropriate individuals so as to corroborate oral with written observations.

The auditors specifically tries to answer the following questions during their visit:

- Is the principal investigator knowledgeable about the study?
- Have ineligible patients been recruited?
- Has the protocol and informed consent been approved by the Ethics Committee? Is there a document that shows the approval?
- Has informed consent been documented for each enrolled patient?
- Is the correct version of ICF being used?
- What process was used to obtain informed consent?
- Have all AEs, SAEs been reported?
- Have all AEs and SAEs been followed up?
- Are study documents stored or filed in an orderly manner?
- Is/was the drug supply stored safely?
- Is/was there any unauthorized use of the study drug?
- Does the information reported on the CFR match the information in the "source document"?
- Does source document contain: every medication being taken by the patient? Every significant medical problem? Every significant exam/test finding?

An auditor usually uses a checklist while conducting the review process *(Template1 checklist)*. In order to answer the above questions they review:

- Protocol, IRB approvals and modifications (if any) to the protocol
- Subject records: source documents are compared with data entered in the CRF. Adverse events, concomitant therapy and intercurrent illness entered or not in the CRF. Consent forms: an auditor usually reviews all of them
- Adverse event recording and reporting
- Investigational product accountability and inspection of storage area
- Laboratory/equipment and associated records (if laboratory at centre used)
- Storage of biological samples (if any)
- Facilities for archiving/storing record.

c. *Audit Observations:* The auditors document all observations. He/she documents all non-conformities referenced with supporting evidence. Ideally they should also mention the standard requirements that have been violated against each non-conformity.

d. *Closing meeting:* This provides an opportunity for most serious findings to be discussed and for suggestions to be made. The auditor discusses the findings of the audits, and possible steps the site could take to rectify the identified problems. He should congratulate the team and the principal investigator on all points of good practice. The investigator should be present for this meeting.

iii. *After the Audit*

Auditors should issue the report within 28 days of the final audit activity. All clinical research personnel should be made aware of findings relevant to their activities. The findings may be presented by level of classification, i.e. critical, major and minor (Template 2: Site Audit Report). Prevention/corrective action list that the monitor/study manager can utilize while responding to the audit should accompany the report.

An executive summary outlining the critical and major findings may be prepared for submission to management (if company policy requires). The responsibility to follow up with the site is usually taken over by the Clinical Research Associate of the respective site. The monitor and study co-coordinator should discuss the audit report and decide how to respond to each finding. After the corrective measures have been taken, or timescale given for implementation, a formal audit response should be prepared and submitted to the concerned personnel.

The audit report is an internal, confidential document. Hence, it should not be shown, or copies given to the investigator or anyone else outside to the company. The audit report should *not* be placed in the study file. The final report and subsequent responses of the audit report are maintained only by the QA department.

Following satisfactory responses to the report the auditor issues an audit certificate (Template 3: Audit Certificate). The certificate should be placed in the in-house investigator file to confirm that an audit has taken place. The audit certificate is also appendiced in the clinical trial report when the same is submitted to the regulatory authorities.

IRB Audit of Investigative Site

Occasionally, the IRB can visit the investigative site. An independent IRB may visit the site to assure itself about the ethical conduct of the trial. It is possible that a proactive IRB could ask one or more people to conduct an audit of the trial. The purpose of the IRB audit program is to ensure that research is being conducted appropriately and that all subjects enrolled have been fully informed through a properly conducted informed consent process. The purpose of such audits is to ensure that the IRB approved plan has been followed, the protection of human subjects has been adhered to, and that proper written documentation exists.

The IRB can also perform different types of audits, which include: administrative, random audit and a for-cause comprehensive audit.

The audit will begin with a review of the IRB files. Based on this review, the team will determine what additional documentation is needed and what activities need to be conducted at the study site. The investigator will be contacted and informed of the pending audit. The investigator will be given a list of documents requested by the team, and will provide the team with a list of all subjects enrolled in the study. The auditors will check for presence or absence of the key documents.

The auditor/team will also review any additional documentation according to the strategy developed for the audit. A subset of subjects may be selected at random by the auditors, and the entire physical record for those subjects will be reviewed.

The audit team will interview the investigator and all key personnel to assess their knowledge of the study, the informed consent process, and human subject protections for this study.

The audit team will then select subjects at random to interview. The interview will be designed to; assess whether the subject has a full understanding of the study, the associated risks and benefits, and their role and rights in the study. The interview may also assess their level of satisfaction with the study, the IRB and the institution associated with the study. The information can be obtained either by verbal interview and/or questionnaire. The audit team will also have the authority to directly observe the consent process. On completion of the audit, a full written report will be prepared and presented to the IRB outlining audit findings and recommending actions, if any.

System Audits of Sponsor/CRO

The purpose is to assess the quality and efficiency of the systems and to evaluate how efficiently the systems are working. The system audits may relate to GCP quality systems established by the sponsor/CRO or to the quality systems in operation by CRO. Policies and procedures that are often audited include:

- Standard Operating Procedures: Since they reveal the intended quality, their review is usually the first activity undertaken in an audit
- Document access control
- Security and validation of computers used in the clinical trial
- Personnel records. This is to look for evidence that staff is appropriately qualified and trained
- Auditors can also interview staff to enquire about their job description and their understanding of job responsibility.

Audit of Clinical Laboratory

Audit of the clinical laboratory is to assure compliance with the trial protocol, analytical plan and standard operating procedures. This involves evaluation of:

- Contracts, financial agreements and delegation
- Facilities and environmental conditions
- Analytical plan, report and results

- Equipments
- Quality control procedures
- Raw data
- Labeling and storage
- Documentation, filing and archiving
- Methodology, specific tests, validation and quality control methods.
- Reference ranges, alerts for out-of-range values.

Audit of Clinical Study Report

The clinical study report is audited to check for compliance with the ICH requirements for study reports, clarity of expression, consistency and accuracy of data. Consistency is judged by comparing the synopsis with the main text and main text with the values mentioned in the tables, graphs, data summaries and statistics. Accuracy of the reported data is verified by comparing statistics and data summaries with pre-processed data tabulations and listings; and further comparing the pre-processed data tabulations and listings with raw data (CRFs and source documents) to identify discrepancies, if any.

Validation of Computer System

Computerized systems are an increasing prevalent feature in the field of clinical research. Confidence needs to be established in the quality and consistency. Thus, for validating the computer system SOPs are specifically looked into. The pertinent SOPs to the use of the computerized system should be available on site. SOPs, which would specifically be looked for, are:

- System setup/installation
- Data collection and handling
- System maintenance
- Data backup, recovery, and contingency plans
- Security
- Change control

The auditor would check for electronic signatures, audit trails and date/time stamps. Section 21 CFR 11.10(e) requires persons who use electronic record systems to maintain an audit trail as one of the procedures to protect the authenticity, integrity, and when appropriate, the confidentiality of electronic records.

INSPECTION

"The act by a regulatory authority(ies) of conducting an official review of documents, facilities, records, and any other resources that are deemed by the authority(ies) to be related to the clinical trial and that may be located at the site of the trial, at the sponsor's and/or contract research organization's (CROs) facilities, or at other establishments deemed appropriate by the regulatory authority(ies)" (ICH GCP Sec 1.29).

The inspection program determines:

i. The degree to which sponsors, monitors, clinical investigators, site staff, IRBs and CROs have fulfilled their trial related obligations and
ii. The acceptability of resultant clinical data in support of a new drug, biologic or device's approval.

The Global Regulatory Officials spearheading drug, biologic, and device bioresearch monitoring programs discussed in this chapter are: US FDAs (Food and Drug Administration) CDER's (Centre for Drug Evaluation and Research) extensive Bioresearch Monitoring Program (BIMO), European Medicines Agency (EMEA), UK's Medicines and Healthcare Products Regulatory Agency (MHRA) GCP Compliance Program and Japan's Ministry of Health, Labour, and Welfare (MHLW).

CDER's Bioresearch Monitoring Program

CDER has a vested interest in the accuracy and validity of clinical and nonclinical study results submitted in INDs (Investigatinoal New Drug), NDAs (New Drug Application) and other applications. Under CDER's Bioresearch Monitoring Program (BIMO), field investigators conduct on-site inspections of laboratories, clinics, and offices where scientific data are developed and stored. BIMO program is a comprehensive program of on-site inspections and data audits designed to monitor all aspects of the conduct and reporting of FDA regulated research. It has become a cornerstone of the FDA pre-approval process for new medicines, medical devices, food and color additives and veterinary products introduced to the U.S. consumer. The program is implemented domestically and internationally through five multi-center compliance programs resulting in over 1000 inspections annually. These five compliance programs address inspections of nonclinical testing laboratories (GLP), clinical investigators (GCP), sponsors/monitors and institutional review boards (IRB) and In- Vivo Bioequivalence.

Through these compliance programs, CDER ensures that:

i. The data submitted in product application is accurate and valid
ii. The research studies and the activities of the parties involved in them meet regulatory requirement.
iii. The rights and welfare of human subjects are protected in clinical studies.

Today, CDER's Bioresearch Monitoring Program comprises five separate compliance inspection programs, each designed to evaluate the activities of a key entity in the conduct of a scientific study:

1. Clinical Investigator Inspection Program
2. Sponsor/Monitor/CRO Inspection Program
3. Institutional Review Board (IRB) Inspection Program
4. Non-clinical Laboratory Inspection Program
5. In- Vivo Bioequivalence Inspection Program

Clinical Investigator Inspection Program

While clinical investigators are the focus of most CDER bioresearch inspections, there are several reasons why the results of such inspections are of great importance to clinical trial sponsors and IRBs as well. First, since drug sponsors are ultimately responsible for the conduct of clinical studies and IRBs are responsible for protecting the rights and welfare of clinical subjects, the FDA's inspections of clinical investigators will, at least in part, provide an indication of how well sponsors and IRBs are performing in their respective roles.

Sponsor/ Monitor / CRO Inspectional Program

Historically, CDER's sponsor/monitor/CRO Compliance program has not been one the center's most active monitoring programs. This was claimed to be due to several factors, including relatively broad regulations on sponsor requirements and CDER's greater concerns about investigator activities and compliance. Since there are so few sponsor /monitor/CRO inspections, CDER adopts a risk-based compliance approach i.e. they audit sponsors/monitors/CROs : involved in high priority applications and those which are the subject of a complaint.

IRB Inspectional Program

Under its human subject protection program, CDER conducts routine inspections of approximately 150 IRBs annually. CDER DSI officials claim that they attempt to focus their limited resources on IRBs, which review the highest volume of studies or the most complex and difficult studies. FDA periodically inspects each IRB which reviews research of FDA regulated products. These inspections are either surveillance or directed (center receives information that call into question the IRB practices). Those IRBs found to be in full compliance or with minor deficiencies are scheduled for reinspection in 5 years while those IRBs found to have major deficiencies are usually assigned for reinspection within one year. The documents which are collected during audits of IRBs are : IRB written procedures, IRB roster for the time period covered by the inspection, copies of IRB minutes and records of tracked studies (protocol, consent form, investigator brochure's and correspondence between IRB and the clinical Investigator). An IRB inspection may reveal significant regulatory deviations, which may lead to clinical investigator and/or sponsor inspection.

In Vivo Bioequivalence Inspection Program

Through its bioequivalence inspection program, the FDA inspects both clinical and analytical facilities to ensure the safety and quality of generic drugs (i.e., by ensuring the validity of bioequivalence data submitted not only in ANDAs (Abbreviated New

Drug Application), but also in some NDAs) as well as the safety of subjects participating in bioequivalence studies.

During these inspections, FDA investigators evaluate how well sponsors, monitors, contract research organizations, IRBs, and clinical and nonclinical investigational site staff have fulfilled their various responsibilities and commitments under GCP, study protocols, and other standards and regulatory requirements. The Establishment Inspection Report (EIR) generated under the BIMO program is:

a. *No Action Indicated (NAI):* No objectionable conditions or practices were found during an inspection (or the objectionable conditions found do not justify further regulatory action). In such a case FDA generally forwards a so-called "untitled letter" indicating that no compliance problems have been discovered.

b. *Voluntary Action Indicated (VAI):* Objectionable conditions or practices were found, but the agency is not prepared to take or recommend any administrative or regulatory action. In these cases the FDA generally forwards an "untitled letter" to identify the areas of non-major compliance problems found during the inspection. In the letter, the FDA encourages the site to address these areas, and may state that the agency will assess the site's activities in such areas during a future inspection.

c. *Official Action Indicated (OAI):* Regulatory and/or administrative actions will be recommended. An OAI classification means that the FDA discovered that a site or investigator was found to have objectionable practices or conditions that represent significant departure from FDA regulations.

Common Inspection Findings

Common problems encountered during inspections include: failure to follow the protocol (43%), record keeping errors (20%) and informed consent problems (25%), drug accountability issues (17%) and adverse event reporting issues (12%). Some of the significant violations include: enrollment of ineligible subjects, protocol deviations affecting safety, inadequate oversight of study personnel, failure to communicate with the IRB and data integrity issues.

The European Medicines Agency (EMEA)

The EMEA coordinates the evaluation and oversight of medicinal products throughout the 25 Member States comprising the European Union, plus the three European Economic Area (EEA) countries of Norway, Iceland, and Lichtenstein. The EMEA is directly involved in the centralized procedure, under which a medicine can gain access to the entire EU market through the submission and approval of a single marketing dossier.

Under the mutual recognition procedure, the EMEA's Committee for Medicinal Products for Human Use (CHMP) the GCP inspection program focuses largely on clinical trials and clinical data used to support marketing applications under the centralized procedure. Presently GCP inspections are conducted by EMEA only at the request of the scientific committee of CHMP for instance where the assessors of the centralized dossier want an inspection to be carried out to confirm information or because they have questions which can only be answered through an inspection.

Majority of the GCP inspections are carried out by inspectors from the relevant member state agencies. The Inspection of ongoing trials in the member states is carried out as part of their national inspection programs. EMEA can request the inspection reports if, for instance, the trials are subsequently included in a marketing authorization application to the centralized procedure.

To determine which inspectorates will actually carry out the inspection, a simple algorithm is followed. If the (Clinical Trial) site or sponsor to be inspected is located within an EU Member State, then the inspectorate of that member state leads the inspection. But, if the site is outside the EU, then mostly the inspectorate of the rapporteur or co-rapporteur agency for the centralized application procedure will carry out the inspection in the third country.

The UK's Medicines and Healthcare Products Regulatory Agency (MHRA)GCP Compliance Program

According to the MHRA, its GCP inspectors "assess compliance with the requirements of applicable GCP regulations and guidelines, by conducting inspections at the sites of pharmaceutical sponsor companies, contract research organizations, non-commercial organizations (hospital trusts, academic institutions, charitable organizations, etc.), investigational trial sites, clinical laboratories, GCP archives and other facilities involved in clinical research".

Interestingly, the MHRAs GCP Compliance Unit does not inspect Institutional Review Boards (IRB)/Research Ethics Committees (REC), although its inspections do ensure that the study related documents used in a study (e.g. informed consent form, protocol) were approved by the relevant IRB/REC. IRB/REC oversight is the responsibility of the Central Office for Research Ethics Committees (COREC), which is part of the National Patient Safety Agency, and a ministerial body called the UK Ethics Committee Authority (UKECA).

Japan's Ministry of Health, Labour, and Welfare (MHLW)

An independent administrative organization that sits outside Japan's Ministry of Health, Labour, and Welfare (MHLW) the Pharmaceutical and Medical Devices Agency (PMDA) is responsible for reviewing and approving new drugs and medical devices, monitoring the reliability of clinical trial and other scientific data submitted in product marketing applications, and consulting with industry on drug and device trials. Founded in April 2004, PMDA comprises 13 offices, including three offices directly involved in the review of new drugs. PMDA also reviews the documentation submitted in all new drug approval, re-examination and re-evaluation applications to ensure that the data comply with GCP, GLP and other relevant standards from both an ethical and scientific perspective.

Specifically, the agency reviews the data to ensure that the applications have been prepared appropriately based on the relevant study results and are consistent with Japan's criteria for reliability of application data. In addition PMDA undertakes on-site GCP reviews of hospitals/clinical study sites (including IRB) and drug sponsors to review the data submitted in support of pending marketing application.

Consequences of inspection

The consequences of problems found during audit can be significant, especially when they have an impact on a large amount of data for a pivotal study. The study at a particular site may be invalidated, if there were significant protocol deviations or underreporting of adverse events or concomitant therapies. Both the sponsor and the investigator would face consequences. These problems could delay the new drug approval or even result in a disapproved application. The investigator may be disqualified or restricted from conducting the clinical trials in future.

Indian Regulations

Presently no separate committee has been created under Drug Controller General of India for conducting Inspections of the clinical trials. But, Schedule-Y does list Audit Certificate as an appendix requirement (if available) under the Appendix II "Structure, Content and Format for Clinical Study reports."

SUMMARY AND CONCLUSION

Audit activities are aimed at independently assuring that the procedures for providing quality data, including QC activities, are being implemented as described in the SOPs. Audits are generally conducted for a sample of studies. However, audits are performed at all stages of the clinical trial process (e.g protocol audit, CRF audit, laboratory audit, CT report audit and investigator site audit, etc.). They provide assurance to management and others involved in the trial process that clinical research activities have resulted in work of the highest quality.

Inspections are the quality assurance activities performed by the regulatory authorities. They usually take place after few years after the trial was run. In addition to US FDA different regulatory authorities "(European, Japan, etc.) Have also begun inspecting clinical trials and other countries are currently putting in place compliance programs. Therefore, the likelihood of regulatory inspections at investigator site is increasing all the time.

ACKNOWLEDGEMENTS

I sincerely thank Ms Radhika for typing assistance and Dr Ravindra Ghooi Principal ICRI (Delhi campus) for reviewing and editing the article.

SUGGESTED READING

1. Nickols PC (2001). *Principles of Clinical Research,* Wrightson Biomedical Publishing Ltd.UK.
2. http://www.fda.gov/ora/compliance_ref/bimo/default.htm,
3. Spilker B (1991). *Guide to Clinical Trials*, Raven Press, New York.
4. The Global GCP Compliance Report 2006: US,EU and Japan.

Template: 1
Site Audit Check List

Protocol Title
Version :
Date of visit:
Study Site Code
Site Staff Present(Name & Designation)
Auditor's Name:
Site Monitor/ CRA:
Sponsor representative

Site Status No. of subjects screened:
No. of subjects enrolled:
No. of subjects withdrawn:
No. of active subjects:
No. of treatment-complete subjects:
No of monitoring visits:
No of monitoring visit follow-up letters:

1.0. INFORMED CONSENT ***(Review all ICFs)***

S.No	*Description*	*Yes*	*No*
1.1	Informed consent document, including amendments, on file for each participating subject?	☐	☐
1.2	Are the subjects given a copy of the signed ICFs, including amendments?	☐	☐
1.3	Current version of ICFs used (EC approved)?	☐	☐
1.4	If two versions of ICFs used in the study, whether filed the previous version in the ISF?	☐	☐
1.5	ICFs signed, dated and witnessed (as applicable)?	☐	☐
1.6	Consent approved prior to study procedures and/or screening, whichever is applicable?	☐	☐
1.7	Consent procedure documented in source documents/ progress notes?	☐	☐

Note: Any "No" requires comments

S. NO	*Comment*

2. ETHICS COMMITTEE (EC)

S.No	*Description*	*Yes*	*No*	*NA*
2.1	Did the EC approval letter list out the minimum quorum to be present during the EC meeting and the voting process?	☐	☐	
2.2	If so, does the quorum constitute the Schedule Y representations?	☐	☐	
2.3	Is the PI member of the EC?	☐	☐	☐
2.4	If so, did the PI abstain from voting process of the EC?	☐	☐	☐
2.5	If advertisements used, were they approved by the EC?	☐	☐	☐
2.6	Were periodic progress reports submitted to EC, if applicable?	☐	☐	☐

Note: Any "No" requires comments

S. No.	Comment

3.0 PROTOCOL ADHERENCE

S.No	*Description*	*Yes*	*No*
3.1	Inclusion/Exclusion (I/E) criteria met as per protocol?	☐	☐
3.2	Procedures performed as per the protocol	☐	☐
3.3	Protocol deviations, if any, documented and reported to IRB?	☐	☐

Note: Any "No" requires comments

Patient Nos. whose CRFs reviewed:

☐☐☐, ☐☐☐, ☐☐☐, ☐☐☐, ☐☐☐, ☐☐☐

Subject No. with protocol deviations:

☐☐☐, ☐☐☐, ☐☐☐, ☐☐☐, ☐☐☐, ☐☐☐

S. No.	Comment

4.0 ADVERSE EVENTS(AEs) and UNEXPECTED AES and SERIOUS ADVERSE EVENTS (UAEs & SAEs)

S.No	*Description*	*Yes*	*No*	*NA*
4.1	All Adverse Events (AEs) reported in the source documents recorded on AE log attached to CRFs?	☐	☐	☐
4.2	Are all Serious Unexpected Adverse Events (SUAEs) reported to IRB and Sponsor as per timeline requirements?	☐	☐	☐
4.3	Was EC notified of all SAEs received from Sponsor?	☐	☐	☐
4.4	Were all SAE Reports submitted to EC acknowledged?	☐	☐	☐

Note: Any "No" requires comments

S. No.	Comment

5.0 TEST ARTICLE(Investigational Product)

S.No	Description	Yes	No	NA
51.	Adequate record of CT Drug supplies receipt present?	☐	☐	☐
5.2.	Adequate record of dispensing, return and/ or destruction present?	☐	☐	☐
5.3.	Are the storage conditions according to protocol?	☐	☐	☐
5.4.	If a blinded study, adequate care taken to protect blind of the IP?	☐	☐	☐
5.5.	If blind broken, justification documented?	☐	☐	☐
5.6.	If the randomization codes are kept at the site, is there 24 hour access to the codes?	☐	☐	☐
5.7.	Are the IPs stored under lock and key and are accessible to designated personnel only?	☐	☐	☐

6.0 LAB REPORTS

S.No	Description	Yes	No	NA
6.1	Are all the lab reports of all the subjects received and filed in the respective subject folder/ file?			
6.2	Are all the lab test requisition forms (site copies) present?			
6.3	Do the dates and patient demographics for all the reports match with the test requisition forms?			
6.4	Are all the lab kits stored according to the labeled storage conditions?			
6.5	Are the lab kits stored under lock and key and access restricted to designated personnel only?			

7.0 INVESTIGATOR SITE FILE(Essential Documents)

S.No	*Description*	*Yes*	*No*	*NA*
7.1	Is copy of regulatory approval placed in file?	☐	☐	☐
7.2	Investigator Undertaking available?	☐	☐	☐
7.3	Signed Confidentiality Disclosure agreement available?	☐	☐	☐
7.4	Investigator's CV	☐	☐	☐
7.6	CVs of other study staff	☐	☐	☐
7.7	Signed Protocol/ amendment(s) signature page(S)?	☐	☐	☐
7.8	EC approved protocol/ amendment(s) present?	☐	☐	☐
7.9	Investigators Brochure/ amendment(s) and safety updates if any present?	☐	☐	☐
7.10	Fully executed Clinical Trial Agreement/ Financial contract present?	☐	☐	☐
7.11	Insurance Certificate present?	☐	☐	☐
7.12	Clinical Laboratory Accreditation/ certification present?	☐	☐	☐
7.13	Clinical Laboratory normal reference ranges present?	☐	☐	☐
7.14	Study site signature and responsibilities log present?	☐	☐	☐
7.15	Participant screen/enrollment/randomization log in study file	☐	☐	☐
7.16	Staff training records in study file present?	☐	☐	☐
7.17	All study related correspondence in study file present?	☐	☐	☐
7.18	Blank CRF	☐	☐	☐
7.19	CRF completion guidelines	☐	☐	☐
7.20	Is the Site Visit Log signed and dated by the CRA on each monitoring visit?	☐	☐	☐
7.21	Do the visit dates on the Site Visit Log match the Monitoring Report Dates?	☐	☐	☐

8.0 MISCELANEOUS

S.No	Description	Yes	No	NA
8.1	Appropriate delegation of authority to study staff?	☐	☐	☐
8.2	Tasks and responsibilities delegated to qualified personnel?	☐	☐	☐
8.3	Adequate investigator involvement in conducting orsupervising trial?	☐	☐	☐
8.4	Are the study documents stored under lock and key and restricted only to authorized personnel only?	☐	☐	☐
8.5	Is the document storage and archival location a secure one?	☐	☐	☐
8.6	Review of local laboratory performed?	☐	☐	☐

S. No.	Comment

Prepared By:

Name of the Auditor	
Signature and Date of Auditor	

Template: 2
Site Audit Report

Audit Date(s):	
Auditor Name:	
Protocol Title:	
Protocol Code:	
Site Code:	
Sponsor Name:	
CRO Name	
Project Manager:	
Name of the CRA:	
Auditees:	
Type of Audit:	
Communication Date:	

S. No. type	*QA Observations*	*Corrective Actions*
critical		
major		
minor		

Sign and Date of the Auditor	
Sign and Date of Head/designated person	

Template: 3
Quality Review Certificate Template

Date of Review
Type of Review
Protocol code
Site Code
Protocol Title:
Investigator Name
Name of QA person
Designation
Signature and Seal
Date __ __ / __ __ / __ __ __ __

25

Fraud and Misconduct in Clinical Research

JK Joshi

INTRODUCTION

Fraud and misconduct in clinical research has received intense attention in medical literature and the media in recent years.[1-6] This is partly due to the large increase in published clinical research in the last few decades; and partly due to the exposure of several 'high-profile' fraudulent reports in medical literature, commercial newsletters, and the lay press. Several cases of fraud have been detected by high index of suspicion, biostatistical incongruity,[7-9] good monitoring, and whistle-blowing.[2,10] Numerous clinical researchers, often persons of excellent repute and academic standing, as well as pharmaceutical medicine specialists committing scientific fraud have been detected, investigated, found guilty, and punished by due process of the law. Others have gone scot-free because their misconduct could not be proven 'beyond doubt' or by a 'preponderance of evidence'; or because they were genuinely unaware of the situation.

It is important for the clinical researcher to be aware of the definitions and the reasons of fraud and misconduct, so that they can more critically analyze published clinical research reports, and avoid accusations of misconduct and fraud in their own research programs due to ignorance of the exact definitions and scope of the terms fraud and misconduct. In view of the large number of clinical trials being planned in India, the subject assumes special importance for clinical researchers in India, so that their research methodology and reports are not tainted by inadvertent or designed fraud and/or misconduct.

The terms fraud and misconduct in clinical research, are difficult to define without attaching significant extra terminology, which would help define the degree of seriousness of the occurrence, and the penalties, which should be applied in cases of proven fraud or misconduct. By their very nature these episodes would pass off as genuine research, unless detected, and investigated either formally or informally. If proven, they must attract penalties according to current thinking on the issue; and if not proven, the investigation reports would certainly result either in a complete exoneration or a lingering doubt. It is therefore necessary that a quantification of the severity of the misconduct be built into its definition; and starting from a broad definition, attempts have been made to provide more specific descriptions of the various shades of fraud and misconduct that have been reported over the years.

The issue has been clouded with debate in recent years, as clinical research and researchers have increasingly been employed by commercially interested sponsors, which has led to questions on the relative rights of the investigator and the sponsor in the design of clinical research experiments, as well as the right to publish both positive as well as negative outcomes of the experiment. Several professional bodies have attempted to define fraud and misconduct in clinical research, and have unanimously ruled that suppression of the results of clinical studies that have failed to find what the sponsors were looking for could also constitute a form of fraud. Thus the definition of fraud and misconduct in clinical research appears to be evolving and this has been aptly summed up by Richard Smith in the Committee of Publication Ethics (COPE) Report 2000[1] where he writes that *"A universally agreed, operational definition of research misconduct is surely unachievable, but this does not mean that definitions should not be attempted. The act of trying to define misconduct will in itself be valuable, deepening our understanding of the issue. Similarly, the debate, which surrounds any definition, will be useful, and the definition can then be modified. But we will not reach the Holy Grail of a universally agreed, operational definition."*

In the six years since he wrote the above words, several occurrences and advances in codifying the issue have occurred, and in this chapter we shall try to put the issue in perspective.

DEFINITIONS OF FRAUD AND MISCONDUCT

While the United States Food and Drugs Administration uses the terms 'fraud' and 'misconduct' interchangeably, it can be argued that the terms "misconduct" and "fraud" constitute a continuum of acts ranging from minor deviations from good scientific practice, through minor or major scientific misconduct, to more extreme cases of fabrication and falsification of data obtained in clinical research.

Broadly, research misconduct is defined as "behavior by a researcher, intentional or not, that falls short of good ethical and scientific standards". However this definition is too rigorous and all inclusive and has been intensely debated and challenged.

The United States Food and Drugs Administration defines uses the terms fraud and misconduct interchangeably and "research fraud" is defined as 'the fabrication, falsification, plagiarism, or deception in proposing, carrying out, or reporting of research; or deliberate, dangerous, or negligent deviations from accepted practices in carrying out research'.

It includes failure to follow established protocols (e.g. consent), including those of the local research ethics committee if this failure results in unreasonable risk or harm to humans, other vertebrates or the environment, and facilitating of misconduct in research by collusion in, or concealment of, such actions by others.

It also includes intentional, unauthorized use, disclosure of or removal of, or damage to research-related property of another, including apparatus, materials, writings, data, hardware or software, or any other substances or devices used in or produced by the conduct of research.

It does not include honest error or honest differences in the design, execution, interpretation or judgment in evaluating research methods or results or misconduct unrelated to the research process. Similarly it also does not include poor research (aim, design, or execution) unless this encompasses the intention to deceive.

Integrity is defined as the use of honest and verifiable methods in proposing, performing, and evaluating research; and reporting research results with particular attention to adherence to rules, regulations, guidelines, and commonly accepted professional codes or norms.

The US Commission of Research Integrity defines research misconduct as "significant misbehavior that improperly appropriates the intellectual property or contributions of others, that intentionally impedes the progress of research, or that risks corrupting the scientific record or compromising the integrity of scientific practices" (Boxes 25.1 and 25.2).

Box 25.1: Consequences of misconduct and fraud in clinical research

Sponsor –	data validity compromised, submission jeopardized, additional costs
Investigator–	disqualification, fines, incarceration, legal expenses, ruined career
Institution –	lawsuits
Subjects –	safety at risk, loss of trust in clinical trial process

Box 25.2: Preliminary taxonomy of research misconduct[1]

1. Fabrication: invention of data or cases
2. Falsification: willful distortion of data
3. Plagiarism: copying of ideas data or words without attribution
4. Failing to get consent from an ethics committee for research
5. Not admitting that some data are missing
6. Ignoring "outliers" without declaring it
7. Not including data on side effects in a clinical trial
8. Conducting research in humans without informed consent or without justifying why consent was not obtained to an ethics committee
9. Publication of *post hoc* analysis without declaration that they were *post hoc*
10. Gift authorship
11. Not attributing other authors
12. Redundant publication
13. Not disclosing a conflict of interest
14. Not attempting to publish completed research
15. Failure to do an adequate search of existing research before beginning new research

Examples of misconduct include but are not limited to the following:

Misappropriation: Includes plagiarism or making use of information in breach of a confidentiality agreement.

Interference: Includes materially damaging any research related property (e.g., data, apparatus, reagents, reports, software, etc.) used or produced in the conduct of the research.

Misrepresentation: Includes the actions or deeds of an investigator who shall with intent to deceive, or in reckless disregard for the truth state or present material that is untrue, omit information/data that when presented as a whole represents inaccurate or false conclusions.

The Nordic countries and Britain have taken a different line from the Americans and opted for broad definitions. The Norwegian Committee on Scientific Dishonesty defines research misconduct as 'all serious deviation from accepted ethical research practice in proposing, performing, and reporting research'. [1]

RECENT HISTORY OF FRAUD CLINICAL RESEARCH

On Wednesday 11 January, 2006 Seoul National University concluded that Hwang Woo-Suk, a pioneer in stem cell research and a national hero in Korea, had fabricated much of his research. His claim in 2005 to have produced stem cells from adult cells had reverberated around the world because it opened up new ways to treat Parkinson's disease and other degenerative diseases. His disgrace was equally high profile, providing one of the most dramatic cases ever of scientific fraud.

The modern history of fraud in clinical research is supposed to have begun with the detection in 1974 of a leading scientist having committed fraud.[11] William Summerlin from the Sloan-Kettering Institute in New York, one of the world's leading biomedical research centres, claimed to have transplanted human corneas into rabbits. He also faked transplantation experiments in white mice by blackening patches of their skin with a pen; an extraordinarily crude form of forgery.

Another famous case is that of John Darsee, who worked in the department of cardiology at Harvard and was observed falsifying data. His boss, Eugene Braunwald, an eminent cardiologist, decided that this misconduct was an isolated incident and so did not fire him. A few months later, however, it became clear that results he had obtained in a study being conducted in several places were very different from those of the others. An investigation was started and went back to when he was an undergraduate. Many of his more than a 100 studies proved to be fraudulent and had to be retracted.

Case after case followed, but scientists were slow to respond. Eventually politicians became involved because much of the fraudulent research had been funded with public money, and after many bitter battles between scientists and politicians the Federal Office of Research Integrity (ORI) was founded. [11]

Between 1993 and 2002, 39 clinical trial staff were investigated for scientific misconduct by the Office of Research Integrity (ORI). Analysis of ORI case records reveals practices regarding workload, training and supervision that enable misconduct. Considering the potential effects on human subjects protection, quality and reliability of data, and the trustworthiness of the clinical research enterprise, regulations or guidance on use of clinical trial staff ought to be available.

Current ORI regulations do not hold investigators or institutions responsible for supervision and training of clinical trial staff. Given the important issues at stake, the definition of research misconduct should encompass the intentional or negligent mismanagement of scientific projects. Individual institutions and professional associations not only can but also should adopt stricter standards of conduct than those reflected in federal regulations.

Two key examples of Indian researchers who have been in the news recently for allegations of fraud include Dr RK Chandra and Dr RB Singh. Dr Chandra, an eminent nutritionist has allegedly produced fraudulent data on the effectiveness of multivitamin in improving cognitive dysfunction in elderly patients.[12] Suspicion of the data presented arose because of values that were abnormal, and a full investigation uncovered the fact that the data was concocted. The study nurse testified before the committee enquiring into the matter. Dr Chandra resigned from the institute and migrated to another. A full investigation of his previous publications appeared to prove that he had a long record of similar fabrications and falsifications.[13]

The *BMJ* published a paper by Ram B Singh in 1992.[14] Doubts were raised about that paper and subsequent manuscripts submitted by the same author. In the absence of answers from the author, the *BMJ* tried to find a legitimate authority to investigate and adjudicate on its concerns, and failed. The *BMJ* decided it had no option other than to publish an article documenting its efforts.[15] However this took more than 10 years, and still there is confusion about whether fraud was committed knowingly or not.

Prevalence

There is little information about the prevalence of research integrity problems in the scientific literature. In a mail survey[16] of 549 authors who had published reports of pharmaceutical clinical trials from 1998 to 2001 that appeared in the Cochrane Database of Systematic Reviews authors were asked about fabricated data or misrepresentations of research in three contexts:

i. The target study (the report from which their name was obtained),
ii. Another study they had participated in, or
iii. A study that they personally knew about.

Replies were received from 64% of authors with valid addresses. Two authors (1%) reported that the target article misrepresented the research. Almost 5% reported fabrication or misrepresentation in a study they had participated in the last 10 years, and 17% of authors personally know about a case of fabrication or misrepresentation in the last 10 years from a source other than published accounts of research misconduct.

It was concluded that fraud and misrepresentation in clinical trials appear to be rare on a per-published report basis. However, they occur sufficiently frequently that scientists have a significant chance of participating in a project affected by fraud or misrepresentation during their research careers. These rates of exposure justify vigorous efforts to prevent research misconduct.

The debates on how best to define research misconduct continue, and so there can be no definitive answer on how commonly it occurs. Minor forms of misconduct are common, but we have less good information on the prevalence of serious misconduct. The USA, which has far more biomedical research than any other country and where the problem has been taken seriously for two decades, has seen hundreds of cases, many of them serious. It has also recently had a series of high profile cases in the physical sciences. The committees of scientific integrity in the Nordic countries have seen dozens of cases, few of them serious.[17] Britain has had about two dozen general practitioners participating in trials conducted by pharmaceutical companies found guilty of serious professional misconduct for research fraud. There have also been about a dozen cases among medical academics. Germany has had a very high profile case in molecular biology, which sent shockwaves through the German academic system. The Dutch have also had a prominent professor found guilty of serious research misconduct, but many countries have had few cases.

Mike Farthing, the chairman of the Committee on Publication Ethics who has been the dean of three medical schools, estimates that major institutions in Britain have roughly one serious case a year. That means about 50 cases a year.

To discover what types of scientific misconduct are most likely to influence the results of a clinical trial a Delphi survey of expert opinion with three rounds of consultation was done.[18] The setting was the non-industry clinical trial "community". Participants were experts identified from invitees to a previous Medical Research Council consultation on clinical trials. 32 out of the 40 experts approached agreed to participate. Thirteen forms of scientific misconduct were identified, for which there was majority agreement (>50%) that they would be likely or very likely to distort the results and majority agreement (>50%) that they would be likely or very likely to occur. Of these, the over-interpretation of 'significant' findings in small trials, selective reporting and inappropriate subgroup analysis were the main themes.

According to this expert group, [18] the most important forms of scientific misconduct in clinical trials are selective reporting and the opportunistic use of the play of chance. Data fabrication and falsification were not rated highly because it was considered that these were unlikely to occur. Registration and publication of detailed clinical trial protocols could make an important contribution to preventing scientific misconduct.

Detection of Fraud and Misconduct in Clinical Research

Despite a widely recognized need, most countries still have no coherent system to deal with scientific misconduct. Committees have been established by the national medical research councils in Denmark (1992), Norway (1994), and Sweden (1997), and by the Ministry of Education in Finland (1994), to deal with scientific misconduct, i.e., to initiate preventive measures, to investigate alleged cases, or both. Each committee includes both scientifically and legally qualified members. Cooperation between the four Nordic committees has shown close agreement on specific issues and cases, despite minor differences in definitions, organization, and procedures.[1]

To detect fraud and misconduct in clinical trials it is necessary to have a high index of suspicion. Several investigative reporters have spotted inconsistencies in clinical reports and with the use of biostatistical expertise it has amply been demonstrated in many studies that fraud occurred at the data record or data entry stage.[7-9] This, is probably the most serious kind of fraud viz. the willful falsification of data; fortunately it appears to be detectable when scrutinized by experts.

A common method of fraud in drug trials conducted in individual or group practices is to use the same subject in several trials without an adequate wash-out period as mandated by the protocol and informed consent form. These have been reported in literature in the past, but no data on actual prevalence of this malpractice is available.

Several instances of doctoring of blots using photoshop have been reported prompting a strongly worded editorial on the prevalence and precautions to be observed against this type of fraud.[4]

Ghost authorship is said to occur when an individual who has contributed substantially to a manuscript is not named in the byline or acknowledgments. Ghost authors are sometimes employed by industry to prepare clinical trial results for publication. A well-known expert is then credited as author so as to lend an air of credibility and neutrality to the manuscript. Ghost authorship is difficult to detect, and in most cases has been revealed as such only after investigative work by lawyers, journalists, or scientists. Ghost authorship is ethically questionable in that it may be used to mask conflicts of interest with industry.

Investigation of Fraud

A finding of research misconduct depends on three requirements. First, there must be 'a significant departure from accepted practices of the relevant research community'. Secondly, the misconduct must be 'committed intentionally or knowingly, or recklessly'. Thirdly, the allegations must be proved 'by a preponderance of evidence'.[19]

Those procedures normally have four stages:

i. An inquiry to determine whether the allegation or related issues warrant further investigation,
ii. When warranted, an investigation to collect and thoroughly examine evidence,
iii. A formal finding, and
iv. Appropriate disposition of the matter.

It is important to note that any new polices and procedures to deal with allegations of violations of the integrity of research must be incorporated into existing institutional polices and procedures for employment and academic conduct. Institutions must be vigilant to provide all parties with appropriate due process. It is reasonable to expect at different situations may require specific accommodations to insure the protection of the rights of all involved individuals. Institutions should be alert to possible harm to any parties throughout the process. An institution may choose, following an investigation, to refer any "findings" to its standing disciplinary procedures, or to develop processes specific to cases of fraud and misconduct in research.

Biostatisticians should be involved in preventing fraud (as well as unintentional errors), detecting it, and quantifying its impact on the outcome of clinical trials. We use the term 'fraud' specifically to refer to data fabrication (making up data values) and falsification (changing data values). Reported cases of such fraud involve cheating on inclusion criteria so that ineligible patients can enter the trial, and fabricating data so that no requested data are missing.[20] Such types of fraud are partially preventable through a simplification of the eligibility criteria and through a reduction in the amount of data requested. These two measures are feasible and desirable in a surprisingly large number of clinical trials, and neither of them in any way jeopardizes the validity of the trial results. With regards to detection of fraud, a brute force approach has traditionally been used, whereby the participating centres undergo extensive monitoring involving up to 100% verification of their case records. The cost-effectiveness of this approach seems highly debatable, since one could implement quality control through random sampling schemes, as is done in fields other than clinical medicine. Moreover, there are statistical techniques available (but insufficiently used) to detect 'strange' patterns in the data including, but no limited to, techniques for studying outliers, inliers, overdispersion, underdispersion and correlations or lack thereof. These techniques all rest upon the premise that it is quite difficult to invent plausible data, particularly highly dimensional multivariate data. The multicentric nature of clinical trials also offers an opportunity to check the plausibility of the data submitted by one centre by comparing them with the data from all other centres. Finally, with fraud detected, it is essential to quantify its likely impact upon the outcome of the clinical trial. Many instances of fraud in clinical trials, although morally reprehensible, have a negligible impact on the trial's scientific conclusions.

Investigations into allegations of fraud may result in various outcomes, including:

i. A finding of fraud
ii. A finding of serious scientific misconduct short of fraud
iii. A finding that no culpable conduct was committed, but serious scientific errors were discovered
iv. A finding that no fraud, misconduct or serious scientific error was committed.

Penalties for Proven Fraud and Misconduct

Responsibility for determining the nature and severity of disciplinary action should be specified in an institution's policy. This may, but need not necessarily, be done through the institution's regular faculty disciplinary or grievance procedures. Many actions may be available to the institution. Examples may include:

- Removal from particular project
- Letter of reprimand
- Special monitoring of future work
- Probation
- Suspension
- Salary reduction
- Rank reduction
- Termination of employment

Consideration also should be given to formal notification of other concerned parties who may not till then have been notified, such as:

- Sponsoring agencies, funding sources
- Co-authors, co-investigators, collaborators
- Editors of journals in which fraudulent research was published
- State professional licensing boards
- Editors of journals or other publications other institutions, sponsoring agencies, and funding sources with which the individual has been affiliated
- Professional societies
- Where appropriate, criminal authorities.

Prevention of Fraud

Ethics and integrity in clinical research is essential and a set of criteria to facilitate rigorous assessment of the integrity of clinical and basic research protocols has been proposed. These include:

- An integrity-focused training of researchers to adhere to specific laboratory procedure and tactics which discourage fraud
- Appointment of external reviewers to detect unusual and suspicious experimental process or data patterns; and
- Encouragement of multicenter trials.

Although it is widely recognized that the sole determinant of scientific misconduct is the individual investigator's integrity, a number of precautions may effectively reduce the prevalence of this event, which may affect the status and trends of biomedical research in general.

Prevention through monitoring and a quality assurance (QA) program is an integral protective mechanism against fraud in the modern clinical trial because it helps identify the problem at an early stage. The key parameters on which a good QA program depends on the desire (on part of all professionals involved in the trial including the IRB) to ensure proper protection of trial subjects. It necessitates the provisions made to ensure that protocol-related procedures are carried out and that monitoring is carried out to the standards prescribed by the regulators.

Most serious pharmaceutical companies ensure that their internal standards are higher than the benchmark set by regulators, because they have a lot more to lose if an unsafe drug is discovered soon after marketing authorization is obtained.

Fraud and misconduct is more common on the part of an individual investigator and there are numerous examples of investigators who have forged data on non-existent patients, duplicated electrocardiograms and X-rays, and collected money for investigations that were never done. It is the task of the clinical trial monitor appointed by the sponsor or funding agency to ensure that adequate safety measures to prevent fraud are in place before beginning clinical research.

Proper selection of investigator is possible in countries where the ratio of clinician to number of research projects available is high. With dwindling patients' pools available for clinical research and a high number of doctors and drug companies seeking to conduct clinical trials, it is often not possible to select an investigator of integrity except by paying high honoraria for conducting the trial. This in turn may bias the investigator towards producing favorable results and therefore properly conducted training in the ethics of clinical research including fraud and misconduct is essential if this (fraud and misconduct) is to be avoided.

RESPONSIBILITIES OF INDIVIDUAL INVESTIGATORS

Research is a self-regulating profession. To be successful, professional self-regulation relies on conscientious participation by all members of the profession. Individual researchers are expected to

- Maintain a high standard of integrity at all times in all of their research activities
- Assume responsibility for their actions
- Take misconduct or alleged misconduct seriously
- Report apparent misconduct by other researchers.

RESPONSIBILITIES OF RESEARCH INSTITUTIONS

Research institutions should foster an environment that discourages all research misconduct. They should develop and use procedures for receiving and investigating reports of research misconduct and inform scientific and administrative staff of the procedures for responding to allegations of research misconduct and of the importance of complying with these procedures. They must take immediate, appropriate action when research misconduct is suspected or alleged to have occurred at the institution and investigate and rule on suspicions or allegations of research misconduct and report both the start of and the results of a formal investigation (not the initial inquiry) into an allegation of research misconduct to the office of research integrity. An annual report on file on possible research misconduct with the designated federal agency.[21,22]

In recent years, regulatory and law enforcement authorities responsible for combating fraud and abuse have focused greater attention on the scientific research process, in particular, the process of seeking reimbursement for research costs, the process of performing clinical research, and the potential improper remuneration of researchers or research subjects. The US Federal False Claims Act allows the government to recover treble damages plus substantial penalties from persons who knowingly submit false claims or make false statements to the government. It has been used to achieve a number of multimillion-dollar settlements with research institutions. There have also been instances of temporary suspension of research activities at a number of prominent institutions and the investigation of illegal "inducements" or "kickbacks" provided by manufacturers to researchers and by research institutions to patients.[22]

A basic tenet of research ethics is that the data from clinical trials should be fully analyzed and published. If the knowledge gained from trials is not shared, subjects have been exposed to risk needlessly. Moreover, participants in future studies may be harmed because earlier results were not available. These principles are reflected in federal regulations regarding the protection of human subjects, which define research as "a systematic investigation designed to develop or contribute to generalizable knowledge." [6]

The spate of publications investigating the phenomenon of fraud and misconduct in clinical research have prompted the International Committee of Medical Journal Editors (IMCJE) and national governmental bodies such as the USFDA, NICE, and the EMEA, as well as private bodies such as the ABPI to issue guidelines regarding what can and should be published and why every clinical trial needs to be registered and its results should be available in the public domain for anyone who wishes to see them.

A group of UK medical journal editors has issued best practice guidelines to help stem research misconduct, a problem characterized by its chairman as "endemic" in the United Kingdom and the United States.[23]

The guidelines, drawn up by the Committee on Publication Ethics (COPE), are intended to promote and safeguard intellectual honesty at all stages in the research and publication cycle, from initial study design onwards.

Ethical approval, data analysis, competing interests, authorship, peer review, redundant publication, and editors' duties are among the key areas addressed. The guidance also advises editors on how to investigate suspected cases and what sanctions may be suitably applied when misdemeanors have been detected.

The review, Scientific Misconduct Investigations 1993-1997, shows that falsification, fabrication, and plagiarism were the most common findings.

COPE was established in 1997 as an ad hoc self help group for medical journal editors. Since then it has grown into a properly constituted international body of editors seeking to improve the integrity of biomedical publications. Its members meet six times a year to advise each other on how to handle anonymized cases that present ethical dilemmas for the editors involved. The cases and the committee's advice are posted on COPE's website, which has now become a fully searchable resource for anyone interested in publication ethics, with an extensive archive covering the whole gamut of issues from redundant publication, undeclared conflicts of interest, authorship disputes, plagiarism, and data fabrication.

From the start, COPE's emphasis has been on the misdemeanors of authors and peer reviewers. But editors behave badly too, or simply make mistakes. COPE's code of conduct for editors, launched at the end of 2004, recognized the need to raise the standards of editorial behavior by setting out broad principles of good conduct. These include:

- Publishing corrections and apologies where necessary
- Retracting fraudulent or erroneous articles[24]
- Publishing cogent criticisms from readers
- Ensuring research articles conform to ethical guidelines
- Keeping editorial and commercial decisions separate
- Declaring their own and other people's conflicts of interest
- Dealing properly with complaints, and,
- Making all reasonable efforts to ensure that allegations of misconduct are properly investigated.

Six main sources of relevant international guidelines on conducting, reporting, and editing research:

- Council of International Organizations for Medical Sciences (CIOMS)
- World Medical Association (WMA)
- Consolidated Standards of Reporting Trials (CONSORT)
- International Committee of Medical Journal Editors (ICJME)
- World Association of Medical Editors (WAME)
- Committee on Publication Ethics (COPE)

A new independent body called the UK Panel for Health and Biomedical Research Integrity was launched recently to tackle biomedical research misconduct in the United Kingdom, but its powers will be limited to providing advice and promoting good practice.[25] This has been initially set up as a three year project, and its first priority will be to develop a code of practice applicable to universities, the NHS, and industry. The panel will also support whistleblowers reporting cases of alleged research fraud in addition to offering training, seminars, and advice on how to investigate suspected cases of research malpractice. Its functions will be "promotional and advisory" as it will not be able to investigate research misconduct, which will remain the responsibility of the employer or research sponsor.

CONCLUSIONS

Misconduct and fraud can take several forms and can be perpetrated at several stages in the clinical trial process. It has been estimated that the probability of this occurrence is higher in commercial institution sponsored clinical trials than in academic research. But it occurs with unfailing certainty in both and is due to the usual reasons ascribed viz. financial gain, and career advancement. Clinical trials involving human subjects face increased scrutiny and regulation by academic councils and governmental bodies are essential to minimize the occurrence of fraud or misconduct. Almost all aspects of clinical trial conduct need to be examined, from how patients are recruited and how they give informed consent, to the relationship between the researchers and the company sponsoring the research if fraud in clinical research is to be discouraged. Further discouragement to commit fraud can be induced by the publication and dissemination of institutional policies regarding what constitutes fraud and how it must be detected, reported, investigated, and the penalties that are possible if fraud is proven.

REFERENCES

1. Smith R. What is Research Misconduct? The Cope Report. Br Med J 2000;317.
2. Ankier SI. Dishonesty, misconduct, and fraud in clinical research: an international problem. J Int Med Res 2002;30:357-65.
3. Eliades T, Athanasiou AE, Papadopulos JS. Ethics and fraud in science: a review of scientific misconduct and applications to craniofacial research. World J Orthodont 2005;6(3):226-32.
4. Neill US. Stop Misbehaving. J Clin Investigation 2006;116(7):1740-1.
5. Smith R. Research misconduct: the poisoning of the well. J Royal Soc Med 2006; 99:232-37.
6. Steinbrook R. Gag clauses in clinical trial agreements. N Engl J Med 2005; 352:2160-2.
7. Akhtar-Danesh N, Dehgan-Kooshkghazi M. How does correlation structure differ between real and fabricated data sets? BMC Medical Research Methodology 2003;3:18-26.
8. Al-Marzouki S, Evans S, Marshal T, Roberts I. Are these data real? Statistical methods for the detection of data fabrication in clinical trials. Br Med J 2005;331:267-70.
9. Buyse M, George SL, Evans S, et al. The role of biostatistics in the prevention, detection and treatment of fraud in clinical trials. Statistical Medicine 1999;18(24):3435-51.
10. Rhodes R, Strain JJ. Whistleblowing in academic medicine. J Med Ethics 2004;30:35-39.
11. Dingell JD. Misconduct in Clinical Research (Shattuck Lecture). N Engl J Med 1993,328(22):-1610-5.
12. Chandra RK. Effect of vitamin and trace element supplementation on cognitive function in elderly subjects. Nutrition 2001;7:709-12.
13. Smith R. Investigating the previous studies of a fraudulent author. Br Med J 2005;331:288-91.
14. Singh RB, Rastogi SS, Verma R, Laxmi B, Singh R, Ghosh S, Niaz MA. Randomised controlled trial of cardioprotective diet in patients with recent acute myocardial infarction: results of one year follow up. Br Med J 1992;304:1015-9.
15. White E. Suspected research fraud: difficulties in getting at the truth. Br Med J 2005;331:281-88.
16. Gardner W, Lidz CW, Hartwig KC. Authors' reports about research integrity problems in clinical trials. Contemporary Clinical Trials 2005; 26(2):244-51.

17. Nylenna M, Andersen D, Dahlquist G, Sarvas M, Aakvaag A. Handling of scientific dishonesty in the Nordic countries. National Committees on Scientific Dishonesty in the Nordic Countries. Lancet 1999;354(9172):57-61.
18. Al-Marzouki S, Roberts I, Marshal T, Evans S. The effects of scientific misconduct on the results of clinical trials: a Delphi Survey. Contemporary Clinical Trials 2005;26(3):331-7.
19. Mello MM, Brennan TA. Due process in investigations of research misconduct. New Engl J Med 2003;349(13):1280-86.
20. Lexchin J, Bero LA, Djulbegovic. Pharmaceutical industry sponsorship and research outcome and quality: a systematic review. Br Med J 2003; 326:1167-70.
21. Association of American Universities, Framework for Institutional Policies and Procedures to Deal With Fraud in Research; 1988.
22. Kalb PE, Koehler KG. Legal issues in scientific research. JAMA 2002; 287(1):85-91.
23. Jones J. UK Watchdog issues guidelines to combat medical research fraud. Br Med J 1999;319:660.
24. Sox HC, Drummond R. Research misconduct, retraction and the cleansing of medical literature: lessons from the Poehlman case. Ann In Med 2006; 144:609-13.
25. Cole A. UK launches panel to tackle research misconduct. Br Med J 2006; 332:871.

26

An Introduction to Medical Writing

Natasha Das

INTRODUCTION

Broadly speaking, medical writing is about communicating medical and other health related data and information to a range of audience in many different formats using both the print and the electronic media. It has evolved from being a rather underappreciated field to an important career choice today. Over the last few years, the market for medical writers has been growing at a steady rate of about 15% per year.[1] The demand for medical writers is thus ever increasing. In the United States, the American Medical Writers Association (AMWA), an organization that sets industry standards for medical writers, has been around since the 1940s. Even in India, medical writers have been around for more than 50 years now.[2] However, it is only recently, with the advent of global clinical trials into the country, that the critical role played by the medical writer, is being appreciated well. A good quality medical writing can often cut short the delays encountered in drug submission and approval by the regulatory authorities.

TYPES OF MEDICAL WRITERS

There are basically two types of medical writers: [3]

- Scientific Medical Writers
- Marketing Medical Writers.

Scientific medical writers are those who may have a degree in medicine, pharmacy or science. A marketing medical writer does not necessarily need to have a strong science background. An English degree or a degree in journalism may suffice for such medical writers. The type of work that the scientific medical writer and the marketing medical writer undertake may differ.

Scientific medical writers usually undertake the following types of work:[4]

- Medical journal abstracts and articles

- Advertising copy for medications and other products
- Medical education material for doctors and other healthcare professionals
- Internet content for healthcare professionals
- Pharmaceutical marketing and advertising
- Product monographs
- Physician speeches
- Physician presentations
- Posters
- Sales training manuals
- Clinical trial documents including
  - Trial protocols
  - Investigator brochures
  - Investigational new drug annual reports
  - Informed consent forms
  - Manuscripts
  - Integrated summary documents
  - Trial reports — draft and final
- Policy documents
- Research grant writing
- Editing.

Examples of work that the marketing medical writers usually take up include:

- Newsletters
- Patient education materials
- Public relations materials
- Proof readings
- Editing
- Training manuals
- Marketing materials
- Advertising copy
- Internet content for the general public
- Magazine articles (both for the popular press and for the professional press)
- Proposal writing

A scientific medical writer can also do much of the work done by a marketing medical writer.

QUALIFICATIONS AND SKILLS REQUIRED

Understanding of Basic Medical Terminologies

Medical writing is all about health and medicine. Hence, a medical writer needs to have basic knowledge of medical terminologies. An Internet search does provide a huge volume of information about any particular term, but it is not always the best thing to do. In order to write an original article or to conduct substantive editing, a medical writer needs to have a clear perception and understanding about the topic he/she is going to work.

Educational Qualification

The term "medical writer" seems to imply that you need to have a medical degree, which is not at all necessary. Most successful medical writers are not doctors. A medical degree is not needed for medical writers in the UK, USA and Australia. However, in some European countries a medical training may be essential.[5] There are no specific requirements for medical writers to possess any specific qualifications or experience.

Many medical writers are scientists who end up writing. Pharmaceutical and biotech companies usually prefer hiring "scientists who can write". In contrast, marketing medical writers, who do not do much technical writing; need not possess a medicine or science degree, though these degrees are always an added advantage.

A good understanding of the human anatomy and physiology is necessary for being a medical writer. It's an advantage to have knowledge about diseases and their treatments. However, in most cases, you gain knowledge about the specific diseases, as you get involved in various medical writing projects.[6] Each new project is a learning experience.

Basic Computer Knowledge

In this new world of IT revolutions, a basic knowledge of computers has become essential for all kinds of writers. Keyboard skills are almost mandatory if you choose to be employed in an agency. Freelance writers do have the freedom of choice, though. They may provide a handwritten manuscript of their writings to the clients. However, even clients who hire freelancers always seem to prefer having a soft copy of the document as well. Proofreading and editing on a soft copy of a write-up using a computer is always easier than getting such things done manually on paper.

Even for a freelance medical writer who chooses to write by hand, computer skill is needed. He/she may need to refer to the Internet at times for her projects. Internet search engines have made information and data access from across the world much faster and easier.

Good Writing and Word Processing Skills

As in case of any writing career, a medical writer too needs to possess good skills in writing and word processing. Most employers today ask for a writing test as part of the interview to judge your writing skills. The format of the test may be variable; depending mainly on the type of writing the employers might be involved in.

The features assessors look for in a good quality medical writing have been discussed later in the chapter.

Ability to Provide Customized Writing

A good medical writer first defines his/her target audience and accordingly pitches the use of language and the style of writing. When writing for a medical journal with medical professionals as the target audience one has to be more practical in the approach using relevant medical terminology. However, when writing a health feature for a popular magazine or newspaper, the medical writer has to be more creative. Excess use of medical terminology must be avoided. An article for a medical journal may require the writer to follow certain uniform guidelines. Moreover, there may be certain specific requirements for different medical journals too. Therefore, a good medical writer should be able to provide customized writing to his/her clients.

Ability to Meet Deadlines

"A deadline is a negative inspiration. Still it's better than having no inspiration at all.[7]" As a medical writer, one shall have to meet very tight deadlines during working on most projects. It is important for a writer to produce a piece that is acceptable to the editor or the client by the publication deadline.

CHARACTERISTICS OF GOOD MEDICAL WRITING

There does not seem to be a slow down in the market for medical writers soon. More and more people are today considering medical writing as a career option. However what clients are looking for today, is a high quality medical writing. The characteristics of good medical writing include:

Thorough Research

Medical and health information is updated constantly. The Internet has made it possible for writers to conduct extensive research before writing on any topic. Articles published in the current issues of journals contain the latest information. A good medical writing is always based on a thorough web search and literature search.

Data Accuracy

Medical writing is all about health and illness. What a medical writer writes should ideally be 100% accurate. The validity of data should be crosschecked with a peer-reviewed and approved database. When in doubt, a more thorough search may be required. A good medical writing always cites the source of medical information.

Conciseness

A high quality medical writing is always concise and to the point. A good medical writer puts in only the information that is relevant to the target audience. The writing should be concise, eliminating excessive wordiness.

Logical Flow of Information

Medical writing is not like creative writing. The text must be logical from the reader's point of view. A good medical writer's manuscript should not have contradictory, redundant and illogical sentences or paragraphs.

Readability

This is perhaps the toughest part for the medical writer to deal with. The medical information is available in various databases. The accuracy of the data can be checked using certain methods. There are also certain guidelines available to follow in order to maintain the logical flow of this information. But the biggest challenge to the medical writer is to keep the reader interested while reading the article. A high quality medical writing should be accessible and comprehensible to the target audience. It should be easy for them to read. The message should be clear.[8]

AVAILABLE TRAINING

Most medical writers get their training on-the-job.[9] Progress is made based on the feedback they receive. Short courses and workshop often provide an insight into the field of medical writing. Some organizations also offer formal training for medical writers. The European Medical Writers Association (EMWA) offers a training program in medical writing. [10] In North America, the American Medical Writers Association (AMWA) provides specialist training and recognized examinations.[11] Other players in the field who offer training in medical writing include. The center for professional innovation and education.[12]

In India, medical writing training is usually sporadic, taught occasionally in pre-conference workshops, and in a handful of institutions.[13] With a huge volume of work from the US and Europe being outsourced to India, it is become increasingly necessary to have well trained medical writers in the country. Some companies that hire medical writers do have a provision of in-house training. But most of the training is still gained on the job from a more experienced medical writer. Extensive reading and constructive criticism of other writers also helps improve the skills of a medical writer.

PRIMARY EMPLOYER

Opportunities of work for medical writers are available at various types of set ups. These include pharmaceutical companies, contract research organizations (CROs), academic medical centers, hospital/healthcare systems and medical communication agencies. Medical writers are also hired to develop content for electronic and audiovisual media. However, many medical writers also work as freelancers.

FREELANCE MEDICAL WRITING

The field of freelance medical writing is growing very fast. The main reason for this is that computers and the Internet allow writers to work from distances more easily. Freelance writers also have a greater control over their jobs, work potential and time. But freelance medical writing is not just a bed of roses.

As a freelancer working from home, one has to be disciplined. He has to attract business on his own and should be ready to face rejection from several companies. There is an uncertainty of work, lack of training opportunities and a limited feedback.

But freelancers do have the independence and opportunity to exercise choice, get a variety of projects to work on and can work at flexible work hours. Those with the necessary experience can think of freelance medical writing as a career option.

CONCLUSIONS

Medical writing is certainly not a new avenue for work opportunities. It has been there for many decades now. However, all these years it had lacked professional status, finesse and recognition. Today, with the deluge of clinical trials, more and more drugs are in the pipeline for regulatory approvals making medical writers much sought after. The market for medical writers in India has been on the increase. Companies in the US and some European countries are outsourcing a part of their medical content development to medical communication agencies and freelance medical writers in India. The long-term future of medical writers in India thus looks bright.

REFERENCES

1. Medical Writing Market Appreciation. The Center Watch Monthly. July 2004;11(7).
2. Journal of Postgraduate Medicine. JPGM GOLD CON: 50 years of Medical Writing. [Homepage on the Internet]. Last accessed on August 24, 2006. Available at URL: http://www.jpgmonline.com/goldcon.asp
3. American Medical Writers Association-The Delaware Valley Chapter. Toolkit for New Medical Writers. [Homepage on the Internet]. Last accessed on August 24, 2006. Available on URL: http://www.amwa-dvc.org/toolkit/index.shtml
4. American Medical Writers Association-The Delaware Valley Chapter. Toolkit for New Medical Writers. [Homepage on the Internet]. Last accessed on August 24, 2006. Available on URL: http://www.amwa-dvc.org/toolkit/index.shtml.
5. Discovering New Medicines: Careers in Pharmaceutical Research and Development, PD Stonier, John Wiley and Sons Ltd. 1994.
6. European Medical Writers Association. Medical Writing. [Homepage on the Internet] ©2002. Last accessed September 1, 2006. Available at URL: http://www.spd.dcu.ie/careersweb/publications/EMWA% 20Careers%20Leaflet%20medical% 20writing.pdf#search=%22MEdical% 20writing%20%2B%20EMWA%22.

7. Brown RM. Study Guides and Strategies. Writing under deadlines. [Homepage on the Internet] Last revised on June 02, 2006. Last accessed on September 1, 2006. Available at URL: http://www.studygs.net/wrtstr12.htm.
8. Words Work. Readability and Medical Writing. [Homepage on the Internet] Last accessed on September 2, 2006. Available at URL: http://wordswork.com/samples/medical/readability.html.
9. Opportunities in Medical Writing. [Homepage on the Internet] Last accessed on September 2, 2006. Available at URL: http://www.abpi-careers.org.uk/htm/medicalwrit_opp.htm.
10. The EMWA Professional Development Programme. [Homepage on the Internet] Last accessed on September 2, 2006. Available at URL: http://www.emwa.org/EPDP.html.
11. Discovering New Medicines: Careers in Pharmaceutical Research and Development, PD Stonier, John Wiley and Sons Ltd. 1994.
12. Introduction to Effective Medical Writing. [Homepage on the Internet] Last accessed on September 2, 2006. Available at URL: http://www.cfpie.com/showitem.aspx?productid= 047.
13. Sriganesh V. Challenges of Bridging the Information Literacy Gap for the Practice of Evidence Based Healthcare In India. [Homepage on the Internet] Last accessed on September 3, 2006. Available at URL: http://www.icml9.org/program/track9/public/documents/Vasumathi%20Sriganesh 105007.doc.

27 Communication Skills

Rajani Mathur

DEFINING COMMUNICATION

Communication is defined as the process through which two or more people exchange ideas and improve the understanding between them. Communication is the exchange of facts, ideas, opinions or emotions by two or more people. Alternatively, business communication may be defined as a process that involves transmission and accurate replication of ideas for the purpose of eliciting actions that will accomplish organizational goals. Communication takes many forms such as oral or written. Effective communication skills such as writing and speaking well, displaying proper etiquette and listening attentively have gained tremendous importance with time, to the extent that they often determine career success. Communication shortcomings of individuals and the importance of communication at professional front explain why one should improve communication skills.

Basically, there are four aspects to communication, namely, something has to be communicated; there must be at least one receiver; ensure that the communication is understood and lastly, feedback of the communication. Communication is a multi-step process involving a sender, message, encoding of the message, channel of transmission of the encoded message, receiver, decoding of the message by the receiver and feedback.

GOALS OF COMMUNICATION

Effective communication helps to achieve the following goals:

1. Planning
2. Effective operations
3. Decision-making
4. Controlling and coordinating
5. Motivation

6. Improving human relations
7. Improving workers' participation
8. Facilitating change
9. Improving public relations.

CATEGORIZING COMMUNICATION

Communication activities in any organization fall into three broad categories: internal-operational, external-operational and personal.

Internal-operational Communication

All communication that occurs in conducting work is classified as internal operational. It is a major part of the formal communication and may take the form of letters, circulars, memos, posters and instructions. This is the communication among the professional workers that is done to implement the operating plan. It is done for conducting work within a set-up. It includes giving orders, oral exchanges among workers about work matters, preparing for changes, discourage misinformation, assembling reports and writing email. Characteristically, internal communication is large in size, often complex and requires cooperation within workers.

External-operational Communication

Work related communication that is conducted with people and groups outside the system is external-operational communication. It includes communication with government agencies, business partners, other organizations, suppliers, service companies, customers and the general public.

Personal Communication

Communication that is not operational or is without operating plan for the business can be classified as personal communication. It is nonbusiness related exchanges of information and feelings among people. Personal communication is important as it affects the attitude of workers towards each other and their assignments. This directly affects their efficiency and productivity. Nature of conversation at workplace is a major determinant of the prevailing attitude. Heated words and flaming tempers affect the productive efforts of the team. Another factor that affects the workplace attitude is the extent of personal communication permitted. Denial of personal communication leads to emotional upset. On the other hand, excessive personal communication interferes with the work done. With regard to personal communication, middle ground is the best.

COMMUNICATION NETWORK OF THE ORGANIZATION

Information flow in an organization forms a complex network. The network represents the pattern of contacts among the members of the organization. The choice of network would depend upon the nature of channels of communication and the number of people involved. It determines the speed, accuracy and smoothness with which the message flows in the organization.

Most of the flow is in the form of 'chain network.' The chain may be 'downward' along formal lines-from top executives down to the workers. Through these formal channels, bulk of the communication that the business needs to operate-orders, instructions, working information, either through intranet, email or portals.

Simultaneously, executive of good organizations understand the utility of open 'upward' communication also. Activity reports, opinions, ideas, suggestions, complaints and grievances constitute upward communication. These channels help to open channels to be better informed of the status of things on the front line. They also have found that information from the lower levels can be important in achieving company goals. Further, they help to demonstrate concern for each employee and create a feeling of belongingness.

Transmission of information among positions of the same level is defined as 'horizontal communication.' It is often a by-product of vertical communication. With increasing specializations of work fields, there are fewer opportunities for horizontal communication. Consequently, since it has fewer implications of authority and status, it poses fewer difficulties.

The secondary or informal network runs parallel to the formal network. It consists of that part of personal communication that follows no set pattern and is ever changing and infinitely complex structure linking all the members of the organization. This form of communication is also regarded as 'circular network.' It is made complex by the fact that people belong to more than one group and the group memberships and the links between and among groups are continually changing. Known as grapevine, in management literature, this communication network is highly effective and often tapped by managers. It is a constructive tool that when utilized optimally, can help to develop effective course of an organization.

BARRIERS IN COMMUNICATION

Anything or anyone that causes breakdowns, distortions and inaccuracy in communication is a 'barrier' in communication. The barriers in communication may be classified and enumerated as below:

1. Relationship: The status or position of an individual in an organization may often pose as an obstacle in communication.
2. Semantic barriers: The same words may mean different things to different people.
3. Filtering: People involved in the communication process may screen or filter out

certain information and pass on only that information that they think is good for them. This sort of weeding at individual level may pose as barrier in complete and effective communication.

4. Perceptual errors: A person's perception is determined by various factors. He tries to comprehend the information from his own perspective, which creates complexities.
5. Closed mind: The inability of the people to be receptive to new or different ideas is referred to as closed mind. It often poses as the biggest challenge almost insurmountable, in effective communication.
6. Lack of ability to communicate: Some people may not have the skills to communicate their ideas or information. Training can overcome this up to a certain extent.

INNATE LIMITATIONS OF COMMUNICATION PROCESS

The process of communication suffers from limitations that are innate to the process. Firstly, the intended meaning is not always perceived. Due to mental filters different meanings sent may differ from meanings received. No two minds have identical storehouses of words, gestures, facial expressions and the meaning attached to these may vary from one individual to another. These differences may lead to errors in communication. Efforts in the direction of developing skilled communication are aimed at reducing these errors.

Secondly, the meaning is in the mind and not in the words or other symbols used. Accuracy in choosing the words, symbols determine only one half of the communication. Their interpretation depends on the mental and sensory abilities of the receiver.

Lastly, the symbols of communication are imperfect. One reason for this is that the symbols or words are at best crude substitutes for the real thing. Communication is also imperfect because communicators vary in their ability to convey their thoughts.

COMMUNICATION SKILLS IN CLINICAL RESEARCH

With regard to clinical research, communication takes centrestage and involves-planning and co-ordination of activities at different centers by the clinical monitor, communication between physician and volunteers, setting and achieving target dates, data compilation, preparing study reports, writing papers for publication, giving presentations, organizing and conducting meetings etc.

Writing for Right Effect

Written communication is a must in science. Written communication requires clarity of thought and understanding. The impact of the work has to be produced in right perspective without either blowing it out of proportion or undermining it. A conscious effort has to be made to cut out the repetitive use of clichés, which at time may become an individual's trademark. These clichés occur when the thought process is looped and is not a favorable reflection of the mental state.

Negative results should also be communicated with equal vigor, because they also lend to the unique meaning and understanding of the puzzle. However, it often becomes imperative to double-check the negative results before communicating them as they may stir up resistance and hurt goodwill.

The written communication process differs from oral in the following ways:

1. It is more likely to involve creative effort on the part of the communicator. This form of communication needs to be well thought out and may even begin in the mind rather than as a reaction to a message received.
2. A second difference is the time between the cycles. Written communication enjoys longer cycles of communication between the sender and the receiver. In face-to-face communication, cycles occur fast, and in rapid succession. In written communication, some delay occurs. Faster modes of written communication include-fax and email.
3. As they provide record, written word has greater weightage than the spoken word, but may communicate over extremely long period of time. Proper conceptualization, presentation and then transmission of reports and records, letters through proper channels of hierarchy may prove to be the obstacles in rapid communication.

The communication process shows the need for adaptation. By adaptation, it is meant that fitting the message to meet the needs of the specific reader. Thus, for effective communication, one should clearly define the person to whom the communication is targeted. It is essential to keep the message simple so as to be understood. The adaptation has to be made keeping in mind the lowest level that the communication needs to reach. Not doing so and only concentrating on the higher levels, is self-defeating. Selecting the right words is a part of adaptation. For this, the basic requirement would be to be conversant with the language, knowledge of the reader and one's own judgement. The stress is on simplicity as:

1. Many people tend to write at a difficult level.
2. The writer usually knows the subject better than the reader.
3. The result of research support simplicity.

Use of familiar everyday words to communicate helps enhance understanding. Generally, short words are better tools of communication and stiff and difficult words should be avoided. Technical words are vital when communicating with circle of people from one's own background and knowledge. But they prove to be barriers in understanding, when used with laypersons. Legal language is often used. Sometimes it is not possible to replace these words with simpler words. To avoid these as becoming stumbling blocks, they may be at first used with caution, taking care to define them at the outset. This may be followed by their more common use. Selection of words needs caution. Strong and emphatic words are helpful in clarifying and removing ambiguity. Inadvertently they may raise hackles and lead to friction with higher ups. Sometimes it is useful to mellow down or tone down the effect and weaker words prove to be useful here. It is always better to be aware of the implications of the words used especially if they are discriminatory in terms of gender, race or nationality. To avoid any misunderstandings arising because of these, some sensitivity has to be practiced in the choice of words. Arousing negative reactions is counter to the whole idea of communication.

Writing Sentences and Paragraphs that Communicate

Sentences should be adapted in accordance to target readers. Short (16-18 words) and simple sentence structures help to communicate the meaning effectively. Short sentences can be achieved in two ways, either by limiting the sentence content or by economizing on the words used.

Limiting the content requires to mentally select thought units and putting them down in separate sentences. However, overdoing this should be avoided, as it may lend a choppy effect. Using alternate shorter words are often useful. It always pays to eliminate surplus words and avoid superfluous language. Words may only be repeated for effect and emphasis not for presenting the matter in a roundabout manner. Every item should be given its due importance, which may require some judgment.

In a paragraph, there should be cohesiveness. It should talk on one aspect and succinctly explain it. Placing unrelated ideas in a sentence violates unity. The sentences should be linked and show relationship. Excessive detailing often leads to off tracking from the main idea. If however, the detail is important, it should be put in separate, small sentence. Paragraphing also helps to show logical thinking, organization. Deciding on the content is again a matter of personal judgment. Ultimately, each paragraph acts as a move towards the goal.

Report Making

Preparing clinical study report should not be considered as a platform to demonstrate great literary skills. Rather, it is a non-ambiguous, technical, well-organized, structured, error-free presentation of data and its underlying concept.

Since July 1996, it has become mandatory for all clinical study reports to follow the guidelines set at International Conference on Harmonization (ICH Guideline, 1995). This uniformity ensures acceptability at all forums. It is part of sponsor's responsibility under good clinical practice (GCP) to ensure that a final clinical study report is written. Most companies issue standard operating procedures (SOPs) and/or guidelines for clinical report writing, which should be consulted at the outset. Writing in accordance with the ICH guidelines, and the use of templates, dispenses with the challenge of working out a report structure.

An 'integrated' clinical study report is a single report incorporating clinical and statistical descriptions, presentations and analyses, with appendices containing the protocol, sample case report forms, investigator-related information etc. It should also identify, describe and clarify any deviations that were made from the protocol.

After submission of the report, it undergoes review and approval process. It is advisable to maintain copies of drafts and final version, for quick reference at a later date.

Scientific Paper Writing

Scientific paper writing is a well-defined task, with out much leeway. It is mandatory to prepare the manuscript in strict accordance with the guidelines defined by the editorial team of the journal and compiled under the heading *Instructions to Authors*.

Every scientific publication can be broadly divided into three parts: Refractory part, Publication proper and Appended parts. The Refractory part of any publication is its first title page. It may contain the title of the report along with the name of the working group members who have contributed towards the compilation of the project report. Briefly the address of the center and contact numbers may also be recorded in the refractory portion. This is usually followed by the publication proper. Most of the publications communicating scientific contents follow the IMRAD pattern that includes-Introduction, Materials and Methods, Results and Discussion.

In general, Introduction of any report should discuss the "origin" of the concept. The available information and facts, historical background and all other details leading towards the development of the study are comprehensively presented. This is followed by a discussion of the existing lacunae and the "need" to conduct the study in context of the existing information. A complete justification of the study design and the objective behind each investigation should be succinctly presented, so that the reader may be in no doubt regarding the importance of the study. The Discussion portion of the report explains the findings of the study and how they help in enhancing the understanding on the subject. However, it would also be apt to discuss the limitations of the study either in design or implementation and possible recommendations for future studies that may be planned in the field. In the end, a short summary and conclusions drawn from the study may be enumerated.

An appended part of any publication includes legends of tables and figures, acknowledgements, financial sponsorship, conflict of interest and bibliography. While writing the references in the bibliography, utmost care needs to be taken. All citations in the text section should be enumerated here. Extra unquoted references should be completely deleted. Most importantly, the references should be in one consistent pattern, usually defined clearly by the journal where the manuscript is intended to be submitted.

Adding Graphics

Any form of illustrations, which may include charts, pictures, diagrams and maps are categorized under the graphic section of the report. The graphics are useful tools, which should be planned appropriately so as to enhance and uplift any report or presentation. The main aim of the graphics is to simplify and present an important point of the study. Comprehending and assimilating text is dependent on the skills of the individual. Hence, it is prone to misunderstanding, missing the punch line or distortions. On the other hand, graphics are not subject to these limitations. Therefore, they help to convey salient points in an easy manner that may be comprehended by all. It is important to lay stress on the content of the graphics, as the main aim of putting one in a report is to supplement the text and not replace. The position, size, shapes, borders and colors of the graphics need special care. Ideally, they should be placed near the reference text in the report.

Common errors seen in graphics are of three type- error of scale, error of format and error of context. Error of scale is where there is a distortion of scale with no uniformity of scale within the graphic. It should be aimed that in one's zeal to prepare beautiful graphics, one does not overdo it such that font, background, grids, shading are garish and distract the viewer's attention from the main content. These errors of format are the most common and should be avoided.

Verbal Communication

A formal oral presentation is one of the commonest albeit the toughest form of communication. The onus of its success usually lies with one individual and completely dependent on his skills. Therefore, it needs to be prepared thoroughly, with special emphasis on organizing the structure, how to hold audience's attention, convey the contents effectively and authentically.

Verbal communication carries greater implications than written communication. Firstly, it is a direct face-to-face communication where the effect can be seen and perceived immediately. The choice of words and the manner of speaking lend a meaning that written form can never achieve. The presentation should have the 3C's of crispness, clarity and conciseness.

Economizing on the use of words does not imply leaving out essentials. Expressing anger or disregard of the audiences' viewpoint/suggestions/query can be blasphemous and is rarely justified. It is self-defeating and kills the spirit of scientific exchange and interaction. A courteous, sincere but strong approach is often found to be most successful.

It is advisable to make any presentation in terms of "we" rather than "I" or "you". Many reasons can be cited in the favor. Firstly, all results in the presentation being presented by an individual is actually the sum total of the collective effort of the entire team in different capacities. Secondly, it indicates joint responsibility and helps to avoid laying the blame on any individual.

Nonetheless, some points common to both verbal and written communication exist. Exaggerated sentences that seem to be overselling reflect insincerity. Emphasizing a point is better achieved by taking care of the four points in the plan of discussion - position, space, structure and mechanical means.

Position

The beginnings and endings of any communication carry more emphasis than the center parts. It may be explained on the basis of fresh mental energy and receptivity of the recipient. Hence, it is important to summarize in the end and highlight the "take home message" so that any points that may have been missed during the course are re-highlighted.

Space

In order to highlight any point, it is necessary to provide it space. The percentage of talk-time devoted in verbal communication, or text space in written communication, inadvertently reflects its importance. To achieve the desired effect, information on each item has to aptly fill the space allocated to it.

Structure

Explaining succinctly is the main aim of communication. A good communicator is one who can explain the complex in simple terms. For this, the utility of short sentences cannot be overemphasized. These factors together define the structure of the verbal communication. Care should be taken to avoid clubbing the more important information with less important one.

Mechanical Device

The use of mechanical device implies any external or physical aid like quotation mark, underscore, italics, boldface, solid capital, lines, arrow and color that may be used to emphasize the content. Pictorial representation, flowchart and diagrams are the most commonly used mechanical aids used in scientific communication.

Visual Aids

Simple flip charts, overhead projector transparencies (acetates), computer-generated slides, video, multimedia presentation constitute commonly used visual aids during an oral presentation. The choice of aid depends on its availability, feasibility, budget, amount of preparation time and most importantly, comfort level of the speaker in using the aid.

Slides prepared using the Microsoft PowerPoint software, have drastically transformed and elevated the standards of oral preparation. They offer the advantage of being cheap, quick and easy to prepare, without much technical assistance and easily conjunct with Internet. The picture quality is digital with no dependence on pixel properties of any printer. Unlike acetates or 35mm slides, this form of aid can be easily and quickly appended according to the fancies of the speaker. There are unlimited styles of slide preparation most speakers maintain their trademarks. Consequently, it is the most commonly used form of visual aid, and provided by most organizers of the meetings, world over.

Shorter Means of Communication

This is a form of communication that is essentially not under the purview of scientific communication, but forms the backbone of all day-to-day communication. It includes communication of ideas, results, problems and their solutions, decisions, memorandums, future directions and targets etc within a system using aids like internet, intranet, email, fax, short messaging service and teleconferencing.

In this era of outsourcing research, multicentric research co-ordination, this mode of communication becomes necessity. Communicating via these modes has transcended into an essential skill from desirable skill. Shorter means of communication are replacing traditional ink and paper as faster, more reliable and cheaper means of communication. These aids find wide use as they help to create a paper-free workplace, allow formal and informal communication, transmission of high security documents and information for general viewing, in the same vein. Use of satellite-aided-teleconferencing helps to conduct interviews and review meetings within a small group without traveling long distances. It reduces the expenses, saves time and manpower.

CONCLUSION

Since, time immemorial, man has been devising means of enhancing the speed and accuracy of communication. From an era when beating drums was considered as an effective means of communication, we have advanced to a system, where at the touch of a button, instant messages can be sent to innumerable people separated by thousands of kilometers. However, these advancements in technology and increasing reliance on machines for communication, have inadvertently lead to a fall in inter-personal skills. Thus, the need of the hour is to rediscover these ingrained skills for achieving effective communication.

SUGGESTED READING

1. Docherty M and Smith R. The case for structuring the discussion of scientific papaers. Br Med J 1999;318:1224-25.
2. Carson A, Gutgesell HP, Pinsky WW, McNamara DG. The 10-minute talk: organization, slides, writing and delivery. Am Heart J 1986; 111: 193-203.
3. ICH guidelines- www.nihs.go.jp/dig/ich/ichindexe.html.

28 Requirements and Guidelines to Undertake Clinical Trials in India

Schedule Y (Amended Version)

S K Gupta

CLINICAL TRIAL

Definition of Clinical trial "Clinical trial" means a systematic study of new drug(s) in human subject(s) to generate data for discovering and/or verifying the clinical, pharmacological (including pharmacodynamic and pharmacokinetic) and/or adverse effects with the objective of determining safety and/or efficacy of the new drug. ".

APPROVAL FOR CLINICAL TRIAL

(i) Clinical trial on a new drug shall be initiated only after the permission has been granted by the Licensing Authority under rule 21 (b), and the approval obtained from the respective Ethics Committee(s). The Licensing Authority as defined shall be informed of the approval of the respective institutional Ethics Comittee(s) as prescribed in Appendix VIII, and the trial initiated at each respective site only after obtaining such an approval for that site. The trial site(s) may accept the approval granted to the protocol by the Ethics Committee of another trial site or the approval granted by an independent Ethics committee (constituted as per Appendix VIII), provided that the approving ethics Committee(s) is/are willing to accept their responsibilities for the study at such trial site(s) and the trial site(s) is/are willing to accept such an arrangement and that the protocol version is same at all trial sites.

(ii) All trial investigator(s) should possess appropriate qualifications, training and experience and should have access to such investigational and treatment facilities as are relevant to the proposed trial protocol. A qualified physician (or dentist, when appropriate) who is an investigator or a sub-investigator for the trial, should be responsible for all trial-related medical (or dental) decisions. Laboratories used for generating data for clinical trials should be compliant with Good Laboratory Practices. If services of a laboratory or a facilities outside the country are to be availed, its/their name(s), address(s) and specific services to be used should be stated in the protocol to avail Licensing Authority's permission to send clinical trial related samples to such laboratory(ies) and/or facility(ies). In all cases, information about laboratory(ies)/facilities to be used for the trial, if other than those at the investigation site(s), should be furnished to the Licensing Authority prior to initiation of trial at such site(s).

(iii) Protocol amendments, if become necessary, before initiation or during the course of a clinical trial, all such amendments should be notified to the Licensing Authority in writing along with the approval by the Ethics Committee which has granted the approval for the study. No deviations from or changes to the protocol should be implemented without prior written approval of the Ethics committee and the Licensing Authority except when it is necessary to eliminate immediate hazards to the trial subject(s) or when change(s) involve(s) only logistic or administrative aspects of the trial. All such exceptions must be immediately notified to the ethics committee as well as to the Licensing Authority. Administrative and/or logistic changes in the protocol should be notified to the Licensing Authority within 30 days.

Responsibilities of Sponsor

(i) The clinical trial sponsor is responsible for implementing and maintaining quality assurance systems to ensure that the clinical trial is conducted and data generated, documented and reported in compliance with the protocol and Good Clinical Practice (GCP) guidelines issued by the Central Drugs Standard Control Organization, Directorate General of Health Services, Government of India as well as with all applicable statutory provisions. Standard operating procedures should be documented to ensure compliance with GCP and applicable regulations.

(ii) Sponsors are required to submit a status report on the clinical trial to the Licensing Authority at the prescribed periodicity.

(iii) In case of studies prematurely discontinued for any reason including lack of commercial interest in pursuing the new drug application, a summary report should be submitted within 3 months. The summary report should provide a brief description of the study, the number of patients exposed to the drug, dose and duration of exposure, details of adverse drug reactions (Appendix XI), if any, and the reason for discontinuation of the study or non-pursuit of the new drug application.

(iv) Any unexpected serious adverse event (SAE) (as defined in GCP guidelines) occurring during a clinical trial should be communicated promptly (within 14 calendar days) by the sponsor to the Licensing Authority and to the other investigator(s) participating in the study (see Appendix XI).

Responsibilities of the Investigator(s)

The investigator(s) shall be responsible for the conduct of the trial according to the protocol and the GCP guidelines and also for compliance as per the undertaking given in Appendix VII. Standard operating procedures are required to be documented by the investigators for the tasks performed by them. During and following a subject's participation in a trial, the investigator should ensure that adequate medical care is provided to the participant for any adverse events. Investigator(s) shall report all serious and unexpected adverse events to the sponsor within 24 hours and to the Ethics Committee that accorded approval to the study protocol within 7 working days of their occurance.

Informed Consent

(i) In all trials, a freely given, informed, written consent is required to be obtained from each study subject. The Investigator must provide information about the study verbally as well as using a patient information sheet, in a language that is non-technical and understandable by the study subject. The Subject's consent must be obtained in writing using an 'Informed Consent Form.' Both the patient information sheet as well as the informed consent form should have been approved by the Ethics Committee and furnished to the Licensing Authority. Any changes in the informed consent documents should be approved by the Ethics Committee and submitted to the Licensing Authority before such changes are implemented.

(ii) Where a subject is not able to give informed consent (e.g. an unconscious person or a minor or those suffering from severe mental illness or disability), the same may be obtained from a legally acceptable representative (a legally acceptable representative is a person who is able to give consent for or authorize an intervention in the patient as provided by the law(s) of India). If the Subject or his/her legally acceptable representative is unable to read/write—an impartial witness should be present during the entire informed consent process who must append his/her signatures to the consent form.

(iii) A checklist of essential elements to be included in the study subject's informed consent document as well as a format for the informed consent form for study subjects is given in Appendix V.

Responsibilities of the Ethics Committee

(i) It is the responsibility of the Ethics Committee that reviews and accords its approval to a trial protocol to safeguard the rights, safety and well being of all trial subjects. The Ethics Committee should exercise particular care to protect the rights, safety and well being of all vulnerable subjects participating in the study, e.g., members of a group with hierarchical structure (e.g., prisoners, armed forces personnel, staff and students of medical, nursing and pharmacy academic institutions), patients with incurable diseases, umemployed or impoverished persons, patients in emergency situation, ethnic minority groups, homeless persons, nomads, refugees, minors or others incapable of personally giving consent. Ethics committee(s) should get document 'standard operating procedures' and should maintain a record of its proceedings.

(ii) Ethics Committee(s) should make, at appropriate intervals, an ongoing review of the trials for which they review the protocol(s). Such a review may be based on the periodic study progress reports furnished by the investigators and/or monitoring and internal audit reports furnished by the sponsor and/ or by visiting the study sites.

(ii) In case an Ethics Committee revokes its approval accorded to a trial protocol, it must record the reasons for doing so and at once communicate such a decision to the investigator as well as to the Licensing Authority.

Human Pharmacology (Phase I)

(i) The objective of studies in this phase is the estimation of safety and tolerability with the initial administration of an investigational new drug into human(s). Studies in this phase of development usually have non-therapeutic objectives and may be conducted in healthy volunteers subjects or certain types of patients. Drugs with significant potential toxicity e.g., cytotoxic drugs are usually studied in patients. Phase I trials should preferably be carried out by Investigators trained in clinical pharmacology with access to the necessary facilities to closely observe and monitor the subjects.

(ii) Studies conducted in Phase I, usually intended to involve one or a combination of the following objectives:

(a) Maximum tolerated dose: To determine the tolerability of the dose range expected to be needed for later clinical studies and to determine the nature of adverse reactions that can be expected. These studies include both single and multiple dose administration.

(b) Pharmacokinetics, i.e., characterization of a drug's absorption, distribution, metabolism and excretion. Although these studies continue throughout the development plan, they should be performed to support formulation development and determine pharmacokinetic parameters in different age groups to support dosing recommendations.

(c) Pharmacodynamics: Depending on the drug and the endpoints studied, pharmacodynamic studies and studies relating to drug blood levels (pharmacokinetic/ pharmacodynamic studies) may be conducted in healthy volunteer subjects or in patients with the target disease. If there are appropriate validated indicators of activity and potential efficacy, pharmacodynamic data obtained from patients may guide the dosage and dose regimen to be applied in later studies.

(d) Early measurement of drug activity: Preliminary studies of activity or potential therapeutic benefit may be conducted in Phase I as a secondary objective. Such studies are generally performed in later phases but may be appropriate when drug activity is readily measurable with a short duration of drug exposure in patients at this early stage.

Therapeutic Exploratory Trials (Phase II)

(i) The primary objective of Phase II trials is to evaluate the effectiveness of a drug for a particular indication or indications in patients with the condition under study and to determine the common short-term side-effects and risks associated with the drug. Studies in Phase II should be conducted in a group of patients who are selected by relatively narrow criteria leading to a relatively homogeneous population. These studies should be closely monitored. An important goal for this phase is to determine the dose(s) and regimen for Phase III trials. Doses used in Phase II are usually (but not always) less than the highest doses used in Phase I.

(ii) Additional objectives of Phase II studies can include evaluation of potential study endpoints, therapeutic regimens (including concomitant medications) and target populations (e.g., mild versus severe disease) for further studies in Phase II or III. These objectives may be served by exploratory analyses, examining subsets of data and by including multiple endpoints in trials.

(ii) If the application is for conduct of clinical trials as a part of multi-national clinical development of the drug, the number of sites and the patients as well as the justification for undertaking such trials in India shall be provided to the Licensing Authority.

Therapeutic Confirmatory Trials (Phase III)

(i) Phase III studies have primary objective of demonstration or confirmation of therapeutic benefit(s). Studies in Phase III are designed to confirm the preliminary evidence accumulated in Phase II that a drug is safe and effective for use in the intended indication and recipient population. These studies should be intended to provide an adequate basis for marketing approval. Studies in Phase III may also further explore the dose-response relationships (relationships among dose, drug concentration in blood and clinical response), use of the drug in wider populations, in different stages of disease, or the safety and efficacy of the drug in combination with other drug(s).

(ii) For drugs intended to be administered for long periods, trials involving extended exposure to the drug are ordinarily conducted in Phase III, although they may be initiated in Phase II. These studies carried out in Phase III complete the information needed to support adequate instructions for use of the drug (prescribing information).

(iii) For new drugs approved outside India, Phase III studies need to be carried out primarily to generate evidence of efficacy and safety of the drug in Indian patients when used as recommended in the prescribing information. Prior to conduct of Phase III studies in Indian subjects, Licensing Authority may require pharmacokinetic studies to be undertaken to verify that the data generated in Indian population is in conformity with the data already generated abroad.

(iv) If the application is for the conduct of clinical trials as a part of multi-national clinical development of the drug, the number of sites and patients as well as the justification for undertaking such trials in India should be provided to the Licensing Authority along with the application.

Post-marketing Trials (Phase IV)

Post-marketing trials are studies (other than routine surveillance) performed after drug approval and related to the approved indication(s). These trials go beyond the prior demonstration of the drug's safety, efficacy and dose definition. These trials may not be considered necessary at the time of new drug approval but may be required by the Licensing Authority for optimizing the drug's use. They may be of any type but should have valid scientific objectives. Phase IV trials include additional drug-drug interaction(s), dose-response or safety studies and trials designed to support use under the approved indication(s), e.g. mortality/morbidity studies, epidemiological studies etc.

Studies in Special Populations

Information supporting the use of the drug in children, pregnant women, nursing women, elderly patients, patients with renal or other organ systems failure, and those on specific concomitant medication is required to be submitted if relevant to the clinical profile of the drug and its anticipated usage pattern. Any claim sought to be made for the drug product that is not based on data submitted under preceding items of this Schedule should be supported by studies included under this item of the Schedule (Appendix I, item 8.3).

***(1) Geriatrics.* Geriatric patients should be included in Phase III clinical trials (and in Phase II trials, at the sponsor's option) in meaningful numbers, if—**

(a) The disease intended to be treated is characteristically a disease of aging; or

(b) The population to be treated is known to include substantial numbers of geriatric patients; or

(c) When there is specific reason to expect that conditions common in the elderly are likely to be encountered; or

(d) When the new drug is likely to alter the geriatric patient's response (with regard to safety or efficacy) compared with that of the non-geriatric patient.

(2) Pediatrics

(i) The timing of pediatric studies in the new drug development program will depend on the medicinal product, the type of disease being treated, safety considerations, and the efficacy and safety of available treatments. For a drug expected to be used in children, evaluations should be made in the appropriate age group. When clinical development is to include studies in children, it is usually appropriate to begin with older children before extending the trial to younger children and then infants.

(ii) If the new drug is for diseases predominantly or exclusively affecting pediatric patients, clinical trial data should be generated in the pediatric population except for initial safety and tolerability data, which will usually be obtained in adults unless such initial safety studies in adults would yield little useful information or expose them to inappropriate risk.

(iii) If the new drug is intended to treat serious or life-threatening diseases, occurring in both adults and pediatric patients, for which there are currently no or limited therapeutic options, pediatric population should be included in the clinical trials early, following assessment of initial safety data and reasonable evidence of potential benefit. In circumstances where this is not possible, lack of data should be justified in detail.

(iv) If the new drug has a potential for use in paediatric patients – paediatric studies should be conducted. These studies may be initiated at various phases of clinical development or after post-marketing survelliance in adults if a safety concern exists. In cases where there is limited paediatric data at the time of submission of application – more data in paediatric patients would be expected after marketing authorisation for use in children is granted.

(v) The pediatric studies should include:
   (a) Clinical trials,
   (b) Relative bioequivalence comparisons of the paediatric formulation with the adult formulation performed in adults, and
   (c) Definitive pharmacokinetic studies for dose selection across the age ranges of pediatric patients in whom the drug is likely to be used. These studies should be conducted in the pediatric patient population with the disease under study.

(vi) If the new drug is a major therapeutic advance for the pediatric population – the studies should begin early in the drug development , and this data should be submitted with the new drug application.

(vii) Pediatric subjects are legally unable to provide written informed consent, and are dependent on their parent(s)/ legal guardian to assume responsibility for their participation in clinical studies. Written informed consent should be obtained from the parent/ legal guardian. However, all paediatric participants should be informed to the fullest extent possible about the study in a language and in terms that they are able to understand. Where appropriate, pediatric participants should additionally assent to enrol in the study. Mature minors and adolescents should personally sign and date a separately designed written assent form. Although a participant's wish to withdraw from a study must be respected, there may be circumstances in therapeutic studies for serious or life-threatening diseases in which, in the opinion of the investigator and parent(s)/legal guardian, the welfare of a pediatric patient would be jeopardized by his or her failing to participate in the study. In this situation, continued parental/legal guardian consent should be sufficient to allow participation in the study.

(viii) For clinical trials conducted in the pediatric population, the reviewing Ethics Committee should include members who are knowledgeable about pediatric, ethical, clinical and psychosocial issues.

(3) Pregnant or nursing women

(i) Pregnant or nursing women should be included in clinical trials only when the drug is intended for use by pregnant/nursing women or foetuses/nursing infants and where the data generated from women who are not pregnant or nursing, is not suitable.

(ii) For new drugs intended for use during pregnancy, follow-up data (pertaining to a period appropriate for that drug) on the pregnancy, fetus and child will be required. Where applicable, excretion of the drug or its metabolites into human milk should be examined and the infant should be monitored for predicted pharmacological effects of the drug.

Post-marketing Surveillance

(i) Subsequent to approval of the product, new drugs should be closely monitored for their clinical safety once they are marketed. The applicants shall furnish Periodic Safety Update Reports (PSURs) in order to:

(a) Report all the relevant new information from appropriate sources;

(b) Relate these data to patient exposure ;

(c) Summarize the market authorization status in different countries and any significant variations related to safety; and

(d) Indicate whether changes should be made to product information in order to optimize the use of the product.

(ii) Ordinarily all dosage forms and formulations as well as indications for new drugs should be covered in one PSUR. Within the single PSUR separate presentations of data for different dosage forms, indications or separate population need to be given.

(iii) All relevant clinical and non-clinical safety data should cover only the period of the report (interval data). The PSURs shall be submitted every six months for the first two years after approval of the drug is granted to the applicant. For subsequent two years – the PSURs need to be submitted annually. Licensing Authority may extend the total duration of submission of PSURs if it is considered necessary in the interest of public health. PSURs due for a period must be submitted within 30 calendar days of the last day of the reporting period. However, all cases involving serious unexpected adverse reactions must be reported to the licensing authority within 15 days of initial receipt of the information by the applicant. If marketing of the new drug is delayed by the applicant after obtaining approval to market, such data will have to be provided on the deferred basis beginning from the time the new drug is marketed.

(iv) New studies specifically planned or conducted to examine a safety issue should be described in the PSURs.

(v) A PSUR should be structured as follows:
   (a) A title page stating: Periodic safety update report for the product, applicant's name, period covered by the report, date of approval of new drug, date of marketing of new drug and date of reporting,
   (b) Introduction,
   (c) Current worldwide market authorization status,
   (d) Update of actions taken for safety reasons,
   (e) Changes to reference safety information,
   (f) Estimated patient exposure,
   (g) Presentation of individual case histories,
   (h) Studies,
   (I) Other information,
   (j) Overall safety evaluation,
   (k) Conclusion,
   (l) Appendix providing material relating to indications, dosing, pharmacology and other related information.

Special Studies: Bioavailability/Bioequivalence Studies

(i) For drugs approved elsewhere in the world and absorbed systemically, bioequivalence with the reference formulation should be carried out wherever applicable. These studies should be conducted under the labeled conditions of administration. Data on the extent of systemic absorption may be required for formulations other than those designed for systemic absorption.

(ii) Evaluation of the effect of food on absorption following oral administration should be carried out. Data from dissolution studies should also be submitted for all solid oral dosage forms.

(iii) Dissolution and bioavailability data submitted with the new drug application must provide information that assures bioequivalence or establishes bioavailability and dosage correlations between the formulation(s) sought to be marketed and those used for clinical trials during clinical development of the product. (See items 8.1, 8.2 and 8.3 of Appendix I,).

(iv) All bioavailability and bioequivalence studies should be conducted according to the guidelines for bioavailability and bioequivance studies as prescribed.

Note. The data requirements stated in this schedule are expected to provide adequate information to evaluate the efficacy, safety and therapeutic rationale of new drugs (as defined under rule 122-E) prior to the permission for sale. Depending upon the nature of new drugs and disease(s), additional information may be required by the Licensing Authority. The applicant shall certify the authencity of the data and documents submitted in support of an application for new drug. The Licensing Authority reserves the right to reject any data or any document(s) if such data or contents of such documents are found to be of doubtful integrity.

Appendices

APPENDIX I: Data to be Submitted along with the Application to Conduct Clinical Trials/Import/Manufacture of New Drugs for Marketing In the Country

1. Introduction
   A brief description of the drug and the therapeutic class to which it belongs.
2. Chemical and pharmaceutical information
   - 2.1. Information on active ingredients
     Drug information (Generic Name, Chemical Name or INN)
   - 2.2. Physicochemical data
     - a. Chemical name and structure
       Empirical formula
       Molecular weight
     - b. Physical properties
       Description
       Solubility
       Rotation
       Partition coefficient
       Dissociation constant
   - 2.3. Analytical data
     Elemental analysis
     Mass spectrum
     NMR spectra
     IR spectra
     UV spectra
     Polymorphic identification
   - 2.4. Complete monograph specification including
     Identification
     Identity/quantification of impurities
     Enantiomeric purity
     Assay

2.5. Validations
  Assay method
  Impurity estimation method
  Residual solvent/other volatile impurities (OVI) estimation method
2.6. Stability studies (for details refer Appendix IX)
  Final release specification
  Reference standard characterization
  Material safety data sheet
2.7. Data on formulation
  Dosage form
  Composition
  Master manufacturing formula
  Details of the formulation (including inactive ingredients)
  In process quality control check
  Finished product specification
  Excipient compatibility study
  Validation of the analytical method
  Comparative evaluation with international brand(s) or approved Indian brands, if applicable
  Pack presentation
    Dissolution
    Assay
    Impurities
    Content uniformity
    pH
  Force degradation study
  Stability evaluation in market intended pack at proposed storage conditions
  Packing specifications
  Process validation

When the application is for clinical trials only, the international non-proprietary name (INN) or generic name, drug category, dosage form and data supporting stability in the intended container-closure system for the duration of the clinical trial (information covered in item nos. 2.1, 2.3, 2.6, 2.7) are required.

3. Animal pharmacology (for details refer Appendix IV)
   3.1. Summary
   3.2. Specific pharmacological actions
   3.3. General pharmacological actions
   3.4. Follow-up and supplemental safety pharmacology studies
   3.5. Pharmacokinetics: absorption, distribution; metabolism; excretion

4. Animal toxicology (for details refer Appendix III)
   4.1. General aspects
   4.2. Systemic toxicity studies
   4.3. Male fertility study
   4.4. Female reproduction and developmental toxicity studies
   4.5. Local toxicity
   4.6. Allergenicity/Hypersensitivity
   4.7. Genotoxicity
   4.8. Carcinogenicity.

5. Human / Clinical pharmacology (Phase I)
   5.1. Summary
   5.2. Specific pharmacological effects
   5.3. General pharmacological effects
   5.4. Pharmacokinetics, absorption, distribution, metabolism, excretion
   5.5. Pharmacodynamics / early measurement of drug activity.
6. Therapeutic exploratory trials (Phase II)
   6.1. Summary
   6.2. Study report(s) as given in Appendix II.
7. Therapeutic confirmatory trials (Phase III)
   7.1. Summary
   7.2. Individual study reports with listing of sites and investigators.
8. Special studies
   8.1. Summary
   8.2. Bio-availability / Bio-equivalence.
   8.3 Other studies, e.g. geriatrics, paediatrics, pregnant or nursing women.
9. Regulatory status in other countries
   9.1. Countries where the drug is
      a. Marketed
      b. Approved
      c. Approved as IND
      d. Withdrawn, if any, with reasons
   9.2. Restrictions on use, if any, in countries where marketed /approved
   9.3. Free sale certificate or certificate of analysis, as appropriate.
10. Prescribing information
    10.1. Proposed full prescribing information
    10.2. Drafts of labels and cartons.
11. Samples and testing protocol/s
    11.1. Samples of pure drug substance and finished product (an equivalent of 50 clinical doses, or more number of clinical doses if prescribed by the Licensing Authority), with testing protocol/s, full impurity profile and release specifications.

NOTES:

(1) All items may not be applicable to all drugs. For explanation, refer text of Schedule Y.

(2) For requrements of data to be submitted with application for clinical trials refer text of this schedule.

APPENDIX I-A: Data Required to be Submitted by an Applicant for Grant of Permission to Import and/or Manufacture a New Drug Already Approved in the Country

1. Introduction
   A brief description of the drug and the therapeutic class.
2. Chemical and pharmaceutical information
   - 2.1 Chemical name, code name or number, if any; non-proprietary or generic name, if any, structure; physicochemical properties.
   - 2.2 Dosage form and its composition.
   - 2.3 Test specifications
     - (a) active ingredients
     - (b) inactive ingredients.
   - 2.4 Tests for identification of the active ingredients and method of tis assay.
   - 2.5 Outline of the method of manufacture of active ingredients.
   - 2.6 Stability data.
3. Marketing information
   - 3.1 Proposed package insert / promotional literature
   - 3.2 Draft specimen of the label and carton.
4. Special studies conducted with approval of Licensing Authority
   - 4.1 Bioavailability / Bioequivalence and comparative dissolution studies for oral dosage forms
   - 4.2 Sub-acute animal toxicity studies for intravenous infusions and injectables.

APPENDIX II: Structure, Contents and Format for Clinical Study Report

1. Title Page
   This page should contain information about the title of the study, the protocol code, name of the investigational product tested, development phase, indication studied, a brief description of the trial design, the start and end date of patient accrual and the names of the sponsor and the participating institutes (Investigators).
2. Study synopsis (1 to 2 pages): A brief overview of the study from the protocol development to the trial closure should be given here. This section will only summarize the important conclusions derived from the study.
3. Statement of compliance with the 'Guidelines for Clinical Trials on Pharmaceutical Products in India – GCP Guidelines' issued by the Central Drugs Standard Control Organization, Ministry of Health, Government of India.
4. List of abbreviations and definitions.
5. Table of contents
6. Ethics Committee:
   This section should document that the study was conducted in accordance with the ethical principles of declaration of Helsinki. A detailed description of the Ethics Committee constitution and date(s) of approvals of trial documents for each of the participating sites should be provided. A declaration should state that EC notifications as per Good Clinical Practice Guidelines issued by Central Drugs Standard Control Organization and Ethical Guidelines for Biomedical Research on Human Subjects, issued by Indian Council of Medical Research have been followed.
7. Study team:
   Briefly describe the administrative structure of the study (Investigators, site staff, Sponsor/ designates, Central laboratory, etc.).
8. Introduction:
   A brief description of the product development rationale should be given here.
9. Study objective:
   A statement describing the overall purpose of the study and the primary and secondary objectives to be achieved should be mentioned here.
10. Investigational plan:
    This section should describe the overall trial design, the subject selection criteria, the treatment procedures, blinding / randomization techniques if any, allowed/ disallowed concomitant treatment, the efficacy and safety criteria assessed, the data quality assurance procedures and the statistical methods planned for the analysis of the data obtained.
11. Trial subjects
    A clear accounting of all trial subjects who entered the study will be given here. Mention should also be made of all cases that were dropouts or protocol deviations. Enumerate the patients screened, randomized, and prematurely discontinued. State reasons for premature discontinuation of therapy in each applicable case.
12. Efficacy evaluation
    The results of evaluation of all the efficacy variables will be described in this section with appropriate tabular and graphical representation. A brief description of the demographic

characteristics of the trial patients should also be provided along with a listing of patients and observations excluded from efficacy analysis.

13. Safety evaluation
    This section should include the complete list
    13.1 all serious adverse events, whether expected or unexpected and
    13.2 unexpected advese events whether serious or not (compliled from data received as per Appendix XI).
    The comparison of adverse events across study groups may be presented in a tabular or graphical form. This section should also give a brief narrative of all important events considered related to the investigational product.
14. Discussion and overall conclusion
    Discussion of the important conclusions derived from the trial and scope for further development.
15. List of references.
16. Appendices
    List of Appendices to the clinical trial report
    a. Protocol and amendments
    b. Specimen of case record form
    c. Investigators' name(s) with contact addresses, phone, e-mail, etc.
    d. Patient data listings
    e. List of trial participants treated with investigational product
    f. Discontinued participants
    g. Protocol deviations
    h. CRFs of cases involving death and life threatening adverse event cases
    i. Publications from the trial
    j. Important publications referenced in the study
    k. Audit certificate, if available
    l. Investigator's certificate that he/she has read the report and that the report accurately describes the conduct and the results of the study.

APPENDIX III: Animal Toxicology (Non-clinical Toxicity Studies)

1. **General Principles**

Toxicity studies should comply with the norms of Good Laboratory Practice (GLP). Briefly, these studies should be performed by suitably trained and qualified staff employing properly calibrated and standardized equipment of adequate size and capacity. Studies should be done as per written protocols with modifications (if any) verifiable retrospectively. Standard operating procedures (SOPs) should be followed for all managerial and laboratory tasks related to these studies. Test substances and test systems *(in vitro or in vivo)* should be properly characterized and standardized. All documents belonging to each study, including its approved protocol, raw data, draft report, final report, and histology slides and paraffin tissue blocks should be preserved for a minimum of 5 years after marketing of the drug.

Toxicokinetic studies (generation of pharmacokinetic data either as an integral component of the conduct of non-clinical toxicity studies or in specially designed studies) should be conducted to assess the systemic exposure achieved in animals and its relationship to dose level and the time course of the toxicity study. Other objectives of toxicokinetic studies include obtaining data to relate the exposure achieved in toxicity studies to toxicological findings and contribute to the assessment of the relevance of these findings to clinical safety, to support the choice of species and treatment regimen in nonclinical toxicity studies and to provide information which, in conjunction with the toxicity findings, contributes to the design of subsequent non-clinical toxicity studies.

1.1 Systemic Toxicity Studies

1.1.1 Single-dose toxicity studies: These studies (see Appendix I item 4.2) should be carried out in 2 rodent species (mice and rats) using the same route as intended for humans. In addition, unless the intended route of administration in humans is only intravenous, at least one more route should be used in one of the species to ensure systemic absorption of the drug. This route should depend on the nature of the drug. A limit of 2 g/kg (or 10 times the normal dose that is intended in humans, whichever is higher) is recommended for oral dosing. Animals should be observed for 14 days after the drug administration, and minimum lethal dose (MLD) and maximum tolerated dose (MTD) should be established. If possible, the target organ of toxicity should also be determined. Mortality should be observed for up to 7 days after parenteral administration and up to 14 days after oral administration. Symptoms, signs and mode of death should be reported, with appropriate macroscopic and microscopic findings where necessary. LD_{10} and LD_{50} should be reported preferably with 95 percent confidence limits. If LD_{50}s cannot be determined, reasons for the same should be stated.

The dose causing severe toxic manifestations or death should be defined in the case of cytotoxic anticancer agents, and the post-dosing observation period should be to 14 days. Mice should first be used for determination of MTD. Findings should then be confirmed in rat for establishing linear relationship between toxicity and body surface area. In case of nonlinearity, data of the more sensitive species should be used to determine the Phase I starting dose. Where rodents are known to be poor predictors of human toxicity (e.g., antifolates), or where the cytotoxic drug acts by a novel mechanism of action, MTD should be established in non-rodent species.

1.1.2 Repeated-dose systemic toxicity studies: These studies (see Appendix I, item 4.2) should be carried out in at least two mammalian species, of which one should be a non-rodent. Dose ranging studies should precede the 14-, 28-, 90- or 180- day toxicity studies. Duration of the final systemic toxicity study will depend on the duration, therapeutic indication and scale of the proposed clinical trial. (see Item 1.8). If a species is known to metabolize the drug in the same way as humans, it should be preferred for toxicity studies.

In repeated-dose toxicity studies the drug should be administered 7 days a week by the route intended for clinical use. The number of animals required for these studies, i.e. the minimum number of animals on which data should be available, is shown in Item 1.9.

Wherever applicable, a control group of animals given the vehicle alone should be included, and three other groups should be given graded doses of the drug. The highest dose should produce observable toxicity; the lowest dose should not cause observable toxicity, but should be comparable to the intended therapeutic dose in humans or a multiple of it . To make allowance for the sensitivity of the species the intermediate dose should cause some symptoms, but not gross toxicity or death, and should be placed logarithmically between the other two doses.

The parameters to be monitored and recorded in long-term toxicity studies should include behavioral, physiological, biochemical and microscopic observations. In case of parenteral drug administration, the sites of injection should be subjected to gross and microscopic examination. Initial and final electrocardiogram and fundus examination should be carried out in the non-rodent species. In the case of cytotoxic anticancer agents dosing and study design should be in accordance with the proposed clinical schedule in terms of days of exposure and number of cycles. Two rodent species may be tested for initiating Phase I trials. A non-rodent species should be added if the drug has a novel mechanism of action, or if permission for Phase II, III or marketing is being sought.

For most compounds, it is expected that single dose tissue distribution studies with sufficient sensitivity and specificity will provide an adequate assessment of tissue distribution and the potential for accumulation. Thus, repeated dose tissue distribution studies should not be required uniformly for all compounds and should only be conducted when appropriate data cannot be derived from other sources. Repeated dose studies may be appropriate under certain circumstances based on the data from single dose tissue distribution studies, toxicity and toxicokinetic studies. The studies may be most appropriate for compounds which have an apparently long half life, incomplete elimination or unanticipated organ toxicity.

Notes:

(i) Single Dose Toxicity Study: Each group should contain at least 5 animals of either sex. At least four graded doses should be given. Animals should be exposed to the test substance in a single bolus or by continuous infusion or several doses within 24 hours. Animals should be observed for 14 days. Signs of intoxication, effect on body weight, gross pathological changes should be reported. It is desirable to include histopathology of grossly affected organs, if any.

(ii) Dose-ranging Study: Objectives of this study include the identification of target organ of toxicity and establishment of MTD for subsequent studies.

(a) Rodents: Study should be performed in one rodent species (preferably rat) by the proposed clinical route of administration. At least four graded doses including control should be given, and each dose group as well as the vehicle control should consist of a minimum of 5 animals of each sex. Animals should be exposed to the test substance daily for 10 consecutive days. Highest dose should be the maximum tolerated dose of single-dose study. Animals should be observed daily for signs of intoxication (general appearance, activity and behavior etc), and periodically for the body weight and laboratory parameters. Gross examination of viscera and microscopic examination of affected organs should be done.

(b) Non-rodents: One male and one female are to be taken for ascending Phase MTD study. Dosing should start after initial recording of cage-side and laboratory parameters. Starting dose may be 3 to 5 times the extrapolated effective dose or MTD (whichever is less), and dose escalation in suitable steps should be done every third day after drawing the samples for laboratory parameters. Dose should be lowered appropriately when clinical or laboratory evidence of toxicity are observed. Administration of test substance should then continue for 10 days at the well-tolerated dose level following which, samples for laboratory parameters should be taken. Sacrifice, autopsy and microscopic examination of affected tissues should be performed as in the case of rodents.

(iii) 14 to 28 day repeated-dose toxicity studies: One rodent (6-10/sex/group) and one non-rodent (2-3/sex/group) species are needed. Daily dosing by proposed clinical route at three dose levels should be done with highest dose having observable toxicity, mid-dose between high and low dose, and low dose. The doses should preferably be multiples of the effective dose and free from toxicity. Observation parameters should include cage-side observations, body weight changes, food/water intake, blood biochemistry, hematology, and gross and microscopic studies of all viscera and tissues.

(iv) 90-day repeated-dose toxicity studies: One rodent (15-30/sex/group) and one non-rodent (4-6/sex/group) species are needed. Daily dosing by proposed clinical route at three graded dose levels should be done. In addition to the control a "high-dose-reversal" group and its control group should be also included. Parameters should include signs of intoxication (general appearance, activity and behavior etc), body weight, food intake, blood biochemical parameters, hematological values, urine analysis, organ weights, gross and microscopic study of viscera and tissues. Half the animals in "reversal" groups (treated and control) should be sacrificed after 14 days of stopping the treatment. The remaining animals should be sacrificed after 28 days of stopping the treatment or after the recovery of signs and/or clinical pathological changes – whichever comes later, and evaluated for the parameters used for the main study.

(v) 180-day repeated-dose toxicity studies: One rodent (15-30/sex/group) and one non-rodent (4-6/sex/group) species are needed. At least 4 groups, including control, should be taken. Daily dosing by proposed clinical route at three graded dose levels should be done. Parameters should include signs of intoxication, body weight, food intake, blood biochemistry, hematology, urine analysis, organ weights, gross and microscopic examination of organs and tissues.

1.2 Male Fertility Study

One rodent species (preferably rat) should be used. Dose selection should be done from the results of the previous 14 or 28-day toxicity study in rat. Three dose groups, the highest one showing minimal toxicity in systemic studies, and a control group should be taken. Each group should consist of 6 adult male animals. Animals should be treated with the test substance by the intended route of clinical use for minimum 28 days and maximum 70 days before they are paired with female animals of proven fertility in a ratio of 1:2 for mating.

Drug treatment of the male animals should continue during pairing. Pairing should be continued till the detection of vaginal plug or 10 days, whichever is earlier. Females getting thus pregnant should be examined for their fertility index after day 13 of gestation. All the male animals should be sacrificed at the end of the study. Weights of each testis and epididymis should be separately recorded. Sperms from one epididymis should be examined for their motility and morphology. The other epididymis and both testes should be examined for their histology.

1.3 Female Reproduction and Developmental Toxicity Studies

These studies (see Appendix I, item 4.4) need to be carried out for all drugs proposed to be studied or used in women of child bearing age. Segment I, II and III studies (see below) are to be performed in albino mice or rats, and segment II study should include albino rabbits also as a second test species. On the occasion, when the test article is not compatible with the rabbit (e.g. antibiotics which are effective against gram positive, anaerobic organisms and protozoas) the Segment II data in the mouse may be substituted.

1.3.1 Female Fertility Study (Segment I): The study should be done in one rodent species (rat preferred). The drug should be administered to both males and females, beginning a sufficient number of days (28 days in males and 14 days in females) before mating. Drug treatment should continue during mating and, subsequently, during the gestation period. Three graded doses should be used, the highest dose (usually the MTD obtained from previous systemic toxicity studies) should not affect general health of the parent animals. At least 15 males and 15 females should be used per dose group. Control and the treated groups should be of similar size. The route of administration should be the same as intended for therapeutic use.

Dams should be allowed to litter and their medication should be continued till the weaning of pups. Observations on body weight, food intake, clinical signs of intoxication, mating behaviour, progress of gestation/ parturition periods, length of gestation, parturition, post-partum health and gross pathology (and histopathology of affected organs) of dams should be recorded. The pups from both treated and control groups should be observed for general signs of intoxication, sex-wise distribution in different treatment groups, body weight, growth parameters, survival, gross examination, and autopsy. Histopathology of affected organs should be done.

1.3.2 Teratogenicity Study (Segment II): One rodent (preferably rat) and one non-rodent (rabbit) species are to be used. The drug should be administered throughout the period of organogenesis, using three dose levels as described for segment I. The highest dose should cause minimum maternal toxicity and the lowest one should be proportional to the proposed dose for clinical use in humans or a multiple of it. The route of administration should be the same as intended for human therapeutic use.

The control and the treated groups should consist of at least 20 pregnant rats (or mice) and 12 rabbits, on each dose level. All foetuses should to be subjected to gross examination, one of the foetuses should be examined for skeletal abnormalities and the other half for visceral abnormalities. Observation parameters should include: (Dams) signs of intoxication, effect on body weight, effect on food intake, examination of uterus, ovaries and uterine contents, number of corpora lutea, implantation sites, resorptions (if any); and for the foetuses, the total number, gender, body length, weight and gross/ visceral/ skeletal abnormalities, if any.

1.3.3 Perinatal Study (Segment III): This study is specially recommended if the drug is to be given to pregnant or nursing mothers for long periods or where there are indications of possible adverse effects on foetal development. One rodent species (preferably rat) is needed. Dosing at levels comparable to multiples of human dose should be done by the intended clinical route. At least 4 groups (including control), each consisting of 15 dams should be used. The drug should be administered throughout the last trimester of pregnancy (from day 15 of gestation) and then the dose that causes low foetal loss should be continued throughout lactation and weaning. Dams should then be sacrificed and examined as described below.

One male and one female from each litter of F_1 generation (total 15 males and 15 females in each group) should be selected at weaning and treated with vehicle or test substance (at the dose levels described above) throughout their periods of growth to sexual maturity, pairing, gestation, parturition and lactation. Mating performance and fertility of F_1 generation should thus be evaluated to obtain the F_2 generation whose growth parameters should be monitored till weaning. The criteria of evaluation should be the same as described earlier (3.4.1).

Animals should be sacrificed at the end of the study and the observation parameters should include (Dams) body weight, food intake, general signs of intoxication, progress of gestation/ parturition periods and gross pathology (if any); and for pups, the clinical signs, sex-wise distribution in dose groups, body weight, growth parameters, gross examination, survival and autopsy (if needed) and where necessary, histopathology.

1.4 Local toxicity

These studies (see Appendix I, item 4.5) are required when the new drug is proposed to be used by some special route (other than oral) in humans. The drug should be applied to an appropriate site (e.g., skin or vaginal mucous membrane) to determine local effects in a suitable species. Typical study designs for these studies should include three dose levels and untreated and/ or vehicle control, preferably use of 2 species, and increasing group size with increase in duration of treatment. Where dosing is restricted due to anatomical or humane reasons, or the drug concentration cannot be increased beyond a certain level due to the problems of solubility, pH or tonicity, a clear statement to this effect should be given. If the drug is absorbed from the site of application, appropriate systemic toxicity studies will also be required.

Notes:

(i) Dermal toxicity study: The study should be done in rabbit and rat. Daily topical (dermal) application of test substance in its clinical dosage form should be done. Test material should be applied on shaved skin covering not less than 10% of the total body surface area. Porous gauze dressing should be used to hold liquid material in place. Formulations with different concentrations (at least 3) of test substance, several fold higher than the clinical dosage form should be used. Period of application may vary from 7 to 90 days depending on the clinical duration of use. Where skin irritation is grossly visible in the initial studies, a recovery group should be included in the subsequent repeated-dose study. Local signs (erythema, edema and eschar formation) as well as histological examination of sites of application should be used for evaluation of results.

(ii) Photo-allergy or dermal photo-toxicity: It should be tested by Armstrong/ Harber test in guinea pig. This test should be done if the drug or a metabolite is related to an agent causing photosensitivity or the nature of action suggests such a potential (e.g., drugs to be used in treatment of leucoderma). Pretest in 8 animals should screen 4 concentrations (patch application for 2 hours ±15 min.) with and without UV exposure (10 J/cm^2). Observations recorded at 24 and 48 hours should be used to ascertain highest nonirritant dose. Main test should be performed with 10 test animals and 5 controls. Induction with the dose selected from pretest should use 0.3 ml/patch for 2 hour ±15 min. followed by 10 J/cm^2 of UV exposure. This should be repeated on day 0, 2,4,7,9 and 11 of the test. Animals should be challenged with the same concentration of test substance between day 20 to 24 of the test with a similar 2-hour application followed by exposure to 10 J/cm^2 of UV light. Examination and grading of erythema and oedema formation at the challenge sites should be done 24 and 48 hours after the challenge. A positive control like musk ambrett or psoralin should be used.

(iii) Vaginal toxicity test: Study is to be done in rabbit or dog. Test substance should be applied topically (vaginal mucosa) in the form of pessary, cream or ointment. Six to ten animals per dose group should be taken. Higher concentrations or several daily applications of test substance should be done to achieve multiples of daily human dose. The minimum duration of drug treatment is 7 days (more according to clinical use), Subject to a maximum of 30 days. Observation parameters should include swelling, closure of introitus and histopathology of vaginal wall.

(iv) Rectal tolerance test: For all preparations meant for rectal administration this test may be performed in rabbits or dogs. Six to ten animals per dose group should be taken. Formulation in volume comparable to human dose (or the maximum possible volume) should be applied once or several times daily, per rectally, to achieve administration of multiples of daily human dose. The minimum duration of application is 7 days (more according to clinical use), Subject to a maximum of 30 days. Size of suppositories may be smaller, but the drug content should be several fold higher than the proposed human dose. Observation parameters should include clinical signs (sliding on backside), signs of pain, blood and/or mucus in faeces, condition of anal region/sphincter, gross and (if required) histological examination of rectal mucosa.

(v) Parenteral drugs: For products meant for intravenous or intramuscular or subcutaneous or intradermal injection the sites of injection in systemic toxicity studies should be specially examined grossly and microscopically. If needed, reversibility of adverse effects may be determined on a case to case basis.

(vi) Ocular toxicity studies (for products meant for ocular instillation): These studies should be carried out in two species, one of which should be the albino rabbit which has a sufficiently large conjunctival sac. Direct delivery of drug onto the cornea in case of animals having small conjunctival sacs should be ensured. Liquids, ointments, gels or soft contact lenses (saturated with drug) should be used. Initial single dose application should be done to decide the exposure concentrations for repeated-dose studies and the need to include a recovery group. Duration of the final study will depend on the proposed length of human exposure Subject to a maximum of 90 days. At least two different concentrations exceeding the human dose should be used for demonstrating the margin of safety. In acute studies, one eye should be used for drug administration and the other kept as control. A separate control group should be included in repeated-dose studies.

Slit-lamp examination should be done to detect the changes in cornea, iris and aqueous humor. Fluorescent dyes (sodium fluorescein, 0.25 to 1.0%) should be used for detecting the defects in surface epithelium of cornea and conjunctiva. Changes in intraocular tension should be monitored by a tonometer. Histological examination of eyes should be done at the end of the study after fixation in Davidson's or Zenker's fluid.

(vii) Inhalation toxicity studies: The studies are to be undertaken in one rodent and one non-rodent species using the formulation that is to be eventually proposed to be marketed. Acute, subacute and chronic toxicity studies should be performed according to the intended duration of human exposure. Standard systemic toxicity study designs (described above) should be used. Gases and vapors should be given in whole body exposure chambers; aerosols are to be given by nose-only method. Exposure time and concentrations of test substance (limit dose of 5 mg/I) should be adjusted to ensure exposure at levels comparable to multiples of intended human exposure. Three dose groups and a control (plus vehicle control, if needed) are required. Duration of exposure may vary subject to a maximum of 6 hours per day and five days a week. Food and water should be withdrawn during the period of exposure to test substance.

Temperature, humidity and flow rate of exposure chamber should be recorded and reported. Evidence of exposure with test substance of particle size of 4 micron (especially for aerosols) with not less that 25% being 1 micron should be provided. Effects on respiratory rate, findings of bronchial lavage fluid examination, histological examination of respiratory passages and lung tissue should be included along with the regular parameters of systemic toxicity studies or assessment of margin of safety.

1.5 Allergenicity/ Hypersensitivity

Standard tests include guinea pig maximization test (GPMT) and local lymph node assay (LLNA) in mouse. Any one of the two may be done.

Notes:

(i) Guinea pig maximization test: The test is to be performed in two steps; first, determination of maximum nonirritant and minimum irritant doses, and second, the main test. The initial study will also have two components. To determine the intradermal induction dose, 4 dose levels should be tested by the same route in a batch of 4 male and 4 female animals (2 of each sex should be given Freund's adjuvant). The minimum irritant dose should be used for induction. Similarly, a topical minimum irritant dose should be determined for challenge. This should be established in 2 males and 2 females. A minimum of 6 male and 6 female animals per group should be used in the main study. One test and one control group should be used. It is preferable to have one more positive control group. Intradermal induction (day 1) coupled with topical challenge (day 21) should be done. If there is no response, re-challenge should be done 7-30 days after the primary challenge. Erythema and edema (individual animal scores as well as maximization grading) should be used as evaluation criteria.

(ii) Local lymph node assay: Mice used in this test should be of the same sex, either only males or only females. Drug treatment is to be given on ear skin. Three graded doses, the highest being maximum nonirritant dose plus vehicle control should be used. A minimum of 6 mice per group should be used. Test material should be applied on ear skin on three consecutive days and on day 5, the draining auricular lymph nodes should be dissected out 5 hours after i.v. ^{3}H-thymidine or bromo-deoxy-uridine (BrdU). Increase in ^{3}H-thymidine or BrdU incorporation should be used as the criterion for evaluation of results.

1.6 Genotoxicity

Genotoxic compounds, in the absence of other data, shall be presumed to be trans-species carcinogens, implying a hazard to humans. Such compounds need not be subjected to long-term carcinogenicity studies. However, if such a drug is intended to be administered for chronic illnesses or otherwise over a long period of time - a chronic toxicity study (up to one year) may be necessary to detect early tumorigenic effects.

Genotoxicity tests are *in vitro* and *in vivo* tests conducted to detect compounds which induce genetic damage directly or indirectly. These tests should enable a hazard identification with respect to damage to DNA and its fixation.

The following standard test battery is generally expected to be conducted:

(i) A test for gene mutation in bacteria.
(ii) An *in vitro* test with cytogenetic evaluation of chromosomal damage with mammalian cells or an *in vitro* mouse lymphoma assay.
(iii) An *in vivo* test for chromosomal damage using rodent hematopoietic cells.

Other genotoxicity tests, e.g. tests for measurement of DNA adducts, DNA strand breaks, DNA repair or recombination serve as options in addition to the standard battery for further investigation of genotoxicity test results obtained in the standard battery. Only under extreme conditions in which one or more tests comprising the standard battery cannot be employed for technical reasons, alternative validated tests can serve as substitutes provided sufficient scientific justification should be provided to support the argument that a given standard battery test is not appropriate.

Both *in vitro* and *in vivo* studies should be done. Invitro studies should include Ames' *Salmonella* assay and chromosomal aberrations (CA) in cultured cells. In-vivo studies should include micronucleus assay (MNA) or CA in rodent bone marrow. Data analysis of CA should include analysis of 'gaps.'

Cytotoxic anticancer agents: Genotoxicity data are not required before Phase I and II trials. But these studies should be completed before applying for Phase III trials.

Notes:

Ames' Test (Reverse mutation assay in *Salmonella*): S. typhimurium tester strains such as TA98, TA100, TA102, TA1535, TA97 or *Escherichia coli* WP2 *uvrA* or *Escherichia coli* WP2 *uvrA* (pKM101) should be used.

(i) *In vitro* exposure (with and without metabolic activation, S9 mix) should be done at a minimum of 5 log dose levels. "Solvent" and "positive" control should be used. Positive control may include 9-amino-acridine, 2-nitrofluorine, sodium azide and mitomycin C, respectively, in the tester strains mentioned above. Each set should consist of at least three replicates. A 2.5 fold (or more) increase in number of revertants in comparison to spontaneous revertants would be considered positive.

(ii) *In vitro* cytogenetic assay: The desired level of toxicity for *in vitro* cytogenetic tests using cell lines should be greater than 50% reduction in cell number or culture confluency. For lymphocyte cultures, an inhibition of mitotic index by greater than 50% is considered sufficient. It should be performed in CHO cells or on human lymphocyte in culture. *In vitro* exposure (with and without metabolic activation, S9 mix) should be done using a minimum of 3 log doses. "Solvent" and "positive" control should be included. A positive control like cyclophosphamide with metabolic activation and mitomycin C for without metabolic activation should be used to give a reproducible and detectable increase clastogenic effect over the background which demonstrates the sensitivity of the test system. Each set should consist of at least three replicates. Increased number of aberrations in metaPhase chromosomes should be used as the criteria for evaluation.

(iii) *In vivo* micronucleus assay: One rodent species (preferably mouse) is needed. Route of administration of test substance should be the same as intended for humans. Five animals per sex per dose groups should be used. At least three dose levels, plus "solvent" and "positive" control should be tested. A positive control like mitomycin C or cyclophosphamide should be used. Dosing should be done on day 1 and 2 of study followed by sacrifice of animals 6 hours after the last injection. Bone marrow from both the femora should be taken out, flushed with fetal bovine serum (20 min.), pelletted and smeared on glass slides. Giemsa-MayGruenwald staining should be done and increased number of micronuclei in polychromatic erythrocytes (minimum 1000) should be used as the evaluation criteria.

(iv) *In vivo* cytogenetic assay: One rodent species (preferably rat) is to be used. Route of administration of test substance should be the same as intended for humans. Five animals/ sex/dose groups should be used. At least three dose levels, plus "solvent" and "positive" control should be tested. Positive control may include cyclophosphamide. Dosing should be done on day 1 followed by intraperitoneal colchicine administration at 22 hours. Animals should be sacrificed 2 hours after colchicine administration. Bone marrow from both the femora should be taken out, flushed with hypotonic saline (20 min.), pelletted and resuspended in Carnoy's fluid. Once again the cells should be pelletted and dropped on clean glass slides with a Pasteur pipette. Giemsa staining should be done and increased number of aberrations in metaPhase chromosomes (minimum 100) should be used as the evaluation criteria.

1.7 Carcinogenicity (see Appendix I, item 4.8)

Carcinogenicity studies should be performed for all drugs that are expected to be clinically used for more than 6 months as well as for drugs used frequently in an intermittent manner in the treatment of chronic or recurrent conditions. Carcinogenicity studies are also to be performed for drugs if there is concern about their carcinogenic potential emanating from previous demonstration of carcinogenic potential in the product class that is considered relevant to humans or where structure-activity relationship suggests carcinogenic risk or when there is evidence of preneoplastic lesions in repeated dose toxicity studies or when long-term tissue retention of parent compound or metabolite(s) results in local tissue reactions or other pathophysiological responses. For pharmaceuticals developed to treat certain serious diseases, Licensing Authority may allow carcinogenicity testing to be conducted after marketing permission has been granted.

In instances where the life-expectancy in the indicated population is short (i.e., less than 2 - 3 years) - no long-term carcinogenicity studies may be required. In cases where the therapeutic agent for cancer is generally successful and life is significantly prolonged there may be later concerns regarding secondary cancers. When such drugs are intended for adjuvant therapy in tumor free patients or for prolonged use in non-cancer indications, carcinogenicity studies may be / are needed. Completed rodent carcinogenicity studies are not needed in advance of the conduct of large scale clinical trials, unless there is special concern for the patient population.

Carcinogenicity studies should be done in a rodent species (preferably rat). Mouse may be employed only with proper scientific justification. The selected strain of animals should not have a very high or very low incidence of spontaneous tumors.

At least three dose levels should be used. The highest dose should be sub-lethal, and it should not reduce the life span of animals by more than 10% of expected normal. The lowest dose should be comparable to the intended human therapeutic dose or a multiple of it, e.g. 2.5x; to make allowance for the sensitivity of the species. The intermediate dose to be placed logarithmically between the other two doses. An untreated control and (if indicated) a vehicle control group should be included. The drug should be administered 7 days a week for a fraction of the life span comparable to the fraction of human life span over which the drug is likely to be used therapeutically. Generally, the period of dosing should be 24 months for rats and 18 months for mice.

Observations should include macroscopic changes observed at autopsy and detailed histopathology of organs and tissues. Additional tests for carcinogenicity (short-term bioassays, neonatal mouse assay or tests employing transgenic animals) may also be done depending on their applicability on a case to case basis.

Note:

Each dose group and concurrent control group not intended to be sacrificed early should contain atleast 50 animals of each sex. A high dose sattelite group for evaluation of pathology other than neoplasia should contain 20 animals of each sex while the sattellite control group should contain 10 animals of each sex. Observation parameters should include signs of intoxication, effect on body weight, food intake, clinical chemistry parameters, hematology parameters, urine analysis, organ weights, gross pathology and detailed histopathology. Comprehensive descriptions of benign and malignant tumour development, time of their detection, site, dimensions, histological typing, etc. should be given.

1.8 Animal toxicity requirements for clinical trials and marketing of a new drug

Systemic Toxicity Studies			
Route of administration	Duration of proposed human administration	Human Phase(s) for which study is proposed to be conducted	Long term toxicity requirements
Oral or Parenteral or Transdermal	Single dose or several doses in one day, Upto 1wk	I,II,III	2 sp,2 wk
	> 1 wk but upto 2 wk	I,II,III	2 sp;4 wk
	> 2 wk but upto 4 wk	I,II,III	2 sp;12 wk
	Over 1mo	I,II,III	2 sp;24 wk
Inhalation (general anesthetics, aerosols)	Upto 2 wk	I,II,III	2 sp;1mo; (Exposure time 3 h/d, 5 d/wk)
	Upto 4 wk	I,II,III	2 sp;12 wk, (Exposure time 6 h/d, 5 d/wk)

Contd...

Contd...

	> 1 4 wk	I,II,III	2 sp;24 wk, (Exposure time 6 h/d, 5 d/wk)
Local Toxicity Studies			
Dermal	Upto 2 wk	I,II	1 sp;4 wk
		III	2 sp;4 wk
	> 2 wk	I,II,III	2 sp;12 wk
Ocular or Otic or Nasal	Upto 2 wk	I,II	1 sp;4 wk
		III	2 sp;4 wk
	> 2 wk	I,II,III	2 sp;12 wk
Vaginal or Rectal	Upto 2 wk	I,II	1 sp;4 wk
		III	2 sp;4 wk
	> 2 wk	I,II,III	2 sp;12 wk

Special toxicity studies

Male Fertility Study:
- Phase I, II, III in male volunteers/patients

Female Reproduction and Developmental Toxicity Studies:

- Segment II studies in 2 species; Phase II, III involving female patients of child-bearing age.· Segment I study; Phase III involving female patients of child-bearing age: Segment III study; Phase III for drugs to be given to pregnant or nursing mothers for long periods or where there are indications of possible adverse effects on foetal development.

Allergenicity/Hypersensitivity:
- Phase I, II, III - when there is a cause of concern or for parenteral drugs (including dermal application)

Photo-allergy or dermal photo-toxicity:
- Phase I, II, III - if the drug or a metabolite is related to an agent causing photosensitivity or the nature of action suggests such a potential.

Genotoxicity:
- *In vitro* studies - Phase I
- Both *in vitro* and *in vivo* - Phase II, III

arcinogenicity:
- Phase III - when there is a cause for concern, or when the drug is to be used for more than 6 months.

Abbreviations: sp-species; mo-month; wk-week; d -day; h-hour; I, II, III - Phases of clinical trial.

Note:

1. Animal toxicity data generated in other countries may be accepted and may not be asked to be repeated/duplicated in India on a case to case basis depending upon the quality of data and the credentials of the laboratory (ies) where such data has been generated.
2. Requirements for fixed dose combinations are given in Appendix VI.

1.9 Number of animals required for repeated-dose toxicity studies

	14-28 days				84-182 days			
	Rodent (Rat)		Non-rodent (Dog or Monkey)		Rodent (Rat)		Non-rodent (Dog or Monkey)	
	M	F	M	F	M	F	M	F
Control	6-10	6-10	2-3	2-3	15-30	15-30	4-6	4-6
Low dose	6-10	6-10	2-3	2-3	15-30	15-30	4-6	4-6
Intermediate dose	6-10	6-10	2-3	2-3	15-30	15-30	4-6	4-6
High dose	6-10	6-10	2-3	2-3	15-30	15-30	4-6	4-6

2. Laboratory Parameters to be Included in Toxicity Studies

Hematological parameters

- Hemoglobin
- Total RBC Count
- Hematocrit Count
- Reticulocyte
- Total WBC Count
- Differential WBC Count
- Platelet count
- Terminal Bone Marrow Examination
- ESR (Non-rodents only)
- General Blood Picture: A special mention of abnormal and immature cells should be made.
- Coagulation parameters (Non-rodents only): Bleeding time, coagulation time, prothrombin time, activated partial thromboplastin time

Urinalysis Parameters

- Color
- Appearance
- Specific gravity
- 24-hour urinary output
- Reaction (pH)
- Albumin
- Sugar
- Acetone
- Bile pigments
- Urobilinogen
- Occult blood
- Microscopic examination of urinary sediment

Blood biochemical parameters

- Glucose
- Cholesterol
- Triglycerides
- HDL Cholesterol (Non-rodents only)
- LDL Cholesterol (Non-rodents only)
- Bilirubin
- SGPT (ALT)
- SGOT (AST)
- Alkaline Phosphatase (ALP)
- GGT (Non rodents only)

Blood Urea Nitrogen

- Creatinine
- Total Proteins
- Albumin
- Globulin (Calculated values)
- Sodium
- Potassium
- Phosphorus
- Calcium

Gross and Microscopic Pathology

- Brain*: Cerebrum, cerebellum, midbrain
- (Spinal cord)
- Eye
- (Middle Ear)
- Thyroid
- (Parathyroid)
- Spleen*
- Thymus
- Adrenal*
- (Pancreas)
- (Trachea)
- Lung*
- Heart*
- Aorta
- Oesophagus
- Stomach
- Duodenum
- Jejunum
- Terminal ileum
- Colon
- (Rectum)
- Liver*
- Kidney*
- Urinary bladder
- Epididymis
- Testis*
- Ovary
- Uterus*
- Skin
- Mammary gland
- Mesenteric lymph node
- Skeletal muscle

* Organs marked with an asterisk should be weighed.

() Organs listed in parenthesis should be examined if indicated by the nature of the drug or observed effects.

Non-clinical toxicity testing and safety evaluation data of an IND needed for the conduct of different phases of clinical trials

Note: Refer Appendix III (Points 1.1 through 1.9) for essential features of study designs of the non-clinical toxicity studies listed below.

For Phase I Clinical Trials

Systemic toxicity studies

i. Single dose toxicity studies
ii. Dose ranging studies
iii. Repeat-dose systemic toxicity studies of appropriate duration to support the duration to support the duration of proposed human exposure.

Male fertility study

In-vitro genotoxicity tests

Relevant local toxicity studies with proposed route of clinical application (duration depending on proposed length of clinical exposure)

Allergenicity/Hypersensitivity tests (when there is a cause for concern or for parenteral drugs, including dermal application)

Photo-allergy or dermal photo-toxicity test (if the drug or a metabolite is related to an agent causing photosensitivity or the nature of action suggests such a potential).

For Phase II Clinical Trials

Provide a summary of all the non-clinical safety data (listed above) already submitted while obtaining the permissions for Phase I trial, with appropriate references.

In case of an application for directly starting a Phase II trial - complete details of the non-clinical safety data needed for obtaining the permission for Phase I trial, as per the list provided above must be submitted.

Repeat-dose systemic toxicity studies of appropriate duration to support the duration of proposed human exposure

In vivo genotoxicity tests

Segment II reproductive/developmental toxicity study (if female patients of child bearing age are going to be involved).

For Phase III Clinical Trials

Provide a summary of all the non-clinical safety data (listed above) already submitted while obtaining the permissions for Phase I and II trials, with appropriate references.

In case of an application for directly initiating a Phase III trial - complete details of the non-clinical safety data needed for obtaining the permissions for Phase I and II trials, as per the list provided above must be provided.

Repeat-dose systemic toxicity studies of appropriate duration to support the duration of proposed human exposure

Reproductive/developmental toxicity studies

Segment I (if female patients of child bearing age are going to be involved), and

Segment III (for drugs to be given to pregnant or nursing mothers or where there are indications of possible adverse effects on foetal development)

Carcinogenicity studies (when there is a cause for concern or when the drug is to be used for more than 6 months).

For Phase IV Clinical Trials

Provide a summary of all the non-clinical safety data (listed above) already submitted while obtaining the permissions for Phase I, II and III trials, with appropriate references.

In case an application is made for initiating the Phase IV trial, complete details of the non-clinical safety data needed for obtaining the permissions for Phase I, II and III trials, as per the list provided above must be submitted.

Application of Good Laboratory Practices (GLP)

The animal studies be conducted in an accredited laboratory. Where the safety pharmacology studies are part of toxicology studies, these studies should also be conducted in an accredited laboratory.

APPENDIX IV: Animal Pharmacology

1. General Principles

Specific and general pharmacological studies should be conducted to support use of therapeutics in humans. In the early stages of drug development enough information may not be available to rationally select study design for safety assessment. In such a situation, a general approach to safety pharmacology studies can be applied. Safety pharmacology studies are studies that investigate potential undesirable pharmacodynamic effects of a substance on physiological functions in relation to exposure within the therapeutic range or above.

1.1 Specific Pharmacological Actions

Specific pharmacological actions are those which demonstrate the therapeutic potential for humans. The specific studies that should be conducted and their design will be different based on the individual properties and intended uses of investigational drug. Scientifically validated methods should be used. The use of new technologies and methodologies in accordance with sound scientific principles should be preferred.

1.2 General Pharmacological Actions

1.2.1 Essential Safety Pharmacology

Safety pharmacology studies need to be conducted to investigate the potential undesirable pharmacodynamic effects of a substance on physiological functions in relation to exposure within the therapeutic range and above. These studies should be designed to identify undesirable pharmacodynamic properties of a substance that may have relevance to its human safety; to evaluate adverse pharmacodynamic and/or pathophysiological effects observed in toxicology and/or clinical studies; and to investigate the mechanism of the adverse pharmacodynamic effects observed and/or suspected.

The aim of the essential safety pharmacology is to study the effects of the test drug on vital functions. Vital organ systems such as cardiovascular, respiratory and central nervous systems should be studied. Essential safety pharmacology studies may be excluded or supplemented based on scientific rationale. Also, the exclusion of certain test(s) or exploration(s) of certain organs, systems or functions should be scientifically justified.

1.2.1.1 Cardiovascular System

Effects of the investigational drug should be studied on blood pressure, heart rate, and the electrocardiogram. If possible *in vitro, in vivo* and/or *ex vivo* methods including electrophysiology should also be considered.

1.2.1.2 Central Nervous System

Effects of the investigational drug should be studied on motor activity, behavioral changes, coordination, sensory and motor reflex responses and body temperature.

1.2.1.3 Respiratory System

Effects of the investigational drug on respiratory rate and other functions such as tidal volume and hemoglobin oxygen saturation should be studied.

1.3 Follow-up and Supplemental Safety Pharmacology Studies

In addition to the essential safety pharmacological studies, additional supplemental and follow-up safety pharmacology studies may need to be conducted as appropriate. These depend on the pharmacological properties or chemical class of the test substance, and the data generated from safety pharmacology studies, clinical trials, pharmacovigilance, experimental *in vitro* or *in vivo* studies, or from literature reports.

1.3.1 Follow-up Studies for Essential Safety Pharmacology

Follow-up studies provide additional information or a better understanding than that provided by the essential **safety pharmacology**.

1.3.1.1 Cardiovascular System

These include ventricular contractility, vascular resistance and the effects of chemical mediators, their agonists and antagonists on the cardiovascular system.

1.3.1.2 Central Nervous System

These include behavioral studies , learning and memory, electrophysiology studies , neurochemistry and ligand binding studies.

1.3.1.3 Respiratory System

These include airway resistance, compliance, pulmonary arterial pressure, blood gases and blood pH.

1.3.2 Supplemental Safety Pharmacology Studies

These studies are required to investigate the possible adverse pharmacological effects that are not assessed in the essential safety pharmacological studies and are a cause for concern.

1.3.2.1 Urinary System

These include urine volume, specific gravity, osmolality, pH, proteins, cytology and blood urea nitrogen, creatinine and plasma proteins estimation.

1.3.2.2 Autonomic Nervous System

These include binding to receptors relevant for the autonomic nervous system, and functional response to agonist or antagonist responses *in vivo* or *in vitro,* and effects of direct stimulation of autonomic nerves and their effects on cardiovascular responses.

1.3.2.3 Gastrointestinal System

These include studies on gastric secretion, gastric pH measurement, gastric mucosal examination, bile secretion, gastric emptying time *in vivo* and ileocecal contraction *in vitro.*

1.3.2.4 Other Organ Systems

Effects of the investigational drug on organ systems not investigated elsewhere should be assessed when there is a cause for concern. For example, dependency potential, skeletal muscle, immune and endocrine functions may be investigated.

1.4 Conditions under which Safety Pharmacology Studies are Not Necessary

Safety pharmacology studies are usually not required for locally applied agents, e.g. dermal or ocular, in cases when the pharmacology of the investigational drug is well known, and/or when systemic absorption from the site of application is low. Safety pharmacology testing is also not necessary, in the case of a new derivative having similar pharmacokinetics and pharmacodynamics.

1.5 Timing of Safety Pharmacology Studies in Relation to Clinical Development

1.5.1 Prior to First Administration in Humans

The effects of an investigational drug on the vital functions listed in the essential safety pharmacology should be studied prior to first administration in humans. Any follow up or supplemental studies identified, should be conducted if necessary, based on a cause for concern.

1.5.2 During Clinical Development

Additional investigations may be warranted to clarify observed or suspected adverse effects in animals and humans during clinical development.

1.5.3 Before Applying for Marketing Approval

Follow-up and supplemental safety pharmacology studies should be assessed prior to approval unless not required, in which case this should be justified. Available information from toxicology studies addressing safety pharmacology endpoints or information from clinical studies can replace such studies.

1.6 Application of Good Laboratory Practices (GLP)

The animal studies be conducted in an accredited laboratory. Where the safety pharmacology studies are part of toxicology studies, these studies should also be conducted in an accredited laboratory. Appendix V.

APPENDIX V: Informed Consent

CHECKLIST FOR STUDY SUBJECT'S INFORMED CONSENT DOCUMENTS

Essential Elements

1. Statement that the study involves research and explanation of the purpose of the research
2. Expected duration of the Subject's participation
3. Description of the procedures to be followed, including all invasive procedures and
4. Description of any reasonably foreseeable risks or discomforts to the Subject
5. Description of any benefits to the Subject or others reasonably expected from research. If no benefit is expected Subject should be made aware of this.
6. Disclosure of specific appropriate alternative procedures or therapies available to the Subject.
7. Statement describing the extent to which confidentiality of records identifying the Subject will be maintained and who will have access to Subject's medical records
8. Trial treatment schedule(s) and the probability for random assignment to each treatment (for randomized trials)
9. Compensation and/or treatment(s) available to the Subject in the event of a trial-related injury
10. An explanation about whom to contact for trial related queries, rights of Subjects and in the event of any injury
11. The anticipated prorated payment, if any, to the Subject for participating in the trial
12. Subject's responsibilities on participation in the trial
13. Statement that participation is voluntary, that the Subject can withdraw from the study at any time and that refusal to participate will not involve any penalty or loss of benefits to which the Subject is otherwise entitled
14. Any other pertinent information

Additional elements, which may be required

a. Statement of foreseeable circumstances under which the Subject's participation may be terminated by the Investigator without the Subject's consent.
b. Additional costs to the Subject that may result from participation in the study.
c. The consequences of a Subject's decision to withdraw from the research and procedures for orderly termination of participation by Subject.
d. Statement that the Subject or Subject's representative will be notified in a timely manner if significant new findings develop during the course of the research which may affect the Subject's willingness to continue participation will be provided.
e. A statement that the particular treatment or procedure may involve risks to the Subject (or to the embryo or fetus, if the Subject is or may become pregnant), which are currently unforeseeable
f. Approximate number of Subjects enrolled in the study.

FORMAT OF INFORMED CONSENT FORM FOR SUBJECTS PARTICIPATING IN A CLINICAL TRIAL

Informed Consent form to participate in a clinical trial
Study Title:
Study Number:
Subject's Initials: ____________________ Subject's Name: ____________________

Date of Birth / Age: ____________________

Please initial box (Subject)

i. I confirm that I have read and understood the information sheet dated ___ for the above study and have had the opportunity to ask questions. [ ]

ii. I understand that my participation in the study is voluntary and that I am free to withdraw at any time, without giving any reason, without my medical care or legal rights being affected. [ ] [ ]

iii. I understand that the Sponsor of the clinical trial, others working on the Sponsor's behalf, the Ethics Committee and the regulatory authorities will not need my permission to look at my health records both in respect of the current study and any further research that may be conducted in relation to it, even if I withdraw from the trial. I agree to this access. However, I understand that my identity will not be revealed in any information released to third parties or published. [ ]

iv. I agree not to restrict the use of any data or results that arise from this study provided such a use is only for scientific purpose(s) [ ]

v. I agree to take part in the above study. [ ]

Signature (or Thumb impression) of the Subject/Legally Acceptable Representative:___________________________________

Date: _____/_____/______

Signatory's Name: ____

Signature of the Investigator: ______________________________ Date: _____/_____/_____

Study Investigator's Name: ____

Signature of the Witness ___________________________________ Date:_____/_____/______

Name of the Witness: ____

APPENDIX VI: Fixed Dose Combinations (FDCs)

Fixed Dose Combinations refer to products containing one or more active ingredients used for a particular indication(s). FDCs can be divided into the following groups and data required for approval for marketing is described below:

a. The first group of FDCs includes those in which one or more of the active ingredients is a new drug. For such FDCs to be approved for marketing data to be submitted will be similar to data required for any new drug (including clinical trials) [see rule 122E, item (a)].

b. (i) The second group FDCs includes those in which active ingredients already approved/marketed individually are combined for the first time, for a particular claim and where the ingredients are likely to have significant interaction of a pharmacodynamic or pharmacokinetic nature [see rule 122E, item (c)]. If clinical trials have been carried out with the FDC in other countries, reports of such trials should be submitted. If the FDC is marketed abroad, the regulatory status in other countries should be stated. (see Appendix I, item 9).

ii. For marketing permission, appropriate chemical and pharmaceutical data will be submitted. In case such a combination is not marketed anywhere in the world but these drugs are already in use concomitantly (not as an FDC but individually) for the said claim, marketing permission may be granted based on chemical and pharmaceutical data. Data showing the stability of the proposed dosage form will also have to be submitted.

iii. For any other such FDCs, clinical trials may be required. For obtaining permission to carry out clinical trials with such FDCs a summary of available pharmacological, toxicological and clinical data on the individual ingredients should be submitted, along with the rationale for combining them in the proposed ratio. In addition, acute toxicity data (LD 50) and pharmacological data should be submitted on the individual ingredients as well as their combination in the proposed ratio.

c. The third group of FDCs includes those which are already marketed, but in which it is proposed either to change the ratio of active ingredients or to make a new therapeutic claim. For such FDCs, the appropriate rationale including published reports (if any) should be submitted to obtain marketing permission. Permission will be granted depending upon the nature of the claim and data submitted.

d. The fourth group of FDC includes those whose individual active ingredients (or drugs from the same class) have been widely used in a particular indication(s) for years, their concomitant use is often necessary and no claim is proposed to be made other than convenience. It will have to be demonstrated that the proposed dosage form is stable and the ingredients are unlikely to have significant interaction of a pharmacodynamic or pharmacokinetic nature.

No additional animal or human data are generally required for these FDCs, and marketing permission may be granted if the FDC has an acceptable rationale.

APPENDIX VII: Undertaking by the Investigator

1. Full name, address and title of the Principal Investigator (or Investigator(s) when there is no Principal Investigator)
2. Name and address of the medical college, hospital or other facility where the clinical trial will be conducted: Education, training and experience that qualify the Investigator for the clinical trial (Attach details including Medical Council registration number, and / or any other statement(s) of qualification(s))
3. Name and address of all clinical laboratory facilities to be used in the study.
4. Name and address of the Ethics Committee that is responsible for approval and continuing review of the study.
5. Names of the other members of the research team (Co- or sub-Investigators) who will be assisting the Investigator in the conduct of the investigation (s).
6. Protocol Title and Study number (if any) of the clinical trial to be conducted by the investigator.
7. Commitments:
   i. I have reviewed the clinical protocol and agree that it contains all the necessary information to conduct the study. I will not begin the study until all necessary Ethics Committee and regulatory approvals have been obtained.
   ii. I agree to conduct the study in accordance with the current protocol. I will not implement any deviation from or changes of the protocol without agreement by the Sponsor and prior review and documented approval / favorable opinion from the Ethics Committee of the amendment, except where necessary to eliminate an immediate hazard(s) to the trial Subjects or when the change(s) involved are only logistical or administrative in nature.
   iii. I agree to personally conduct and/or supervise the clinical trial at my site.
   iv. I agree to inform all Subjects, that the drugs are being used for investigational purposes and I will ensure that the requirements relating to obtaining informed consent and ethics committee review and approval specified in the GCP guidelines are met.
   v. I agree to report to the Sponsor all adverse experiences that occur in the course of the investigation(s) in accordance with the regulatory and GCP guidelines.
   vi. I have read and understood the information in the Investigator's brochure, including the potential risks and side effects of the drug.
   vii. I agree to ensure that all associates, colleagues and employees assisting in the conduct of the study are suitably qualified and experienced and they have been informed about their obligations in meeting their commitments in the trial.
   viii. I agree to maintain adequate and accurate records and to make those records available for audit/ inspection by the Sponsor, Ethics Committee, Licensing Authority or their authorized representatives, in accordance with regulatory and GCP provisions. I will fully cooperate with any study related audit conducted by regulatory officials or authorized representatives of the Sponsor.
   ix. I agree to promptly report to the Ethics Committee all changes in the clinical trial activities and all unanticipated problems involving risks to human Subjects or others.
   x. I agree to inform all unexpected serious adverse events to the Sponsor as well as the Ethics Committee within seven days of their occurance.
   xi. I will maintain confidentiality of the identification of all participating study patients and assure security and confidentiality of study data.
   xii. I agree to comply with all other requirements, guidelines and statutory obligations as applicable to clinical Investigators participating in clinical trials
8. Signature of Investigator with date

APPENDIX VIII: Ethics Committee

1. The number of persons in an Ethics Committee should have atleast seven members. Ethics Committee should appoint, from among its members, a Chairperson (who is from outside the institution) and a Member Secretary. Other members should be a mix of medical/non-medical, scientific and non-scientific persons, including lay public, to reflect the different viewpoints.

For review of each protocol the quorum of Ethics Committee should be atleast 5 members with the following representations:

a basic medical scientists (preferably one pharmacologist).
b. clinicians
c. legal expert
d social scientist / representative of non-governmental voluntary agency/philosopher / ethicist/ theologian or a similar person
e. lay person from the community.

In any case, the ethics committee must include at least one member whose primary area of interest / specialization is nonscientific and at least one member who is independent of the institution / trial site. Besides, there should be appropriate gender representation on the Ethics Committee. If required, Subject experts may be invited to offer their views. Further, based on the requirement of research area, e.g. HIV AIDS, genetic disorders, etc. specific patient groups may also be represented in the Ethics Committee as far as possible.

Only those Ethics Committee members who are independent of the clinical trial and the Sponsor of the trial should vote / provide opinion in matters related to the study.

2. Format for Approval of Ethics Committee

To
Dr.

Dear Dr. ____________________________

The Institutional Ethics Committee / Independent Ethics Committee (state name of the committee, as appropriate) reviewed and discussed your application to conduct the clinical trial entitled "............................." on .... (date).

The following documents were reviewed:

a. Trial Protocol(including protocol amendments), dated ______________________ Version no (s).______________________________
b. Patient information sheet and informed consent form (including updates if any) in English and/or vernacular language.
c. Investigator's Brochure, dated ______________, Version no.______________
d. Proposed methods for patient accrual including advertisement (s) etc. proposed to be used for the purpose.
e. Principal Investigator's current CV.
f. Insurance Policy / Compensation for participation and for serious adverse events occurring during the study participation.
g. Investigator's Agreement with the Sponsor.
h. Investigator's Undertaking (Appendix VII).

The following members of the ethics committee were present at the meeting held on (date, time, place).

______________ Chairman of the Ethics Committee
______________ Member secretary of the Ethics Committee
______________ Name of each member with designation

We approve the trial to be conducted in its presented form.

The Institutional Ethics Committee / Independent Ethics Committee expects to be informed about the progress of the study, any SAE occurring in the course of the study, any changes in the protocol and patient information/informed consent and asks to be provided a copy of the final report.

Yours sincerely,

Member Secretary, Ethics Committee.

APPENDIX IX: Stability Testing of New Drugs

Stability testing is to be performed to provide evidence on how the quality of a drug substance or formulation varies with time under the influence of various environmental factors such as temperature, humidity and light, and to establish shelf life for the formulation and recommended storage conditions.

Stability studies should include testing of those attributes of the drug substance that are susceptible to change during storage and are likely to influence quality, safety, and/or efficacy. In case of formulations the testing should cover, as appropriate, the physical, chemical, biological, and microbiological attributes, preservative content (e.g., antioxidant, antimicrobial preservative), and functionality tests (e.g., for a dose delivery system).

Validated stability-indicating analytical procedures should be applied. For long term studies, frequency of testing should be sufficient to establish the stability profile of the drug substance.

In general, a drug substance should be evaluated under storage conditions that test its thermal stability and, if applicable, its sensitivity to moisture. The storage conditions and the length of studies chosen should be sufficient to cover storage, shipment and subsequent use.

Stress testing of the drug substance should be conducted to identify the likely degradation products, which in turn establish the degradation pathways, evaluate the intrinsic stability of the molecule and validate the stability indicating power of the analytical procedures used. The nature of the stress testing will depend on the individual drug substance and the type of formulation involved.

Stress testing may generally be carried out on a single batch of the drug substance. It should include the effect of temperatures), humidity where appropriate, oxidation, and photolysis on the drug substance.

Data should be provided for (a) Photostability on at least one primary batch of the drug substance as well as the formulation, as the case may be and (b) the susceptibility of the drug substance to hydrolysis across a wide range of pH values when in solution or suspension.

Long-term testing should cover a minimum of 12 months' duration on at least three primary batches of the drug substance or the formulation at the time of submission and should be continued for a period of time sufficient to cover the proposed shelf life. Accelerated testing should cover a minimum of 6 months duration at the time of submission.

In case of drug substances, the batches should be manufactured to a minimum of pilot scale by the same synthetic route and using a method of manufacture that simulates the final process to be used for production batches. In case of formulations, two of the three batches should be at least pilot scale and the third one may be smaller. The manufacturing process(es) used for primary batches should simulate that to be applied to production batches and should provide products of the same quality and meeting the same specifications as that intended for marketing.

The stability studies for drug substances should be conducted either in the same container - closure system as proposed for storage and distribution or in a container - closure system that simulates the proposed final packaging. In case of formulations, the stability studies should be conducted in the final container - closure system proposed for marketing.

Stability testing of new drug substances and formulations

i. Study conditions for drug substances and formulations intended to be stored under general conditions

Study	*Study conditions*	*Duration of study*
Long term	30°C ± 2°C/65% RH ± 5% RH	12 months
Accelerated	40°C ± 2°C/75% RH ± 5% RH	6 months

If at any time during 6 months' testing under the accelerated storage condition, such changes occur that cause the product to fail in complying with the prescribed standards, additional testing under an intermediate storage condition should be conducted and evaluated against significant change criteria.

ii. Study conditions for drug substances and formulations intended to be stored in a refrigerator

Study	*Study conditions*	*Duration of study*
Long term	5°C ± 3°C	12 months
Accelerated	25°C ± 2°C/60% RH ± 5% RH	6 months

iii. Study conditions for drug substances and formulations intended to be stored in a freezer

Study	*Study conditions*	*Duration of study*
Long term	- 20°C ± 5°C	12 months

iv. Drug substances intended for storage below -20°C shall be treated on a case-by-case basis.

v. Stability testing of the formulation after constitution or dilution, if applicable, should be conducted to provide information for the labeling on the preparation, storage condition, and in-use period of the constituted or diluted product. This testing should be performed on the constituted or diluted product through the proposed in-use period.

APPENDIX X: Contents of the Proposed Protocol for Conducting Clinical Trials

Title Page

a. Full title of the clinical study,
b. Protocol / Study number, and protocol version number with date
c. The IND name/number of the investigational drug
d. Complete name and address of the Sponsor and contract research organization if any
e. List of the Investigators who are conducting the study, their respective institutional affiliations and site locations
f. Name(s) of clinical laboratories and other departments and/or facilities participating in the study.

Table of Contents

A complete Table of Contents including a list of all Appendices.

1. **Background and Introduction**
   a. Preclinical experience
   b. Clinical experience.
   Previous clinical work with the new drug should be reviewed here and a description of how the current protocol extends existing data should be provided. If this is an entirely new indication, how this drug was considered for this should be discussed. Relevant information regarding pharmacological, toxicological and other biological properties of the drug/biologic/medical device, and previous efficacy and safety experience should be described.
2. **Study Rationale:** This section should describe a brief summary of the background information relevant to the study design and protocol methodology. The reasons for performing this study in the particular population included by the protocol should be provided.
3. Study Objective(s) (primary as well as secondray) and their logical relation to the study design.
4. **Study Design:**
   a. Overview of the Study Design: Including a description of the type of study (i.e., double-blind, multicenter, placebo controlled, etc.), a detail of the specific treatment groups and number of study Subjects in each group and investigative site, Subject number assignment, and the type, sequence and duration of study periods.
   b. Flow chart of the study
   c. A brief description of the methods and procedures to be used during the study.
   d. Discussion of Study Design: This discussion details the rationale for the design chosen for this study.
5. **Study Population:** The number of Subjects required to be enrolled in the study at the investigative site and by all sites along with a brief description of the nature of the Subject population required is also mentioned.
6. **Subject Eligibility**
   a. Inclusion criteria
   b. Exclusion criteria.
7. **Study Assessments:** Plan, procedures and methods to be described in detail.
8. Study Conduct stating the types of study activities that would be included in this section would be: medical history, type of physical examination, blood or urine testing, electrocardiogram (ECG),

diagnostic testing such as pulmonary function tests, symptom measurement, dispensation and retrieval of medication, Subject cohort assignment, adverse event review, etc.

Each visit should be described separately as Visit 1, Visit 2, etc.

Discontinued Subjects: Describes the circumstances for Subject withdrawal, dropouts, or other reasons for discontinuation of Subjects. State how drop outs would be managed and if they would be replace.

Describe the method of handling of protocol waivers, if any. The person(s) who approves all such waivers should be identified and the criteria used for specific waivers should be provided.

Describes how protocol violations will be treated, including conditions where the study will be terminated for non-compliance with the protocol.

9. Study Treatment

a. Dosing schedule (dose, frequency, and duration of the experimental treatment) Describe the administration of placebos and/or dummy medications if they are part of the treatment plan. If applicable, concomitant drug(s), their doses, frequency, and duration of concomitant treatment should be stated.

b. Study drug supplies and administration: A statement about who is going to provide the study medication and that the investigational drug formulation has been manufactured following all regulations Details of the product stability, storage requirements and dispensing requirements should be provided.

c. Dose modification for study drug toxicity: Rules for changing the dose or stopping the study drug should be provided.

d. Possible drug interactions

e. Concomitant therapy: The drugs that are permitted during the study and the conditions under which they may be used are detailed here. Describe the drugs that a Subject is not allowed to use during parts of or the entire study. If any washout periods for prohibited medications are needed prior to enrollment, these should be described here.

f. Blinding procedures: A detailed description of the blinding procedure if the study employs a blind on the Investigator and/or the Subject

g. Unblinding procedures: If the study is blinded, the circumstances in which unblinding may be done and the mechanism to be used for unblinding should be given.

10. Adverse Events (See Appendix XI): Description of expected adverse events should be given. Procedures used to evaluate an adverse event should be described.

11. Ethical Considerations: Give the summary of:

a. Risk/benefit assessment:

b. Ethics Committee review and communications

c. Informed consent process

d. Statement of Subject confidentiality including ownership of data and coding procedures

12. Study Monitoring and Supervision: A description of study monitoring policies and procedures should be provided along with the proposed frequency of site monitoring visits, and who is expected to perform monitoring.

Case Record Form (CRF) completion requirements, including who gets which copies of the forms and any specifics required in filling out the forms CRF correction requirements, including who is authorized to make corrections on the CRF and how queries about study data are handled and how errors, if any, are to be corrected should be stated.

Investigator study files, including what needs to be stored following study completion should be described.

13. Investigational Product Management

a. Give Investigational product description and packaging (stating all Ingredients and the formulation of the investigational drug and any placebos used in the study)

b. The precise dosing required during the study
c. Method of packaging, labeling, and blinding of study substances
d. Method of assigning treatments to Subjects and the Subject identification code numbering system
e. Storage conditions for study substances
f. Investigational product accountability: Describe instructions for the receipt, storage, dispensation, and return of the investigational products to ensure a complete accounting of all investigational products received, dispensed, and returned/destroyed.
g. Describe policy and procedure for handling unused investigational products.

14. **Data Analysis:** Provide details of the statistical approach to be followed including sample size, how the sample size was determined, including assumptions made in making this determination, efficacy endpoints (primary as well as secondary) and safety endpoints.
    Statistical analysis: Give complete details of how the results will be analyzed and reported along with the description of statistical tests to be used to analyze the primary and secondary endpoints defined above. Describe the level of significance, statistical tests to be used, and the methods used for missing data; method of evaluation of the data for treatment failures, non-compliance, and Subject withdrawals; rationale and conditions for any interim analysis if planned.
    Describe statistical considerations for Pharmacokinetic (PK) analysis, if applicable.
15. **Undertaking by the Investigator (see Appendix VII)**
16. **Appendices:** Provide a study synopsis, copies of the informed consent documents (patient information sheet, informed consent form, etc.); CRF and other data collection forms; a summary of relevant pre-clinical safety information and any other documents referenced in the clinical protocol.

APPENDIX XI: Data Elements for Reporting Serious Adverse Event Occurring in a Clinical Trial

Patient Details

- Initials and other relevant identifier (hospital/OPD record number etc.)*
- Gender
- Age and/or date of birth
- Weight
- Height.

Suspected Drug(s)

- Generic name of the drug*
- Indication(s) for which suspect drug was prescribed or tested
- Dosage form and strength
- Daily dose and regimen (specify units - e.g., mg, ml, mg/kg)
- Route of administration
- Starting date and time of day
- Stopping date and time, or duration of treatment.

Other Treatment(s)

Provide the same information for concomitant drugs (including non prescription/OTC drugs) and non-drug therapies, as for the suspected drug(s).

Details of Suspected Adverse Drug Reaction(s)

Full description of reaction(s) including body site and severity, as well as the criterion (or criteria) for regarding the report as serious. In addition to a description of the reported signs and symptoms, whenever possible, describe a specific diagnosis for the reaction.*

- Start date (and time) of onset of reaction
- Stop date (and time) or duration of reaction
- Dechallenge and rechallenge information
- Setting (e.g., hospital, out-patient clinic, home, nursing home).

Outcome

Information on recovery and any sequelae; results of specific tests and/or treatment that may have been conducted .

For a fatal outcome, cause of death and a comment on its possible relationship to the suspected reaction; Any postmortem findings.

Other information: anything relevant to facilitate assessment of the case, such as medical history including allergy, drug or alcohol abuse; family history; findings from special investigations, etc.

Details about the Investigator*

Name
Address
Telephone number
Profession (specialty)

Date of reporting the event to Licensing Authority:
Date of reporting the event to Ethics Committee overseeing the site:

Signature of the Investigator
Note: Information marked * must be provided."

(F.No. X-11014/1/2003-DMS and PFA)

(RITA TEOTIA),
JOINT SECRETARY, GOVERNMENT OF INDIA

Foot Note :- The Prinicipal Rules were published in the Official Gazette vide notification No. F. 28-10/45-H(I), dated the 21st December, 1945 and last amended vide GSR (E) dated the

SUGGESTED READING AND REFERENCES

This chapter has been incorporated from: www.cdsco.nic.in/html/Schedule-Y%20(Amended%20Version-2005)%20original.htm – 764k

INDEX

A

B

C